# Immuno Systems Biology

# Immuno Systems Biology

Editor: Jim Wang

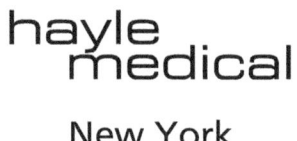

hayle
medical

New York

Hayle Medical,
750 Third Avenue, 9th Floor,
New York, NY 10017, USA

Visit us on the World Wide Web at:
www.haylemedical.com

ISBN 978-1-64647-571-1 (Hardback)

**Cataloging-in-publication Data**

Immuno systems biology / edited by Jim Wang.
    p. cm.
Includes bibliographical references and index.
ISBN 978-1-64647-571-1
1. Immune system. 2. Systems biology. 3. Immunology.
4. Immune response--Molecular aspects. I. Wang, Jim.
QR181 .I46 2023
616.079--dc23

# Contents

**Permissions**

**List of Contributors**

**Index**

# Preface

The immune system refers to the network of biological processes that protect an organism from diseases. It recognizes and reacts to a wide range of pathogens including cancer cells, viruses and parasitic worms. The immune system is divided into two main subsystems, namely, the adaptive immune system and the innate immune system. The adaptive immune system recognizes the unique components of individual pathogens, whereas innate immune system recognizes the components shared by all pathogens. Antigens are the type of substances that are identified by the immune system and can subsequently trigger an immune response. A dysfunctional immune system can lead to cancer, autoimmune diseases, and inflammatory diseases. Immunodeficiency is caused when the immune system is not active, which leads to persistent and potentially fatal infections. This book is compiled in such a manner, that it will provide in-depth knowledge about immuno systems biology. It will prove to be immensely beneficial to students and researchers in this area of study.

This book unites the global concepts and researches in an organized manner for a comprehensive understanding of the subject. It is a ripe text for all researchers, students, scientists or anyone else who is interested in acquiring a better knowledge of this dynamic field.

I extend my sincere thanks to the contributors for such eloquent research chapters. Finally, I thank my family for being a source of support and help.

**Editor**

# Modulating the T Lymphocyte Immune Response via Secretome Produced miRNA: From Tolerance Induction to the Enhancement of the Anticancer Response

*Mark D. Scott, Duncheng Wang, Wendy M. Toyofuku and Xining Yang*

## Abstract

T cells are key mediators of graft tolerance/rejection, development of autoimmunity, and the anticancer response. Consequently, differentially modifying the T cell response is a major therapeutic target. Most immunomodulatory approaches have focused on cytotoxic agents, cytokine modulation, monoclonal antibodies, mitogen activation, adoptive cell therapies (including CAR-T cells). However, these approaches do not persistently reorient the systemic immune response thus necessitating continual therapy. Previous murine studies from our laboratory demonstrated that the adoptive transfer of polymer-grafted (PEGylated) allogeneic leukocytes resulted in the induction of a persistent and systemic tolerogenic state. Further analyses demonstrated that miRNA isolated from the secretome of polymer- modified or control allogeneic responses effectively induced either a tolerogenic (TA1 miRNA) or proinflammatory (IA1 miRNA) response both *in vitro* and *in vivo* that was both systemic and persistent. In a murine Type 1 diabetes autoimmune model, the tolerogenic TA1 therapeutic effectively attenuated the disease process via the systemic upregulation of regulatory T cells while simultaneously downregulating T effector cells. In contrast, the proinflammatory IA1 therapeutic enhanced the anticancer efficacy of naïve PBMC by increasing inflammatory T cells and decreasing regulatory T cells. The successful development of this secretome miRNA approach may prove useful treating both autoimmune diseases and cancer.

**Keywords:** T lymphocyte, miRNA, polymer, secretome, tolerance, Treg, proinflammatory, Teff, autoimmunity, cancer, adoptive cell transfer

## 1. Introduction

Biologically, and clinically, the concept of "self" is of crucial importance in protection against foreign biologicals (e.g., viruses and bacteria), abnormal autologous cells (e.g., cancers) and more recently developed "diseases" (i.e., the purposeful introduction of "nonself") such as enzyme-replacement therapy and transfusion and transplantation medicine. The immune system is tasked with preserving "self" and rejecting "nonself" and has multiple components-any of which will be of variable importance depending on the context of the immunological assault. Immunological "self" of most tissues is imparted by the major histocompatibility complex (MHC) which encodes a variety of proteins that provide a means for identifying, targeting, and eliminating foreign invaders and diseased cells while preserving normal "self" tissue. The MHC proteins themselves consist of three classes. MHC Class I molecules are expressed on virtually all nucleated cells while Class II molecules are expressed exclusively on antigen presenting cells (APC; e.g., monocytes, macrophages, dendritic cell, B lymphocytes, and endothelial cells) and activated T lymphocytes. MHC Class III genes encode components of the complement system. The human MHC is referred to as the Human Leukocyte Antigen (HLA) complex while the murine equivalent is referred to as the Histocompatibility-2 (H2) complex. In the context of MHC-mediated immune recognition, the T lymphocyte (T cell) is of particular importance. T cells themselves consist of a diverse array of subsets that fall into two general categories: 1) Regulatory T cells (Treg) which modulate the strength of an immune response and maintain "self"; and effector T

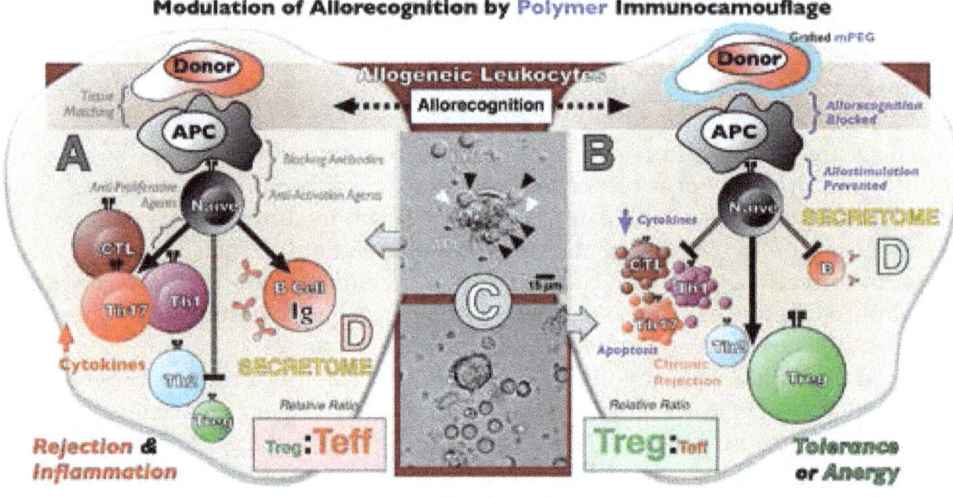

**Figure 1.**

*Immune modulation via pharmacologic and immunocamouflage therapy. (A) Current pharmacologic therapy almost exclusively targets T cell activation and proliferation consequent to allorecognition. Response to nonself is in large part mediated by cell-cell interactions between antigen presenting cells (APC; e.g., dendritic cells) and naive T cells. This cell-cell interaction is characterized by essential adhesion, allorecognition and co-stimulation events. Consequent to allorecognition, a proliferation of proinflammatory T cells (e.g., cytotoxic T lymphocyte, CTL; Th17, IL-17⁺; Th1, IFN-γ⁺; and IL-2⁺ populations) and decrease in regulatory T cells (Treg, Foxp3⁺ and CD25⁺) is observed. Current therapeutic agents are primarily cytotoxic agents preventing T cell activation (e.g., cyclosporine and rapamycin) or T cell proliferation (e.g., methotrexate, corticosteroids and azathioprine). Additionally, blocking antibodies have been investigated. Gray text indicates current techniques to prevent/limit alloimmune responses. (B) In contrast, immunocamouflage of donor cells by methoxy(polyethylene) glycol (mPEG) results in the disruption of the essential cell-cell interactions decreasing T cell proliferation and altering differentiation patterns (decreased Th17 and increased Treg). In aggregate, the polymer induced changes induces a tolerogenic/anergic state both in vitro and in vivo. Size of T cell population denotes increase or decrease in number. Size of B cell indicates antibody response. Blue text represents the consequences of polymer-mediated immunocamouflage of the alloresponse. (C) As shown in photomicrographs, in a control mixed lymphocyte reaction (MLR), significant and persistent interactions (black arrows) occur between allogeneic lymphocytes (LYM) and dendritic cells (APC). The lymphocyte adhesion and antigen presentation interactions typically occur at pseudopodal extensions from the APC (white arrows). PEGylation of either allogeneic PBMC population decreases the stability and duration of initial cell:cell interactions between lymphocytes due to the global charge and steric camouflage of membrane proteins. (D) Importantly, the secretomes derived from the MLR and mPEG-MLR exert potent effects on a secondary MLR encompassing fresh PBMC from the same or different donors. The key component of the secretome are soluble (free and exosome) miRNA. Data derived from Refs [32–43].*

cells (Teff) that mediate the inflammatory response and consists, in part, of Th1, Th17 and Th2 subsets. Hence, the functional ratio of Treg to Teff (Treg:Teff) cells is critical and an imbalance of this ratio from the norm can induce either an autoim-mune (excess Teff or decreased Treg) state or impaired response to "nonself" (e.g., cancer) consequent to biologically ill-advised tolerance (too many Treg or weak Teff response). Indeed, the T cell response plays a (the) central role in autoimmune diseases, transplant rejection, graft versus host disease (GVHD), graft versus leukemia (GVL), cancer and, more recently, cancer therapy. Hence, consequent to the central role of T cells as a key cellular component in the development of autoimmune diseases, graft tolerance or rejection, and the anticancer response, the T cell response has been a major focus in the development of clinical therapies (**Figure 1A**) [1].

## 2. Immunomodulation of the T cell response in autoimmunity and cancer

Autoimmune diseases arise when the immune system recognizes the individual's own tissues or organs as "foreign" and targets them for destruction. Autoimmune diseases can affect virtually all tissues and organ systems and encompass such diverse diseases as Type 1 Diabetes (T1D; pancreas), Idiopathic Thrombocytopenic Purpura (ITP; platelet destruction), Crohn's disease (CD; bowel), Multiple Sclerosis (MS; brain) and Rheumatoid Arthritis (RA; joints). Despite the diversity of tissues affected, extensive research has demonstrated that Treg are downregulated while Teff are upregulated (i.e., leading to a reduced Treg:Teff ratio) leading to a chronic proin-flammatory state. Current therapeutic approaches to managing autoimmune diseases are typically focused on symptom relief and the use of immunosuppressive agents capable of inhibiting the proinflammatory response arising from "self-recognition." Most commonly, treatment for chronic autoimmune disease is via administration of systemic steroids (e.g., dexamethasone), cytotoxic anti-proliferative/activation agents (e.g., cyclosporine) that induce a general immunosuppression, and/or IVIG (pooled, polyvalent, IgG purified from the plasma of >1000 blood donors) [2–6]. Other experimental approaches to the treatment of autoimmune diseases include blocking monoclonal antibodies directed against the TCR, CD4, costimulatory ligands and receptors, adhesion molecules, and cytokine receptors [7–9]. A more recent approach has been to interrupt the cytokine signals necessary for the activation and prolifera-tion of autoreactive T cells. The current gold standard for this approach is Enbrel® (etanercept), a solubilized TNF-α receptor fragment that intercepts and sequesters the TNF-α cytokine thereby inhibiting the proliferation of proinflammatory T cells [10–15]. However, Enbrel® has been given a USA FDA "Black Box" warning due to significantly increased risks of serious infections that may lead to hospitalization or death [16–22]. Common to all of these approaches is an attempt to increase the Treg:Teff ratio by either directly increasing Treg or selectively decreasing Teff populations. However, despite their importance in clinical medicine, many of these agents have been plagued by both significant toxicity/adverse events and an inability to adequately eliminate or inhibit reactive T cells [8].

In contrast to autoimmune diseases, an insufficient/inefficient immune response may underlie the proliferation and dissemination of abnormal cells (i.e., cancer cells). While this may occur for a number of reasons, immunosuppression is a known risk factor. Indeed, acquired or inherited T cell defects as well as long-term therapy with immunosuppressive drugs are clearly associated with an increased risk of neoplasia. The impaired immune response to cancer cells can arise, at least in part, from an increase in the Treg:Teff ratio (too many Treg and/or insufficient Teff cell production). To address this imbalance in the Treg:Teff ratio, experimental therapies are currently focused on the *ex vivo* expansion and subsequent transfusion of autologous Teff capable of killing the cancer cells [23–31]. However, these current immune enhancing methods, while promising, are expensive, complicated to accomplish (e.g., insertion of specific target cancer genes in APC) and requires weeks of tissue culture expansion to meet the threshold for cell infusion.

Perhaps most importantly, current tolerogenic or proinflammatory therapeutic approaches fail to persistently reorient the systemic T cell immune response thus necessitating continual therapy. Moreover, despite the importance of the Treg:Teff ratio, in both autoimmune diseases and cancer, there are a paucity of pharmacologic tools that can directly, and in tandem, target the regulation of both the Treg and Teff subsets. Hence, to diminish or overcome the need for chronic administration of immunotherapeutic agents, new approaches capable of persistently reorienting the endogenous immune (Treg:Teff) response would be of value.

## 3. Immunomodulation via immunocamouflage and differential miRNA production

Previous studies from our laboratory demonstrated that a persistent and systemic reorientation of the animal (murine; or *in vitro* human) immune response towards a tolerogenic response could be induced via the adoptive transfer of immunocamouflaged allogeneic leukocytes to a recipient animal [32–43]. Immunocamouflage of cells is mediated by the covalent grafting of methoxypoly(ethylene glycol) (mPEG) to the leukocyte membrane surface. Consequent to mPEG-grafting (PEGylation), MHC-mediated T cell alloproliferation is dramatically inhibited due to consequent to impaired cell:cell interaction and weak allostimulation (**Figure 1A** and **B**). These studies demonstrated that the PEGylated allogeneic leukocytes diminished intracellular communication preventing a Teff response while simultaneously inducing the generation of Treg cells skewing the Treg:Teff ratio towards a tolerogenic state (**Figure 1B** and **C**) [36, 38–43]. Further *in vitro* and *in vivo* studies demonstrated that, using MLR-based secretome biomanufacturing systems, distinct acellular microRNA (miRNA) based therapeutics could be manufactured from control and PEGylated allorecognition reactions that systemically and persistently reorient the immune response to either a proinflammatory (IA1) or tolerogenic (TA1) state (**Figure 1**) [40, 43]. In this chapter, we will demonstrate how these miRNA-based therapeutics can inhibit the progression of T cell mediated autoimmune diseases (TA1) or conversely enhance the proinflammatory anticancer T cell response (IA1).

## 4. Production of miRNA therapeutics via the alloresponse pathway

Since their discovery in 1996, the role of circulating (cell-free) miRNA in disease processes has become an active research area and recent findings suggest that they may be biomarkers, or possibly mediators, of cancers as well as autoimmune diseases such as T1D [44–46]. To understand mechanistically how the TA1 and IA1 miRNA biologics function, an appreciation of the biological role and regulatory complexity of miRNA is needed. Recent studies have demonstrated that miRNA are key epigenetic regulators of cellular processes including immune responses, inflammation, proliferation, survival, and cellular differentiation [47, 48]. miRNA are short (~22 nucleotides) single-stranded RNA molecules found in all eukaryotes and it is estimated that ~60% of mammalian genes are targeted by one or more miRNA [49, 50]. Moreover, because of their evolutionary importance in gene regulation, miRNA and their sequence and processing are highly conserved between mammalian species (e.g., mouse and human) [49]. While miRNA are most commonly found intracellularly, significant amounts of stable miRNA are also found in the serum of mammals suggesting an important messenger/regulatory role. While the nomenclature of miRNAs is relatively straightforward it is important to note that similarities in miRNA number designation is not indicative of similarity in functionality (**Figure 2**). Moreover, the literature is replete with conflicting claims for the specific actions of a single miRNA.

Indeed, there is a significant lack of clarity regarding the function of a single miRNA. This lack of functional clarity likely arises consequent to the complexity and low fidelity of the miRNA bioregulatory process. Of note, a single miRNA can potentially affect tens to hundreds of genes and individual genes can be regulated by multiple miRNA [50]. Hence, the effect of modifying the expression of a single miRNA on protein regulation and bioregulatory networks is unpredictable. Because of this regulatory complexity, most studies have focused on miRNA as disease biomarkers, not as therapeutic agents as there is a low probability that altered expression of a single, or even a few, miRNA would exert a potent and definitive biological response [51–54]. From a bioregulatory approach, it is more probable that multiple miRNA control protein expression, proliferation and differentiation and it is this "pattern of miRNA expression" (encompassing increased, decreased and static levels) that must be mimicked to achieve pharmacologically effective miRNA-based therapeutics. To achieve this goal our laboratory approach has been purposefully chosen to biologically manufacture relatively complex miRNA preparations mimicking normal biology in order to achieve maximal biological functionality.

Using a Mixed Lymphocyte Reaction (MLR) production model the T cell centric proinflammatory IA1 and tolerogenic TA1 therapeutics can be reproducibly manufactured using the control-MLR and mPEG-MLR (respectively; **Figure 1**). As demonstrated, the allogeneic PBMC populations within the control- and mPEG-MLR express significantly different patterns of miRNA expression relative to resting

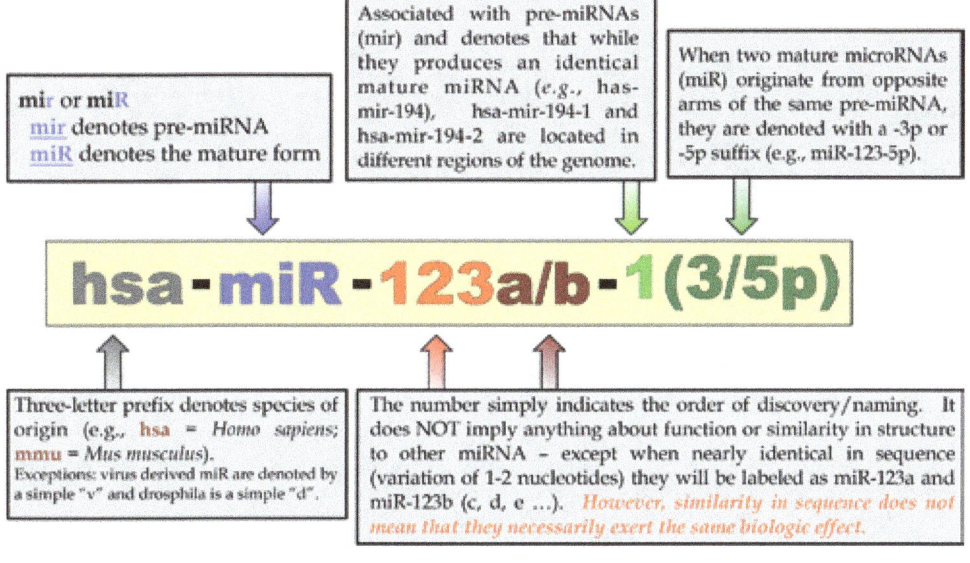

**Figure 2.**
*miRNA nomenclature explained. An important concept to understand is that the miRNA number (e.g., 123 as shown) has no relationship to function or structure. For example, "hsa-miR-123" has no implied structural or functional similarity to "hsa-miR-128." However, because of the highly conserved nature of miRNA, human "hsa-miR-123" has very similar structure and function to murine "mmu-miR-123."*

PBMC as evidenced via clustergram (**Figure 3A**), volcano plot (**Figure 3B**) and Log2 Fold (**Figure 3C**) miRNA expression analyses. Importantly, as shown in **Figure 3C**, the control- and mPEG-MLRs show unique patterns of expression. While there are some similarities in the pattern of expression there are significant disparity in miRNAs expressed as well (not shown are the miRNA unchanged from resting cells).

Importantly, the differences in miRNA expression between the Control- and mPEG-MLR leukocyte yield secretomes that exert dramatically different effects when used to treat resting human PBMC or murine splenocytes. Collection of the secretome produced (**Figure 4A**) during the control and polymer modified allorecognition-based MLR yields a reproducible, acellular, miRNA-rich, material that is stable and can be frozen and thawed with minimal decrement to its activity. As schematically presented (**Figure 4B**), TA1 upregulates regulatory T cell populations (e.g., Treg) while simultaneously downregulating Teff (e.g., Th17 and Th1) cells. In contrast, the proinflammatory IA1 increases Teff while decreasing Treg cells. Of note, the secretome from resting cells (SYN) has minimal to no effect on human or mouse immune cells. Moreover, due to the conserved nature of mammalian miRNA, cross species efficacy is observed with both TA1 and IA1. As shown in **Figure 4C**, murine splenocyte produced TA1 and IA1 exerted dose-dependent effects on a human MLR with murine-sourced TA1 reducing $CD3^+CD4^+$ T cell proliferation and the murine IA1 enhancing $CD3^+CD4^+$ T cell proliferation. Hence, a polymer-based, alloresponse manufacturing system may provide a unique avenue for more effectively, and safely, modulating the Treg:Teff cell ratio via the production of therapeutically effective TA1 and IA1 miRNA-based therapeutics [32–43]. Importantly, the effects of TA1 and IA1 immunotherapy was persistent. In murine studies, a single dosing of TA1 to mice resulted in significant increase in Treg cells within the spleen of normal mice that persisted to ≥270 days post treatment (**Figure 4D**).

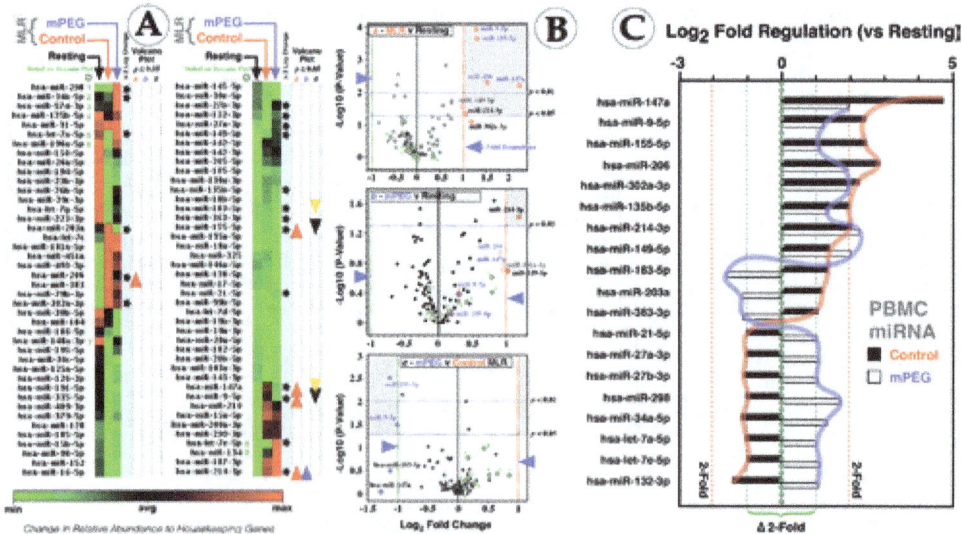

**Figure 3.**
*Partial qPCR characterization of the miRNA expression in the Control- and mPEG-MLR. (A–C) Clustergram (A), Volcano Plot (B) and Log2 Fold (C) analyses of the miRNA expression in the mPEG-MLR and Control-MLR relative to resting cells. (C) Because of the complexity of miRNA regulation of genes, we have consciously chosen to produce a relatively complex miRNA preparations mimicking normal biology in order to achieve maximal biological functionality. Multiple miRNA changes are noted in the hTA1 miRNA compared to either resting cells (green dashed line = 0) or the proinflammatory hIA1 miRNA preparation. Using miRNA expressing a net ΔLog2 Fold change, significantly different "patterns of expression" are noted between the hTA1 and hIA1 miRNA. This pattern of expression, comprising both INCREASED and DECREASED miRNA species is essential for effective immunomodulation of recipient animals. Values derived from a minimum of 3 independent biological replicates. Unpublished data.*

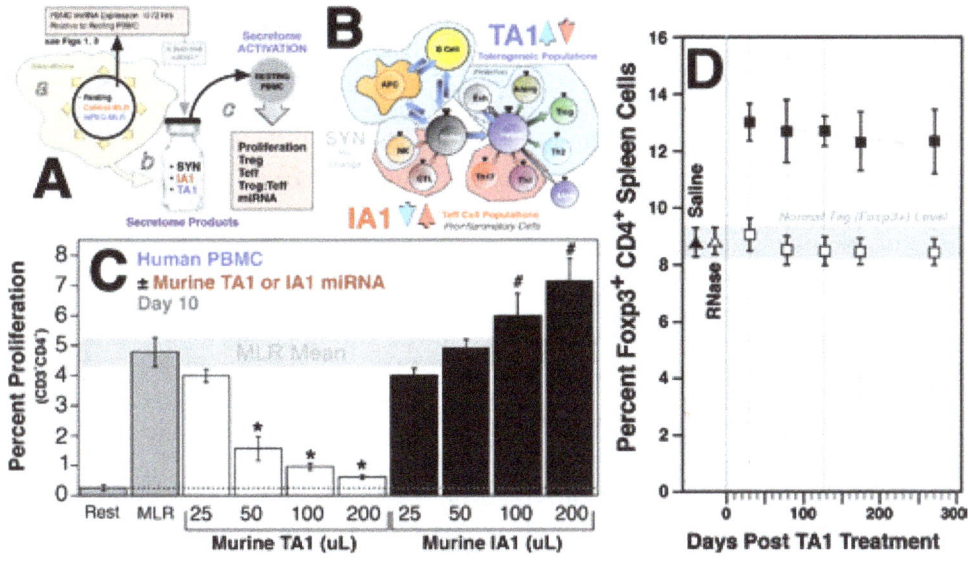

**Figure 4.**
*Differential effects of TA1 and IA1 on the immune system. (A and B): Secretome production (A) of SYN (resting), IA1 (MLR) and TA1 (mPEG-MLR) gave rise to unique immunomodulatory activity (B). While IA1 enhanced proinflammatory subsets and reduced Treg cells, TA1 enhanced Treg while reducing Teff subpopulations. (C) Attesting to the conserved nature of miRNA, murine TA1 and IA1 exerted significant, dose-dependent, immunomodulatory effects on resting human PBMC. The SYN secretome product had no substantive effects on T cell proliferation and differentiation. Data derived from Refs: [32–43] TA1 administration induces a persistent tolerogenic state in immunocompetent mice. (D) As shown, CD4+Foxp3+ Treg cells remain elevated for ≥270 days following a SINGLE TA1 administration at age 7–8 weeks. In contrast, RNase-treated TA1 (to degrade the miRNA) had no immunomodulatory effect. Results shown are from a minimum of 8 animals per group Unpublished data.*

## 5. Tolerogenic TA1: immunomodulation of autoimmune disease

Autoimmune destruction of pancreatic islets gives rise to T1D and occurs via T cell dependent pathways [55–57]. Elucidation of the role of T cells in T1D has been most effectively examined in the nonobese diabetic (NOD) mouse model. In the NOD mouse, evidence suggests that a deficit in Treg control over diabetogenic Teff cells leads to the development of insulitis and disease [56–66]. Indeed, changes in the Treg:Teff ratio (i.e., balance) can be observed as early as 3–4 weeks of age and becomes more pronounced with disease progression (**Figure 5**) [56]. Human studies have similarly demonstrated that T1D Treg exhibit an impaired ability to suppress Teff [67]. Thus, the emergence of an aggressive diabetogenic lymphocyte response in NOD mice, and likely humans, is dependent upon a change in the Treg:Teff ratio.

As demonstrated in **Figure 5**, the Treg:Teff ratio (defined as the ratio of Foxp3+ to Th17+ T cells) in control (saline treated) NOD mice decreased with disease progression from 103 in nondiabetic 7 week old mice to only 4.7 in diabetic mice at time of sacrifice (15–30 week). Moreover, control NOD mice exhibited a rapid onset of diabetes with 75% (12 of 16) of the mice becoming diabetic by week 19. Subsequent to week 19, no additional mice became diabetic. In contrast, a single dosing (3 injections at 2 days intervals) of the TA1 therapeutic at 7 weeks of age dramatically altered both the incidence and rate of progression of the T1D in the NOD mouse. By week 19 only 13% (2 of 15) of the TA1 treated mice became diabetic with an additional 4 mice becoming diabetic between weeks 21 and 23 (total diabetic 6/15; 40%). Mechanistically, these findings were associated with a systemic alteration of the immune system as noted in **Figure 5**. In control NOD mice, the progression to diabetes was characterized by significantly elevated levels of most proinflammatory Teff (e.g., INF-$\gamma^+$, Th17$^+$, and IL-2$^+$) lymphocytes and a corresponding decrease in regulatory subsets. In contrast, TA1 therapy dramatically and significantly blunted the expansion of Teff cells (as exemplified by INF-$\gamma^+$, Th17$^+$, and IL-2$^+$ lymphocytes; **Figure 5A**) relative to diabetic or nondiabetic control NOD mice coupled with a simultaneous increase in a broad range of tolerogenic/anergic regulatory T cell subsets (e.g., foxp3$^+$, IL-10$^+$, TGF-$\beta^+$; **Figure 5B**) in the pancreatic lymph node. These studies also demonstrated that TA1 treated NOD mice had significant numbers of histologically normal pancreatic islets while no normal islets were identified in the untreated mice [40]. It is worth noting that all diabetic mice (control and TA1-treated) exhibited significantly lower levels of these tolerogenic cells than did the 30 week old nondiabetic (control or TA1) mice. Moreover, the effects of TA1-miRNA therapy were not localized to the pancreatic lymph node microenvironment. Analyses of the T cell subsets present in the spleen and brachial lymph node of control and TA1 treated NOD mice (diabetic and nondiabetic) similarly demonstrated dramatic changes in the

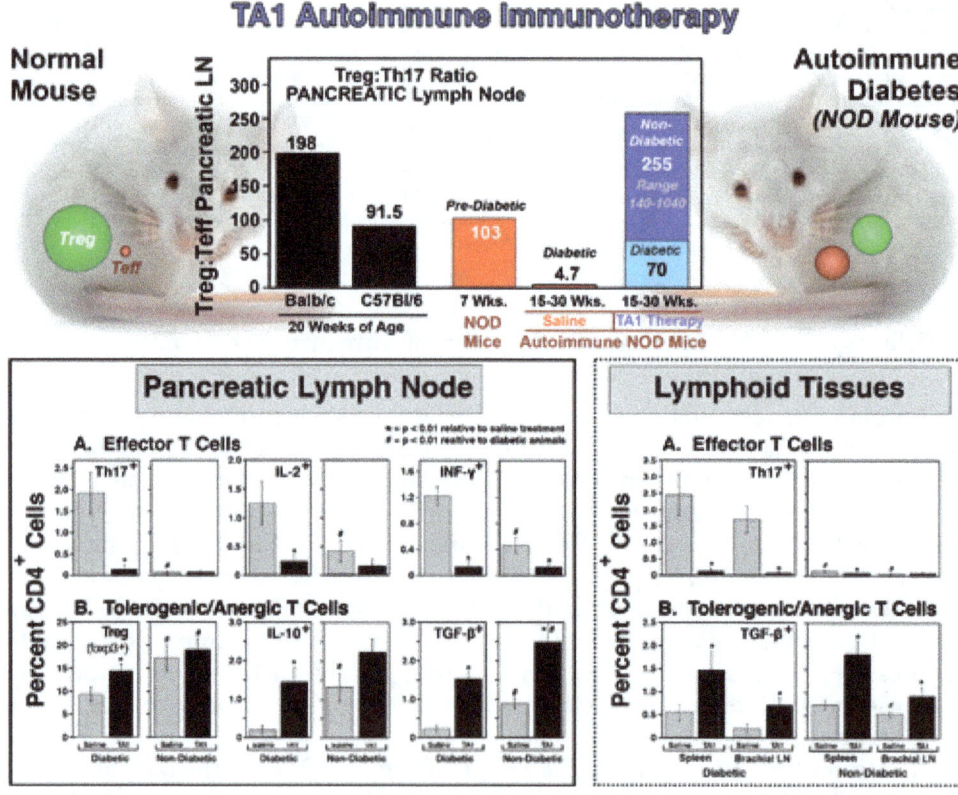

**Figure 5.**
*The autoimmune disease of T1D process is mediated by a decrease in the Treg:Teff ratio and can be prevented by TA1 administration (top). Treatment with the TA1 miRNA product prevents the decrease and, in fact, significantly increases the Treg:Teff ratio. The increased Treg:Teff ratio is protective as evidenced by the finding that the majority of TA1 treated animals remained normoglycemic. Shown in the blue bars are the Treg:Teff ratio for TA1 treated mice who were diabetic (ratio of 70) and nondiabetic (ratio of 255). Mechanistically, TA1 immunotherapeutic significantly altered the expression of multiple proinflammatory (A) and tolerogenic/anergic (B) T cell subsets. These changes were systemic in nature as shown by changes in not only the pancreatic lymph node but in other immune tissues (spleen and brachial lymph node). Diabetic tissues were harvested at time of conversion, nondiabetic tissues were harvested at week 30. Diabetic values are the mean ± SD of 12 saline and 6 TA1 treated NOD mice. Nondiabetic results are the mean ± SD of 4 saline and 9 TA1 treated NOD mice. Derived from Ref. [40].*

Teff cell populations (**Figure 5A**, right) and tolerogenic T cells (**Figure 5B**, right). These findings demonstrate that miRNA-based TA1 therapeutic, directly targets the Treg:Teff ratio yielding a systemic protolerogenic state both *in vivo* (mouse) and *in vitro* (human and mouse) suggesting that this approach would be of utility in a broad range of autoimmune diseases. Furthermore, due to the persistence of the immunomodulatory activity in mice (**Figure 4**), TA1-like drugs could, potentially, dramatically reduce the need for chronic administration of drugs.

## 6. Proinflammatory IA1: enhancing the immune response to cancer

T cells plays a critical role in the anticancer inflammatory responses. An effective anticancer proinflammatory T cell response is dependent upon the activation of Teff cells. Normally, T cells are activated upon ligation of their antigen receptors with specific cognate antigens [68]. However, because of the low frequency of cancer antigen-specific lymphocytes, the immune response to cancers can be initially, and all too often remains, weak. While previous studies have attempted to enhance the anticancer T cell response using pan T cell mitogens (e.g., phytohemagglutinin; PHA), cytokines (e.g., IL-2), or monoclonal antibodies (e.g., anti-CD3 and anti-CD28) the overly robust T cell response arising from these approaches often induced significant systemic toxicity leading to the suspension or abrogation of multiple clinical trials [69–74]. In contrast, in an allorecognition response only 1–10% of T cells are alloreactive [75]. Hence, the IA1 therapeutic, derived from a bioreactor allorecognition response (MLR), is expected to activate endogenous T cells in a more controlled manner, with less toxicity.

To assess IA1's ability to enhance the anticancer activity of resting PBMC, cells were treated for 24 hours with IA1 and overlaid on HeLa and SH-4 cancers cells. Cancer cell proliferation was then followed for 168 hours. Importantly, IA1 exerted no toxicity to resting PBMC but, as shown in **Figure 4**, induced significant activation (e.g., proliferation) of resting CD3$^+$ (CD4$^+$ and CD8$^+$) skewed towards proinflammatory subsets thus decreasing the Teff:Treg ratio. However, as predicted by the biology of the alloresponse, IA1-mediated T cell proliferation was much more restrained than that induced by the anti-CD3/anti-CD28 or PHA stimulation [43]. This finding suggests that the systemic toxicity, relative to pan T cell activators, should be greatly reduced. Crucially, IA1-activated PBMC demonstrated a potent inhibition of cancer cell (HeLa and SH-4 melanoma) proliferation relative to the resting PBMC (**Figure 6**). The anti-proliferation effect of IA1-activated PBMC was noted within ~12 hours vs. 4–5 days for resting cells. These findings demonstrate that miRNA-enriched therapeutics can be biomanufactured from the secretome and can induce a potent proinflammatory, anticancer, effect on resting lymphocytes.

The potential utility and use of IA1 in Adoptive Cell Therapy (ACT) is diagrammatically shown in **Figure 6**. The bioproduction of IA1 is both inexpensive and rapid (5 days) and the IA1 can be stored for long periods (several months frozen in the laboratory; data not shown). Moreover, neither IA1 or TA1 production actually requires donor specific tissues (PBMC) making these secretome-based therapeutics an "off-the-shelf" immune adjuvant. Most importantly for patient care, *ex vivo* activation of lymphocytes is rapid (24 hours). The rapidity of this approach is in stark contrast to the weeks to months necessary for production and expansion of CAR-T cells. Hence, IA1 activation of autologous PBMC could be employed as a first line therapy or, potentially, be used as an immunotherapeutic bridge while CAR-T cells are produced. Due to the simplicity and low cost of the approach, multiple rounds could be used as necessary with large numbers of autologous PBMC employed. Indeed, due to the ability to infuse large numbers of IA1 treated autologous cells, enhanced recognition

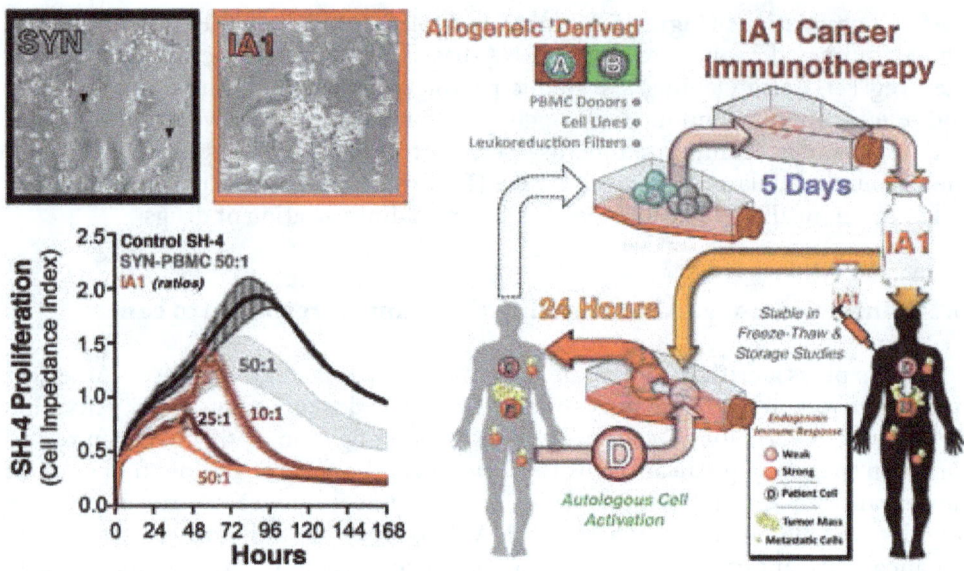

**Figure 6.**
*Schematic presentation of use and efficacy of the IA1 secretome therapeutic. Left panels: the enhanced efficacy of treated PBMC is supported by photomicrographs of allogenic PBMC responding to HeLa cells. As shown, after 72 hours incubation, resting (weak responders; left) PBMC show limited interaction when overlaid on HeLa cells. In contrast, the same PBMC, when treated for 24 hours with IA1, show a robust enhanced interaction (right) with the HeLa cell monolayer. Moreover, when IA1-treated PBMC are overlaid on SH-4 melanoma cells a greatly enhanced anti-cancer effect is noted relative to untreated PBMC. Shown are the growth profiles (as measured by electrical impedance) of SH-4 treated with either the SYN (derived from the secretome of resting PBMC) or IA1therapeutics. PBMC:SH-4 ratios included 50:1, 25:1 and 10:1. Right panels: bioreactor production of IA1 secretome is readily accomplished using an allogeneic MLR. Potential source materials include PBMC donors (A and B), autologous cells (dotted arrow), lymphocytic cell lines, or leukoreduction filters from blood collection bags. The secretome is collected at day 5 for processing into IA1 (**Figure 4**). IA1 is stable for months when aliquoted and frozen. Weak to absent immune response to both the primary tumor and metastatic sites allows for cancer progression. PBMC (D) from the patient can be treated ex vivo for 24 hours with IA1 and then reinfused into the individual where they show enhanced recognition and killing of the primary tumor and, potentially, improved immune surveillance at metastatic sites. Derived from Ref. [43].*

of not only the primary tumor but metastatic sites as well could be achieved thus improving long-term survival. Of note, similarly to our use of the tolerogenic TA1 in NOD mice (**Figures 4** and **5**), IA1 could be directly injected into the recipient yielding a systemic proinflammatory reset of the immune system [40].

## 7. Conclusions

The immunomodulation of the endogenous immune system has become a major focus in treating a broad range of clinical conditions ranging from tissue/organ engraftment, autoimmune disease and cancer therapy. While significant clinical advancements have been made in immunotherapy, substantial challenges remain. One target of interest is the biologic/clinical desire to induce a persistent systemic immunological reset that could reduce both the need for chronic therapy and reduce the potential toxicities associated with current immunomodulatory approaches. Recent studies have demonstrated that miRNA are key regulators of cellular processes involved in both tolerogenic and proinflammatory immune responses and mediate immune cell proliferation and differentiation. Using an alloresponse bioreactor secretome system we have demonstrated that miRNA-based therapeutics can be reproducibly manufactured that can systemically reorient the immune system to either a tolerogenic or proinflammatory state by simultaneously modulating both regulatory and effector T cell subsets thus skewing the Treg:Teff cell ratio to favor tolerance or inflammation. The tolerogenic TA1 therapeutic is derived from polymer-mediated immunocamouflage of the alloresponse reaction while the inflammatory IA1 preparation is derived from the alloresponse itself. The secretomes from these reactions are processed to maintain the miRNA within the secretome. In contrast to most miRNA therapeutic tactics, our approach has been to mimic the "complex pattern of miRNA expression" seen in protolerogenic or proinflammatory states. This "complex" approach was predicated by the inherent nature of miRNA bioregulation in that there is a low probability that altered expression of a single, or even a few, miRNA would exert a potent and definitive biological response. As shown, this approach successfully results in significant and, in mice, systemic and persistent changes to the immune system. The tolerogenic TA1 proved useful in reducing the onset and incidence of autoimmune diabetes in the NOD mouse while the proinflammatory IA1 therapeutic greatly enhanced the efficacy of human T cells to recognize and kill cancer cells without inducing the systemic inflammatory response seen with mitogens or monoclonal antibody (e.g., anti-CD3/CD28) therapies. Moreover, this approach can simultaneously modulate both regulatory and effect T cell subtype. The successful development of this miRNA-immunomodulatory approach may prove useful in facilitating organ engraftment, treating autoimmune disease and enhancing the endogenous anticancer response.

## Acknowledgements

This work was supported by grants from the Canadian Institutes of Health Research (Grant no. 123317; MDS), Canadian Blood Services (MDS) and Health Canada (MDS). The views expressed herein do not necessarily represent the view of the federal government of Canada. We thank the Canada Foundation for Innovation and the Michael Smith Foundation for Health Research for infrastructure funding at the University of British Columbia Centre for Blood Research. The funders had no role in study design, data collection and analysis, decision to publish, or preparation of the manuscript.

## Author details

Mark D. Scott[1,2,3]*, Duncheng Wang[4], Wendy M. Toyofuku[1,2] and Xining Yang[1,2,3]

1 Centre for Innovation, Canadian Blood Services, University of British Columbia, Vancouver, BC, Canada

2 Centre for Blood Research, University of British Columbia, Vancouver, BC, Canada

3 Department of Pathology and Laboratory Medicine, University of British Columbia, Vancouver, BC, Canada

4 MD Anderson Cancer Center, Houston, Texas, USA

*Address all correspondence to: mdscott@mail.ubc.ca

# References

[1] Kaufmann SHE. Immunology's coming of age. Frontiers in Immunology. 2019;**10**:684. DOI: 10.3389/fimmu.2019.00684

[2] Barrat FJ, Cua DJ, Boonstra A, Richards DF, Crain C, Savelkoul HF, et al. In vitro generation of interleukin 10-producing regulatory CD4(⁺) T cells is induced by immunosuppressive drugs and inhibited by T helper type 1 (Th1)- and Th2-inducing cytokines. The Journal of Experimental Medicine. 2002;**195**:603-616. DOI: 10.1084/jem.20011629

[3] Crow AR, Lazarus AH. The mechanisms of action of intravenous immunoglobulin and polyclonal anti-D immunoglobulin in the amelioration of immune thrombocytopenic purpura: What do we really know? Transfusion Medicine Reviews. 2008;**22**:103-116. DOI: 10.1016/j.tmrv.2007.12.001

[4] Imbach P, Lazarus AH, Kuhne T. Intravenous immunoglobulins induce potentially synergistic immunomodulations in autoimmune disorders. Vox Sanguinis. 2010;**98**:385-394. DOI: 10.1111/j.1423-0410.2009.01264.x

[5] Lazarus AH. Adoptive-transfer effects of intravenous immunoglobulin in autoimmunity. Journal of Clinical Immunology. 2010;**30**(Suppl 1):S20-S23. DOI: 10.1007/s10875-010-9410-9

[6] Anthony RM, Kobayashi T, Wermeling F, Ravetch JV. Intravenous gammaglobulin suppresses inflammation through a novel T(H)2 pathway. Nature. 2011;**475**:110-113. DOI: 10.1038/nature10134

[7] Blazar BR, Jenkins MK, Taylor PA, White J, Panoskaltsis-Mortari A, Korngold R, et al. Anti-CD3 epsilon F(ab')2 fragments inhibit T cell expansion in vivo during graft-versus-host disease or the primary immune response to nominal antigen. The Journal of Immunology. 1997;**159**:5821-5833

[8] Delmonico FL, Cosimi AB. Monoclonal antibody treatment of human allograft recipients. Surgery, Gynecology & Obstetrics. 1988;**166**:89-98

[9] Blazar BR, Korngold R, Vallera DA. Recent advances in graft-versus-host disease (GVHD) prevention. Immunological Reviews. 1997;**157**: 79-109. DOI: 10.1111/j.1600-065x.1997.tb00976.x

[10] Toussirot E, Wendling D. The use of TNF-alpha blocking agents in rheumatoid arthritis: An overview. Expert Opinion on Pharmacotherapy. 2004;**5**:581-594. DOI: 10.1517/eoph.5.3.581.27357

[11] Nam JL, Ramiro S, Gaujoux-Viala C, Takase K, Leon-Garcia M, Emery P, et al. Efficacy of biological disease-modifying antirheumatic drugs: A systematic literature review informing the 2013 update of the EULAR recommendations for the management of rheumatoid arthritis. Annals of the Rheumatic Diseases. 2014;**73**:516-528. DOI: 10.1136/annrheumdis-2013-204575

[12] Ramiro S, Gaujoux-Viala C, Nam JL, Smolen JS, Buch M, Gossec L, et al. Safety of synthetic and biological DMARDs: A systematic literature review informing the 2013 update of the EULAR recommendations for management of rheumatoid arthritis. Annals of the Rheumatic Diseases. 2014;**73**:529-535. DOI: 10.1136/annrheumdis-2013-204575

[13] Arora A, Mahajan A, Spurden D, Boyd H, Porter D. Long-term drug survival of TNF inhibitor therapy in RA patients: A systematic

review of European National Drug Registers. International Journal of Rheumatology. 2013;**2013**:764518. DOI: 10.1155/2013/764518

[14] Berard RA, Laxer RM. Etanercept (Enbrel) in the treatment of juvenile idiopathic arthritis. Expert Opinion on Biological Therapy. 2013;**13**:1623-1630. DOI: 10.1517/14712598.2013.840580

[15] Morgan CL, Emery P, Porter D, Reynolds A, Young A, Boyd H, et al. Treatment of rheumatoid arthritis with etanercept with reference to disease-modifying anti-rheumatic drugs: Long-term safety and survival using prospective, observational data. Rheumatology (Oxford). 2014;**53**:186-194. DOI: 10.1093/rheumatology/ket 333

[16] Blumenauer B, Judd M, Cranney A, Burls A, Coyle D, Hochberg M, et al. Etanercept for the treatment of rheumatoid arthritis. Cochrane Database of Systematic Reviews. 2003:CD004525. DOI: 10.1002/14651858.cd004525.pub2

[17] Chong BF, Wong HK. Immunobiologics in the treatment of psoriasis. Clinical Immunology. 2007;**123**:129-138. DOI: 10.1016/j.clim.2007.01.006

[18] Langley RG, Strober BE, Gu Y, Rozzo SJ, Okun MM. Benefit-risk assessment of tumour necrosis factor antagonists in the treatment of psoriasis. The British Journal of Dermatology. 2010;**162**:1349-1358. DOI: 10.1111/j.1365-2133.2010.09707.x

[19] Romero-Mate A, Garcia-Donoso C, Cordoba-Guijarro S. Efficacy and safety of etanercept in psoriasis/psoriatic arthritis: An updated review. American Journal of Clinical Dermatology. 2007;**8**:143-155. DOI: 10.2165/00128071-200708030-00002

[20] Sanchez Carazo JL, Mahiques Santos L, Oliver Martinez V. Safety of etanercept in psoriasis: A critical review. Drug Safety. 2006;**29**:675-685. DOI: 10.2165/00002018-200629080-00004

[21] Inoue Y, Kaifu T, Sugahara-Tobinai A, Nakamura A, Miyazaki J, Takai T. Activating Fc gamma receptors participate in the development of autoimmune diabetes in NOD mice. Journal of Immunology. 2007;**179**:764-774. DOI: 10.4049/jimmunol.179.2.764

[22] Shoda LK, Young DL, Ramanujan S, Whiting CC, Atkinson MA, Bluestone JA, et al. A comprehensive review of interventions in the NOD mouse and implications for translation. Immunity. 2005;**23**:115-126. DOI: 10.1016/j.immuni.2005.08.002

[23] Bachanova V, Miller JS. NK cells in therapy of cancer. Critical Reviews in Oncogenesis. 2014;**19**:133-141. DOI: 10.1615/critrevoncog.2014011091

[24] Forget MA, Malu S, Liu H, Toth C, Maiti S, Kale C, et al. Activation and propagation of tumor-infiltrating lymphocytes on clinical-grade designer artificial antigen-presenting cells for adoptive immunotherapy of melanoma. Journal of Immunotherapy. 2014;**37**:448-460. DOI: 10.1097/cji.0000000000000056

[25] Liu S, Lizee G, Lou Y, Liu C, Overwijk WW, Wang G, et al. IL-21 synergizes with IL-7 to augment expansion and anti-tumor function of cytotoxic T cells. International Immunology. 2007;**19**:1213-1221. DOI: 10.1093/intimm/dxm093

[26] Miller JS. Therapeutic applications: Natural killer cells in the clinic. Hematology. American Society of Hematology. Education Program. 2013;**2013**:247-253. DOI: 10.1182/asheducation-2013.1.247

[27] Peng BG, He Q, Liang LI, Xie BH, Hua YP, Chen ZB, et al. Induction of cytotoxic T-lymphocyte responses

using dendritic cells transfected with hepatocellular carcinoma mRNA. British Journal of Biomedical Science. 2006;**63**:123-128. DOI: 10.1080/09674845.2006.11732731

[28] Sangiolo D. Cytokine induced killer cells as promising immunotherapy for solid tumors. Journal of Cancer. 2011;**2**:363-368. DOI: 10.7150/jca.2.363

[29] Savage P, Millrain M, Dimakou S, Stebbing J, Dyson J. Expansion of CD8+ cytotoxic T cells *in vitro* and *in vivo* using MHC class I tetramers. Tumour Biology. 2007;**28**:70-76. DOI: 10.1159/000099152

[30] Symes JC, Siatskas C, Fowler DH, Medin JA. Retrovirally transduced murine T lymphocytes expressing FasL mediate effective killing of prostate cancer cells. Cancer Gene Therapy. 2009;**16**:439-452. DOI: 10.1038/cgt.2008.96

[31] Wu JY, Ernstoff MS, Hill JM, Cole B, Meehan KR. Ex vivo expansion of non-MHC-restricted cytotoxic effector cells as adoptive immunotherapy for myeloma. Cytotherapy. 2006;**8**:141-148. DOI: 10.1080/14653240600620218

[32] Murad KL, Gosselin EJ, Eaton JW, Scott MD. Stealth cells: Prevention of major histocompatibility complex class II-mediated T-cell activation by cell surface modification. Blood. 1999;**94**:2135-2141

[33] Chen AM, Scott MD. Current and future applications of immunological attenuation via pegylation of cells and tissue. BioDrugs. 2001;**15**:833-847. DOI: 10.2165/00063030-200115120-00005

[34] Chen AM, Scott MD. Immunocamouflage: Prevention of transfusion-induced graft-versus-host disease via polymer grafting of donor cells. Journal of Biomedical Materials Research. Part A. 2003;**67**:626-636. DOI: 10.1002/jbm.a.10146

[35] Chen AM, Scott MD. Comparative analysis of polymer and linker chemistries on the efficacy of immunocamouflage of murine leukocytes. Artificial Cells, Blood Substitutes, and Immobilization Biotechnology. 2006;**34**:305-322. DOI: 10.1080/10731190600683845

[36] Wang D, Toyofuku WM, Chen AM, Scott MD. Induction of immunotolerance via mPEG grafting to allogeneic leukocytes. Biomaterials. 2011;**32**:9494-9503. DOI: 10.1016/j.biomaterials.2011.08.061

[37] Wang D, Toyofuku WM, Scott MD. The potential utility of methoxypoly(ethylene Glycol)-mediated prevention of rhesus blood group antigen RhD recognition in transfusion medicine. Biomaterials. 2012;**33**:3002-3012. DOI: 10.1016/j.biomaterials.2011.12.041

[38] Wang D, Toyofuku WM, Kyluik DL, Scott MD. Use of flow cytometry in the in vitro and in vivo analysis of tolerance/anergy induction by immunocamouflage. In: Schmid I, editor. Flow Cytometry-Recent Perspectives. Croatia: InTech; 2012. pp. 133-150. DOI: 10.5772/37797

[39] Kyluik-Price DL, Li L, Scott MD. Comparative efficacy of blood cell immunocamouflage by membrane grafting of methoxypoly(ethylene glycol) and polyethyloxazoline. Biomaterials. 2014;**35**:412-422. DOI: 10.1016/j.biomaterials.2013.09.016

[40] Wang D, Shanina I, Toyofuku WM, Horwitz MS, Scott MD. Inhibition of autoimmune diabetes in NOD mice by miRNA therapy. PLoS ONE. 2015;**10**:e0145179. DOI: 10.1371/journal.pone.0145179

[41] Kyluik-Price DL, Scott MD. Effects of methoxypoly (ethylene glycol) mediated immunocamouflage on leukocyte surface marker detection,

cell conjugation, activation and alloproliferation. Biomaterials. 2016;**74**:167-177. DOI: 10.1016/j.biomaterials.2015.09.047

[42] Kang N, Toyofuku WM, Yang X, Scott MD. Inhibition of allogeneic cytotoxic T cell (CD8($^+$)) proliferation via polymer-induced Treg (CD4($^+$)) cells. Acta Biomaterialia. 2017;**57**:146-155. DOI: doi.org/10.1016/j.actbio.2017.04.025

[43] Yang X, Kang N, Toyofuku WM, Scott MD. Enhancing the pro-inflammatory anti-cancer T cell response via biomanufactured, secretome-based, immunotherapeutics. Immunobiology. 2019;**224**:270-284. DOI: 10.1016/j.imbio.2018.12.003

[44] Wei B, Pei G. MicroRNAs: Critical regulators in Th17 cells and players in diseases. Cellular & Molecular Immunology. 2010;**7**:175-181. DOI: 10.1038/cmi.2010.19

[45] Guay C, Roggli E, Nesca V, Jacovetti C, Regazzi R. Diabetes mellitus, a microRNA-related disease? Translational Research. 2011;**157**:253-264. DOI: 10.1016/j.trsl.2011.01.009

[46] Nielsen LB, Wang C, Sorensen K, Bang-Berthelsen CH, Hansen L, Andersen ML, et al. Circulating levels of microRNA from children with newly diagnosed type 1 diabetes and healthy controls: Evidence that miR-25 associates to residual beta-cell function and glycaemic control during disease progression. Experimental Diabetes Research. 2012;**2012**:896362. DOI: 10.1155/2012/896362

[47] Lewis BP, Burge CB, Bartel DP. Conserved seed pairing, often flanked by adenosines, indicates that thousands of human genes are microRNA targets. Cell. 2005;**120**:15-20. DOI: 10.1016/j.cell.2004.12.035

[48] Chen K, Rajewsky N. The evolution of gene regulation by transcription factors and microRNAs. Nature Reviews. Genetics. 2007;**8**:93-103. DOI: 10.1038/nrg1990

[49] Friedman RC, Farh KK, Burge CB, Bartel DP. Most mammalian mRNAs are conserved targets of microRNAs. Genome Research. 2009;**19**:92-105. DOI: 10.1101/gr.082701.108

[50] Bartel DP. MicroRNAs: Target recognition and regulatory functions. Cell. 2009;**136**:215-233. DOI: 10.1016/j.cell.2009.01.002

[51] Bhardwaj A, Singh S, Singh AP. MicroRNA-based cancer therapeutics: Big hope from small RNAs. Molecular and Cellular Pharmacology. 2010;**2**:213-219. DOI: 10.4255/mcpharmacol.10.27

[52] Braicu C, Calin GA, Berindan-Neagoe I. MicroRNAs and cancer therapy-from bystanders to major players. Current Medicinal Chemistry. 2013;**20**:3561-3573. DOI: 10.2174/0929867311320290002

[53] Jopling CL, Yi M, Lancaster AM, Lemon SM, Sarnow P. Modulation of hepatitis C virus RNA abundance by a liver-specific MicroRNA. Science. 2005;**309**:1577-1581. DOI: 10.1126/science.1113329

[54] Liu C, Kelnar K, Liu B, Chen X, Calhoun-Davis T, Li H, et al. The microRNA miR-34a inhibits prostate cancer stem cells and metastasis by directly repressing CD44. Nature Medicine. 2011;**17**:211-215. DOI: 10.1038/nm.2284

[55] Roep BO. The role of T-cells in the pathogenesis of Type 1 diabetes: From cause to cure. Diabetologia. 2003;**46**:305-321. DOI: 10.1007/s00125-003-1089-5

[56] Anderson MS, Bluestone JA. The NOD mouse: A model of immune dysregulation. Annual Review of

Immunology. 2005;**23**:447-485. DOI: 10.1146/annurev.immunol.23.021704. 115643

[57] Richer MJ, Lavallee DJ, Shanina I, Horwitz MS. Immunomodulation of antigen presenting cells promotes natural regulatory T cells that prevent autoimmune diabetes in NOD mice. PLoS ONE. 2012;7:e31153. DOI: 10.1371/journal.pone.0031153

[58] Salomon B, Lenschow DJ, Rhee L, Ashourian N, Singh B, Sharpe A, et al. B7/CD28 costimulation is essential for the homeostasis of the CD4+CD25+ immunoregulatory T cells that control autoimmune diabetes. Immunity. 2000;**12**:431-440. DOI: 10.1016/s1074-7613(00)80195-8

[59] Gregori S, Giarratana N, Smiroldo S, Adorini L. Dynamics of pathogenic and suppressor T cells in autoimmune diabetes development. Journal of Immunology. 2003;**171**:4040-4047. DOI: 10.4049/jimmunol.171.8.4040

[60] You S, Belghith M, Cobbold S, Alyanakian MA, Gouarin C, Barriot S, et al. Autoimmune diabetes onset results from qualitative rather than quantitative age-dependent changes in pathogenic T-cells. Diabetes. 2005;**54**:1415-1422. DOI: 10.2337/diabetes.54.5.1415

[61] Tritt M, Sgouroudis E, d'Hennezel E, Albanese A, Piccirillo CA. Functional waning of naturally occurring CD4+ regulatory T-cells contributes to the onset of autoimmune diabetes. Diabetes. 2008;**57**:113-123. DOI: 10.2337/db06-1700

[62] Richer MJ, Straka N, Fang D, Shanina I, Horwitz MS. Regulatory T-cells protect from type 1 diabetes after induction by coxsackievirus infection in the context of transforming growth factor-beta. Diabetes. 2008;**57**:1302-1311. DOI: 10.2337/db07-1460

[63] D'Alise AM, Auyeung V, Feuerer M, Nishio J, Fontenot J, Benoist C, et al. The defect in T-cell regulation in NOD mice is an effect on the T-cell effectors. Proceedings of the National Academy of Sciences of the United States of America. 2008;**105**:19857-19862. DOI: 10.1073/pnas.0810713105

[64] Feuerer M, Shen Y, Littman DR, Benoist C, Mathis D. How punctual ablation of regulatory T cells unleashes an autoimmune lesion within the pancreatic islets. Immunity. 2009;**31**:654-664. DOI: 10.1016/j.immuni.2009.08.023

[65] Nishio J, Feuerer M, Wong J, Mathis D, Benoist C. Anti-CD3 therapy permits regulatory T cells to surmount T cell receptor-specified peripheral niche constraints. The Journal of Experimental Medicine. 2010;**207**: 1879-1889. DOI: 10.1084/jem.20100205

[66] Thayer TC, Wilson SB, Mathews CE. Use of nonobese diabetic mice to understand human type 1 diabetes. Endocrinology and Metabolism Clinics of North America. 2010;**39**:541-561. DOI: 10.1016/j.ecl.2010.05.001

[67] Lindley S, Dayan CM, Bishop A, Roep BO, Peakman M, Tree TI. Defective suppressor function in CD4(+)CD25(+) T-cells from patients with type 1 diabetes. Diabetes. 2005;**54**:92-99. DOI: 10.2337/diabetes.54.1.92

[68] Cantrell DA. T-cell antigen receptor signal transduction. Immunology. 2002;**105**:369-374. DOI: 10.1046/j.1365-2567.2002.01391.x

[69] Larsson EL, Coutinho A. The role of mitogenic lectins in T-cell triggering. Nature. 1979;**280**:239-241. DOI: 10.1038/280239a0

[70] Swingler S, Mann A, jacque JM, Brichacek B, Sassaville VG, Williams K, et al. HIV-1 Nef mediates lymphocyte chemotaxis and activation by infected macrphages. Nature Medicine. 1999;**5**:997-1003. DOI: 10.1038/12433

[71] Trickett A, Kwan YL. T cell stimulation and expansion using anti-CD3/CD28 beads. Journal of Immunological Methods. 2003;**275**:251-255. DOI: 10.1016/s0022-1759(03)00010-3

[72] Suntharalingam G, Perry MR, Ward S, Brett SJ, Castello-Cortes A, Brunner MD, et al. Cytokine storm in a phase 1 trial of the anti-CD28 monoclonal antibody TGN1412. The New England Journal of Medicine. 2006;**355**:1018-1028. DOI: 10.1056/nejmoa063842

[73] Han T, Takita H. Immunologic impairment in bronchogenic carcinoma: A study of lymphocyte response to phytohemagglutinin. Cancer. 1972;**30**:616-620. DOI: 10.1002/1097-0142(197209)30:3%3C616::aid-cncr2820300304%3E3.0.co;2-q

[74] Maciel RM, Miki SS, Nicolau W, Mendes NF. Peripheral blood T and B lymphocytes, *in vitro* stimulation with phytohemagglutinin, and sensitization with 2,4-dinitrochlorobenzene in Grave's disease. The Journal of Clinical Endocrinology and Metabolism. 1976;**42**:583-587. DOI: 10.1210/jcem-42-3-583

[75] Nisbet NW, Simonsen M, Zaleski M. The frequency of antigen-sensitive cells in tissue transplantation. A commentary on clonal selection. The Journal of Experimental Medicine. 1969;**129**:459-467. DOI: 10.1084/jem.129.3.459

# 2

# KLF4-Mediated Plasticity of Myeloid-Derived Suppressor Cells (MDSCs)

*Daping Fan, Samir Raychoudhury and Walden Ai*

## Abstract

Robustness of tissues refers to their capability to maintain normal functions despite perturbation such as injuries. Recent studies suggest a key role of the immune system in injury repair. In this process, several immune cell lineages exhibit considerable plasticity as they migrate toward the site of damage and contribute to repair. For example, myeloid-derived suppressor cells (MDSCs) are a heterogeneous group of immature cells and possess phenotypic plasticity in cancer, a pathological status that is considered as "wounds that do not heal." They are characterized by their potent ability to suppress immune responses. In cutaneous wound healing, MDSCs not only execute their immunosuppressive function to inhibit inflammation but also stimulate cell proliferation once they adopt a fate of a totally different cell type. At a molecular level, we found that Krüppel-like factor 4 (KLF4), a transcription factor with multiple roles in homeostasis and disease development plays a critical role in regulating MDSCs. In this review, KLF4-mediated plasticity of MDSCs and the underlying mechanisms are discussed.

**Keywords:** KLF4, FSP-1, myeloid-derived suppressor cells (MDSCs), plasticity, cancer, wound healing

## 1. Introduction

KLF4 is a member of the Krüppel-like factor family, a group of zinc finger-containing transcription factors that are highly homologous with the Drosophila Krüppel protein [1–4]. It has important functions in a variety of cellular processes that include cell proliferation, differentiation, development, and maintenance of normal tissue homeostasis [5]. KLF4 has also been shown to act either as a tumor suppressor or an oncoprotein in a context-dependent manner [6–8]. Moreover, KLF4 is critical to barrier function of the skin and promotes physiological and pathological wound healing [9–11].

MDSCs are bone marrow-derived cells present in bone marrow, spleen, and circulation. They are a heterogeneous collection of immature myeloid cells. These immature cells possess typical CD11b$^+$Ly6G$^+$ markers in mice with a wider range of markers in humans. The main function of MDSCs is their potent ability to suppress the host immune responses, especially T-cell proliferation and cytokine production [12]. They possess phenotypic plasticity in cancer [13, 14], a pathological status that is considered as "wounds that do not heal." However, while the involvement of MDSCs in wound healing has been shown by their recruitment to the wound sites [15], the role of their plasticity in wound healing has not been fully examined. On the other hand, two immune cell lineages closely related to MDSCs, namely neutrophils and macrophages, demonstrated their phenotypical and functional plasticity in wound repair [16]. In addition, we showed that in wound healing MDSCs not only execute their immunosuppressive function to inhibit inflammation, but also stimulate cell proliferation once they adopt a fibrocyte fate [11]. Collectively, these observations support a key role of MDSC plasticity in wound healing leading to tissue robustness, though the underlying cellular and molecular mechanisms are not clear.

We recently reported that KLF4 promotes cancer development by regulating the recruitment and function of MDSCs [8, 17, 18]. In addition, we found that KLF4 regulates generation of fibrocytes, emerging effector cells in chronic inflammation [19, 20], from MDSCs in cancer [8], wound healing [11], allergic asthma [21]. Given the importance of plasticity of macrophages, a highly relevant cell type to MDSCs, in tissue repair and regeneration [22], we postulate that KLF4 also regulates myeloid plasticity in wound healing. In this review, the role of KLF4 in regulating plasticity of MDSCs in wound healing and the underlying molecular mechanisms will be discussed.

## 2. Plasticity of MDSCs in cancer and wound healing

MDSCs represent a group of heterogeneous monocytes during myeloid cell development with a major attribute of immunosuppressive activities. The population of these cells increases in a number of conditions associated with chronic inflammation, autoimmune diseases, and cancer. These heterogeneous cells are now further divided into two major subgroups including polymorphonuclear (PMN) and monocytic (M)-MDSCs [23]. Although non-immunosuppressive MDSCs exist in tumor-bearing hosts or in conditions of chronic inflammation [24], in which MDSCs can be classified as MDSC-like cells (MDSC-LC), demonstration of immunosuppressive activities is required to accurately define MDSCs after the initial phenotypical characterization by cell surface markers. In term of immunosuppressive activities of MDSCs, different mediators were reported, such as arginases, nitric oxide (NO), reactive oxygen species (ROS), indoleamine 2,3-dioxygenase (IDO), transforming growth factor-$\beta$1 (TGF-$\beta$1), and prostaglandin E2 (PGE2) among others, depending on specific conditions. As MDSCs are heterogeneous and suppress immune functions with different mechanisms, it is not surprising that they possess phenotypical and functional plasticity [25], reflecting their adaptation to varied environmental conditions. Note that immune cell plasticity could be understood from two different and important senses [16]. The first one is *intra-lineage cell plasticity*, that is, changes in cell function within a given cell lineage. This is also known as functional plasticity. The second sense is *trans-lineage cell plasticity*, that is, the switch from one lineage to another. Alternatively, this can be called "transdifferentiation" or "phenotypical plasticity." We will mainly use "phenotypical plasticity" and "functional plasticity" to discuss MDSC functions in this chapter.

### 2.1 MDSC plasticity in cancer

Immunotherapies against cancer rely on activated T cells or NK cells to recognize and eliminate tumor cells. However, the effector cells in the tumor microenvironment encounter a wide array of factors that limit their activities. MDSC-mediated immune suppression represents one of the major mechanisms by which the functions of immune effector cells are blocked in cancer. In addition, MDSCs are implicated not only in regulating tumor immune response, but also in tumor angiogenesis, tumor cell invasion, and formation of pre-metastatic niches [26].

Phenotypical plasticity of MDSCs in cancer could be first understood from the capacity of myeloid regulatory cells to convert from each other under certain conditions. Such plasticity could explain confusing observations on the role of MDSCs in tumor growth or tumor inhibition [13]. For example, while MDSCs are well known for their tumor promoting function because of their immunosuppressive activities against T cells, they can be converted to dendritic cells (DCs) in the presence of nature killer T (NKT) cells and α-galactosylceramide, leading to an anti-tumor immune response against HER2/CT26 tumor [27]. Mechanistically, it was proposed that NKT cells interact with MDSCs. This interaction leads to the conversion of MDSCs to DCs by increasing gene expression of CD80, CD86 and CD70. Consequently, interactions of CD80 and CD70 on newly converted DCs with CD28 and CD27 on T cells support these T cell responses to the tumor cells resulting in elimination of MDSC-mediated immune suppression [13].

Phenotypical plasticity of MDSCs could also be understood from the existence of MDSC subtypes and their differentiation into macrophages under normal and abnormal conditions. Because PMN-MDSCs are short lived, M-MDSCs have been studied in a more detail. In addition, most studies did not correlate M-MDSCs with monocytes expressing high levels of Ly-6C (Ly-6C$^{hi}$ cells). These Ly-6C$^{hi}$ cells are frequently referred to inflammatory monocytes. Given their elevated function at the tumor site and their potent immunosuppressive activities, Ly-6C$^{hi}$ monocytes in the tumor microenvironment most likely represent *bona fide* M-MDSCs [14]. M-MDSCs have been shown to differentiate into tumor-associated macrophages (TAMS) after they are recruited to the tumor site [28]. It was shown that the CD45-mediated inhibition of STAT3 in MDSCs promotes TAM differentiation [29]. Besides TAMs and DCs as we discussed earlier, MDSCs differentiate into fibrocytes, an emerging group of cells with multiple functions in inflammation and cancer [19, 20, 30, 31].

Functional plasticity of MDSCs could be understood by their intrinsic features especially their immunosuppressive activities. It is known that immunosuppressive activities of MDSCs are mainly detected in tumors, but rarely in other tissues or organs including bone marrow or spleen. However, MDSCs in tumor and other chronic inflammatory conditions may not always be immunosuppressive. For example, in the initiation stage of chronic inflammation or early stage tumors, there are cells with MDSC phenotypical markers but without potent immunosuppressive activities. Moreover, even in advanced stage tumors, not all cells with a MDSC phenotype possess immune suppressive activity. For example, recent studies showed that in chronic inflammation, cells with an MDSC phenotype lacking suppressive activity actually contribute to the early stages of tumor inflammation [32]. However, the exact nature and the mechanism of how MDSCs acquire their immune suppressive activities are not entirely clear.

## 2.2 Potential role of MDSC plasticity in tissue repair

Though immunologists generally consider the immune system as a system of defense, recent studies suggest a key role of the system in tissue robustness, the capability of an organism to maintain its function and performance despite perturbations [33, 34]. One of the major ways by which the immune system contributes to robustness is through immune cell plasticity. Most studies of tissue repair have focused on the innate immune system, which may reflect the evolutional conservation of the repair-mediated robustness. Although plasticity of γδT cells [35, 36], innate lymphoid cells [37], and regulatory T cells [38] is also involved in tissue repair, we will mainly discuss the role of neutrophils, macrophages, and MDSCs in the process. Neutrophils are the major innate cells recruited to the damage site and are considered as the first line of defense against infection [39]. However, these cells can switch phenotypes, display distinct subpopulations, and produce a large variety of cytokines and chemokines [40]. In tissue repair, neutrophils can show their intra-lineage or functional plasticity by pro- or anti-inflammation, during the early stage of a typical wound repair. In addition, in an inflammatory and pro-type 2 microenvironment of a lesion, neutrophils transdifferentiate into antigen presenting cells (APCs) [41]. Such transdifferentiation into APCs has also been studied in rheumatism, where it could drive sustained inflammation, thereby preventing normal repair [42]. Besides neutrophils, macrophages fulfill roles that change over the duration of wound healing [43]. Initially they are bactericidal, and voraciously phagocytose cell and matrix debris, particularly red blood cells and any spent neutrophils at the wound site. These early stage macrophages are called M1 macrophages, and they are pro-inflammatory. Later in the repair process, macrophages develop the pro-repair capacity. These macrophages are called M2 macrophages, and they are anti-inflammatory and pro-reparative. The resting macrophages are called M0 macrophages. Not surprisingly, the plasticity of macrophages, namely the changeable cellular phenotypes and the range of differentiation and activation states, helps to explain the pleiotropic nature of these cells and their complex functions in wound repair [22, 44]. Beside their role in the early inflammatory stage of wound healing, macrophages contribute to tissue remodeling in wound healing by transdifferentiation, notably into endothelial cells [45, 46], a phenotypical plasticity.

When compared to those of neutrophils and macrophages, the role of MDSCs and their plasticity in wound healing are less studied [47]. However, there is ample evidence supporting a critical role of MDSC plasticity in repair. For example, as a heterogeneous and immature population of myeloid cells, recruited MDSCs at wound sites can differentiate into macrophages, DCs, and neutrophils [25]. In addition, because of their immunosuppressive function, MDSCs appear to dampen inflammation at the early stage but then promote healing after inflammation wanes by adopting a fate of fibrocytes [11], a cell type that can further differentiate into myofibroblasts that produce extracellular matrix in wound closure [48, 49]. In cancer, a pathological condition considered as "wounds that do not heal," fibrocytes are viewed as a subpopulation of MDSCs [50, 51], further highlighting a dynamic and plastic nature of MDSCs in wound healing.

## 3. KLF4-mediated plasticity of MDSCs

### 3.1 KLF4 promotes cancer development through regulating plasticity of M-MDSCs

KLF4 is expressed in many tissues and cells types. Besides in epithelial cells, it is also expressed in bone marrow-derived cells and is key to inflammation [52, 53] and monocyte differentiation [54, 55]. However, it was not clear whether and how immune cell-expressing KLF4 is involved in the development of tumor. It is our hypothesis that the overall function of KLF4 depends on its expression in immune cells and in the resident epithelial cells. In the following discussion, we will focus on the role of MDSC-expressing KLF4 in cancer.

To study the function of KLF4 in MDSCs, we used a 4T1 mammary tumor model. This model is unique due to its similar characteristics with human breast cancer, particularly the ability to spontaneously metastasize to lungs. Based on 4T1 cells, we generated stable KLF4 knockdown cells and control cells using siRNA technology. They were designated as siKLF4 and siCon, respectively. We found that in siCon cell-inoculated BALB/c mice tumors were observed as early as Day 9 and the tumor size reached to 18.2 ± 1.6 mm in diameter. However, in siKLF4 cell-inoculated mice the primary mammary tumors became visible on Day 14 and the tumor size was only 11.3 ± 1.4 mm in diameter [18]. These data were in agreement with our previous results showing that KLF4 knockdown delayed the onset of mammary tumor development and inhibited lung metastasis in immunocompromised NOD/SCID mice inoculated with MDA-MB-231 human breast cancer cells [56]. We then tested whether MDSCs were involved in KLF4-mediated tumor development. We examined MDSCs in bone marrow, spleen, and tumor by flow cytometry. We found that after implantation of 4 T1 cells, KLF4 knockdown significantly reduced the numbers of MDSCs in bone marrow and spleen when compared to siCon counterparts [18]. As a critical control, we examined the immunosuppressive activities of MDSCs from control cell- and KLF4 knockdown cell-inoculated mice [57, 58]. As expected, MDSCs from siKLF4 cell-inoculated mouse inhibited proliferation of CD4+ and CD8+ T-cell significantly less than their siCon counterparts. The same assay using MDSCs purified from mouse tumors confirmed this observation. Moreover, consistent with higher T cell proliferation upon KLF4 knockdown, the arginase activities in MDSCs from siKLF4 cell-inoculated mice were lower when compared to those in siCon counterparts. Furthermore, we examined the infiltration of T cells into tumor sites by CD3 immunofluorescence staining. We found that there were more T cells accumulated in siKLF4 cell-inoculated mice than in siCon group.

Consistently, in a mouse B16-F10 implantation melanoma model, we showed that KLF4 deficiency in bone marrow drastically reduced lung metastasis accompanied by decreased recruitment of monocytic CCR2+ MDSCs (M-MDSCs) in the lungs. Interestingly, bone marrow KLF4 deficiency was linked with significantly reduced numbers of fibrocytes and myofibroblasts in metastatic lungs [8]. We further performed a cause-effect study to exclude the effect of KLF4-mediated development of MDSCs and to test the direct effect of KLF4-regulated fibrocyte generation from M-MDSCs on tumor metastasis. We sorted M-MDSC subset from the lungs of mice bearing B16-F10 melanoma. They were mixed with B16-F10 tumor cells and then injected wild-type mice with the mixture intravenously. We then induced KLF4 knockout in these mice by tamoxifen injection. In the control mice, they only received B16-F10 tumor cells, but were still injected with tamoxifen or sunflower seed oil as controls. Mice were sacrificed at Day 7 after tumor cell inoculation. We found that no difference was observed in the incidence of lung metastasis between the mice administrated with tamoxifen or sunflower seed oil. However, in the KLF4$^{-/-}$ and control groups, metastatic nodules in the pulmonary were drastically fewer than those in the KLF4$^{+/+}$ group. The results strongly suggest that KLF4 controls the process in which M-MDSCs facilitate the seeding and growth of pulmonary metastatic nodules. We also took advantage of the EGFP marker in the transplanted M-MDSCs. We examined MDSC differentiation in the lung by immunofluorescence using COL1A1 and α-SMA antibodies. We found that although there was no difference in the total number of EGFP$^+$ cells between the KLF4$^{+/+}$ and KLF4$^{-/-}$ group, in KLF4 deficient mice the number of COL1A1$^+$EGFP$^+$ cells decreased significantly when compared to that in the KLF4$^{+/+}$ mice. Similarly, α-SMA$^+$EGFP$^+$ cells also decreased in KLF4$^{-/-}$ mice, further supporting our speculation that KLF4 regulates the differentiation of M-MDSCs into fibrocytes and myofibroblasts after they are recruited to the lungs *in vivo*.

### 3.2 KLF4 deficiency compromised cutaneous wound healing depending on functional MDSCs

A pressure ulcer (PU) is defined as an injury caused by unrelieved pressure that results in damage to the skin and underlying tissue [59, 60]. They are thought to be caused by local tissue ischemia, interstitial and lymphatic blockage, reperfusion injury, and mechanical deformation of cells by compressive forces [61]. PUs are detrimental to the patients by prolonging their hospital stay, affecting social life-styles, and contributing to negative psychological consequences [62, 63]. Generally, wound healing includes the early inflammatory phase and the later proliferative and remodeling phases [64–66]. However, this process in PU is frequently stalled in the inflammatory stage [67]. This is the reason why PU has been considered a chronic wound [68].

We have reported that KLF4 ablation delayed cutaneous wound healing in KLF4-CreER/KLF4(flox) [69] and RosaCreER/KLF4(flox) double transgenic mice [11], in which KLF4 was knocked out upon tamoxifen induction. To further test the possibility that KLF4 deficiency-induced delay of cutaneous wound healing may be attributed to bone marrow cells, we transplanted bone marrow cells from RosaCreER/KLF4(flox)/β-actin-EGFP triple transgenic mice into wild type C57BL/6 mice and used these chimeric mice to perform full-thickness wound healing experiments. The wound-closure kinetics showed that wound healing was significantly delayed upon KLF4 knockout in bone marrow. In addition, M-MDSCs but not total MDSCs in the skin wounding bed significantly decreased in the KLF4$^{-/-}$ group compared to those in the KLF4$^{+/+}$ group. By flow cytometric analysis, after we gated EGFP+ cells and analyzed COL1A1$^+$CD45$^+$CD11b$^+$ populations to examine bone marrow-derived fibrocytes in the skin wounding bed, we showed that fibrocytes decreased in KLF4$^{-/-}$ group compared to those in KLF4$^{+/+}$ group. This finding was further confirmed by immunofluorescent staining of the wounding bed, as demonstrated by significantly reduced numbers of COL1A1/EGFP and α-SMA/EGFP co-expressing cells in KLF4$^{-/-}$ group. Moreover, we transplanted bone marrow cells from KLF4/EGFP transgenic mice, in which KLF4-expressing cells are labeled with EGFP [69], to the wild type mice and performed full thickness wound healing experiments. Four days after the wound placement, the wound healing tissues were collected and slides prepared, followed by immunofluorescent staining. We found that KLF4 expressing EGFP cells in the wound bed adapted elongated morphology and were co-localized with those expressing α-SMA, a marker of myofibroblasts that play a critical role in wound healing [70, 71].

KLF4 was highly expressed in M-MDSCs, and we postulated that KLF4 in M-MDSCs may directly regulate the cutaneous wound healing. Because of the highest expression level of FSP-1 in M-MDSCs among all MDSC subpopulations, to test our hypothesis, we used FSP-1-Cre/KLF4(flox) mice to produce PUs [72]. The dorsal skin of WT and FSP-1-Cre/KLF4(flox) (KLF4 null) mice were shaved, gently pulled up and placed between two cylinders of magnets (12 mm in diameter and 5 mm in thickness), producing a compressive pressure of 50 mmHg between the two magnets according to the established PU model [72–74]. A single ischemia-reperfusion cycle (I/R) consisted of a period of magnet placement for 16 h followed by a release or rest of 8 h. Three I/R cycles were used in each animal to initiate decubitus ulcer formation. Ulcers were typically formed at Day 3 (at the end of third I/R cycle) accompanied by full-thickness loss of skin. To assess the wound healing of PU, the detached full-thickness skin (ulcered skin) was removed at Day 3 right after the third I/R cycle, and the closure of open ulcer area in each mouse was monitored and photographed consecutively for 10 days. We found that 1 day after the ulcered skin was removed, the opening areas were increased in both WT and KLF4 null mice, probably because of the acute responses. From Day 2 to Day 10, wounds were gradually healed in WT mice, but the healing was delayed in KLF4 null mice as also indicated by an unclosed wound at Day 10. H&E staining showed an increased suprabasal layer of the skin and decreased hair follicle densities. The infiltrated lymphocytes were almost doubled in granule tissue of the skin in KLF4 null mice. These results suggest an elevated inflammatory status in KLF4 null mice. In agreement with reduced numbers of M-MDSCs and fibrocytes upon KLF4 knockout in bone marrow in our full-thickness wound healing model, these populations were also decreased in FSP-1-Cre/KLF4(flox) mice in the PU model. Interestingly, we found that the populations of CD11b+Ly6C++ cells, which may represent inflammatory monocytes [75], in both blood and skin wounding beds were increased when compared to those in wild type mice. This observation is consistent with the increased inflammation in KLF4 null mice.

### 3.3 Mechanisms of KLF4-mediated MDSC plasticity

MDSC plasticity, and in general, myeloid plasticity, is regulated by the local microenvironment. These cells are environmental sensors and adapters [25]. In tumor, myeloid cells are the most abundant immune cells, and signals within the tumor microenvironment instruct these cells to change their dynamics and plasticity. There are many potential factors/mechanisms in these processes, including hypoxia, tumor ER stress, exosomes, and tumor-derived soluble factors [76]. In the following discussion, we will focus on KLF4-mediated plasticity of MDSCs in cancer and wound healing based on our recent studies.

#### 3.3.1 KLF4 regulates FSP-1 in fibrocyte generation from MDSCs

FSP-1, also known as S100A4, is widely accepted as a fibroblast-specific marker [77, 78]. Given the fact that FSP-1 is expressed in more than 90% of monocytes of the host immune system [79] and that it has a "specific" expression in fibroblasts, it is challenging to reconcile the function of FSP-1 at the cellular level between these two very different cell types. On the other hand, fibrocytes are bone marrow-derived progenitor cells that can differentiate into myofibroblasts and promote cutaneous would healing and cancer development [20, 51, 80, 81]. Therefore, fibrocytes are very good candidates for carrying the expression/function of FSP-1 from the host immune cells such as MDSCs to fibroblasts.

It has been reported that fibrocytes can be generated from bone marrow-derived cells such as MDSCs [82]. We postulated that KLF4 controls MDSC-mediated generation of fibrocytes. To test this hypothesis and to examine the underlying mechanisms, we isolated spleen cells from KLF4 inducible knockout Rosa26CreER/KLF4(flox) mice and examined fibrocyte differentiation using an *ex vivo* assay with murine IL-13 and M-CSF [83]. We found that the application of IL-13 and M-CSF resulted in $58 \pm 7$ fibrocytes per $1 \times 10^5$ cells (**Figure 1A**) in the control group. However, the same treatment decreased the number of fibrocytes to $5 \pm 2$ cells per $1 \times 10^5$ splenocytes when KLF4 was knocked out by induction of 5 μM 4-OH tamoxifen (**Figure 1B**). Furthermore, we examined KLF4 and FSP-1 expression in the process of fibrocyte generation by quantitative RT-PCR analysis. As shown in **Figure 1C**, both KLF4 and FSP-1 mRNA levels were significantly elevated after the application of IL-13 and M-CSF, which was consistent with *ex vivo* generation of fibrocytes. The induction of KLF4 deficiency by 4-OH tamoxifen correlates with a significant decrease in FSP-1 expression, suggesting a KLF4-mediated regulation of FSP-1 in the process. Since splenocytes are a mixed group of cells, we proceeded to examine KLF4 and FSP-1 expression in different subsets of MDSCs from the wild type mouse splenic tissues (**Figure 1D**). Highest levels of KLF4, FSP-1, and CCR2 expression were found in the CD11b$^+$Ly6G$^{Int}$ subpopulation of MDSCs (P2 in **Figure 1D** and **E**), known as M-MDSCs [84, 85]. Note that these M-MDSCs had the highest potential for fibrocyte generation (**Figure 1F**), thus supporting the observation that KLF4 deficiency led to significant decrease in FSP-1 expression and fibrocyte generation (**Figure 1A–C**) in the MDSC pool. To test whether KLF4 directly regulates FSP-1 gene expression, we first using two different KLF4 antibodies to perform a chromatin

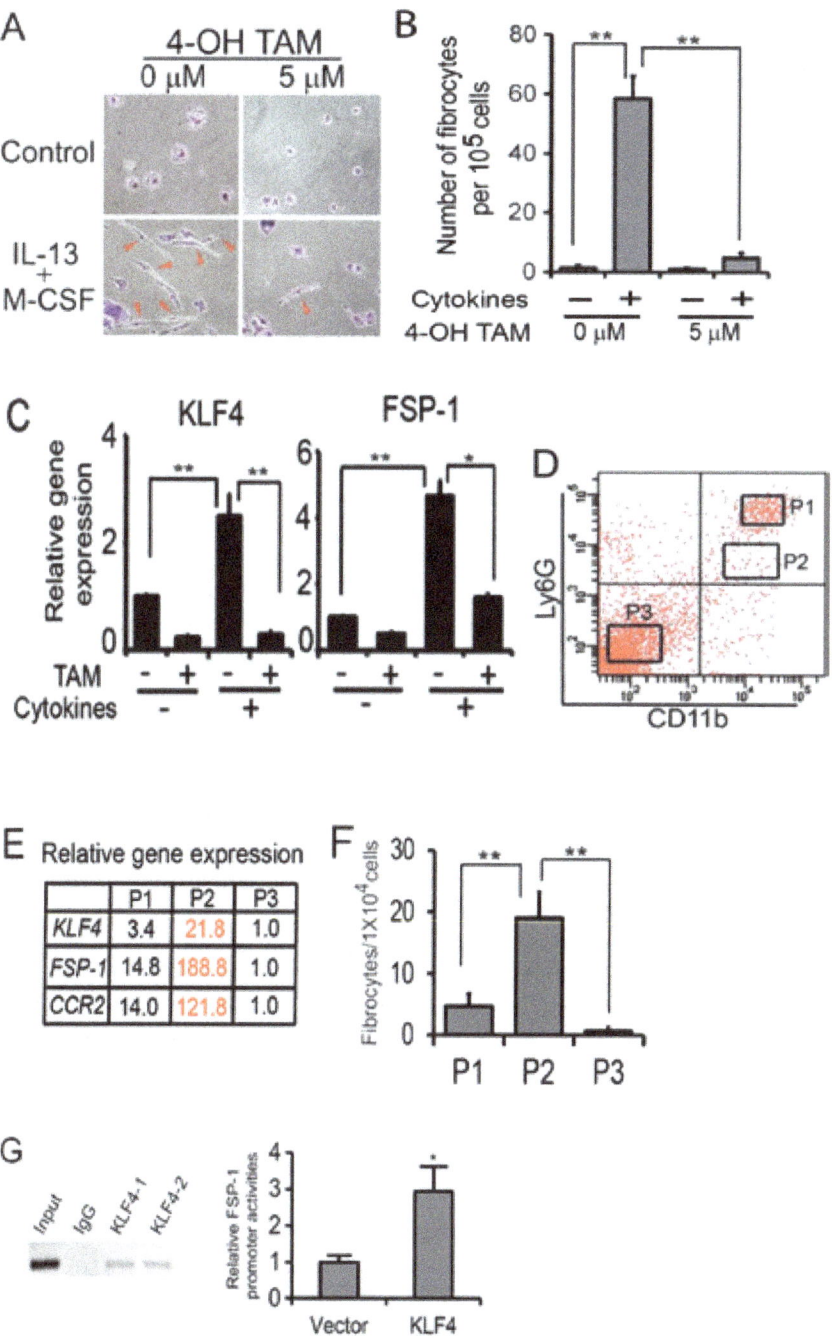

**Figure 1.**
*KLF4 regulates FSP-1 gene expression in fibrocyte generation. (A) Representative photographs of morphological fibrocyte generation from splenocytes in the absence and presence are indicated by red arrows. KLF4 deficiency was induced by 4-OH tamoxifen (TAM). (B) Quantification of the data from (A). (C) Relative levels of KLF4 and FSP-1 mRNA in fibrocyte generation as assessed by qRT-PCR. (D) Different MDSC subsets in mouse splenocytes measured by flow cytometry. (E) Relative levels of KLF4, FSP-1 and CCR2 mRNA in different MDSC subsets by qRT-PCR. (F) Potential of fibrocyte generation from MDSC subsets in mouse spleen. (G) Left—binding of KLF4 to the FSP-1 promoter as assessed by chromatin immunoprecipitation assay using two KLF4 antibodies (KLF4-1 and KLF4-2). IgG was used as a negative control. Right—the effect of KLF4 overexpression on FSP-1 promoter activities, as examined by transient transfection and dual luciferase assays, *P < 0.05, **P < 0.01.*

immunoprecipitation (CHIP) assay. We found that KLF4 directly bound to the FSP-1 proximal promoter region (**Figure 1G** left). Then we constructed a FSP-1 promoter luciferase reporter containing ~2.3 kb of the FSP-1 promoter region. By transient transfection and dual luciferase assays, we found that KLF4 overexpression resulted in three fold increase of the FSP1 promoter activity (**Figure 1G** right), suggesting a direct regulation of FSP-1 by KLF4 at the transcriptional level.

### 3.3.2 Epigenetic control of MDSC plasticity

The studies of epigenetics, heritable changes to gene expression without changes to DNA, are significantly advancing our knowledge of the inflammatory conditions [86]. They include DNA modifications mainly methylation, histone tail modifications, and non-coding RNA-mediated gene regulation. Recent data revealed that epigenetic mechanisms could provide novel strategies for modulating wound healing [87–89].

Critical functions of KLF4 have been shown in the generation of induced pluripotent stem cells and in cancer development through epigenetic mechanisms [90, 91]. In addition, there are numerous reports showing that microRNAs regulate KLF4 [92–94] or KLF4 regulate microRNAs [95, 96] in varied pathological conditions. KLF4-mediated DNA methylation have also been reported in hTert promoter [97] and methylation of KLF4 promoter is associated with urothelial cancer progression and early recurrence [98]. Moreover, the correlation of KLF4 and histone modifications has also been reported. For example, histone methyltransferase KMT2D, a frequently aberrant epigenetic modifier in various cancer, sustains prostate carcinogenesis and metastasis via epigenetically activating KLF4 [99]. From the perspective of MDSCs, epigenetic regulation of their differentiation and function is not completely understood. However, there is evidence to indicate the importance of epigenetic regulation. Shang et al. showed that long non-coding RNA retinal non-coding RNA3 (RNCR3) promotes C/EBP homologous protein (Chop) expression by sponging microRNA 185-5p during MDSC differentiation [100]. In addition, although histone modifications related to myeloid differentiation have been extensively studied [101], currently there is no clear indication about epigenetic markers that can discriminate specific MDSC subsets. Given the role of KLF4 in epigenetic regulation and the importance of MDSC plasticity in cancer and wound healing, it will be very interesting to examine how KLF4 is involved in epigenetic control of MDSC subsets or plasticity.

### 3.3.3 Is there potential molecular plasticity of KLF4 in cancer and wound healing?

KLF4 is a transcription factor with multiple functions in different physiological and pathological conditions, notably in cancer development. For example, KLF4 is well known for its tumor suppressive effect on tumor development in the gastrointestinal tract [102]. However, high expression of KLF4 is associated with skin cancer and breast cancer development [56, 103, 104], suggesting a tumor promoting function of KLF4 in these tissues. Recently, a tumor suppressive function of KLF4 was also reported in breast cancer [105]. These contradictory reports suggest context-dependent functions of KLF4 in cancer development [106]. At a molecular level, different KLF4 transcripts were found in testis [107], and alternative splicing of KLF4 has been proposed to explain context-dependent functions of KLF4 [108]. Consistently, an oncogenic KLF4 isoform, named KLF4α, has been found in both pancreatic cancer [109] and breast cancer [110]. In line with these observations, there is dynamic expression of KLF4 isoforms in mouse embryogenesis [111].

Interestingly, another human KLF4 isoform with an additional 34 amino acid-fragment in the C-terminal region has been reported in leukemia patients [112] and in myeloid cells [113], which further supports the importance of differential expression of KLF4 in different conditions.

We speculate that the existence of different isoforms of KLF4 and possibly relative ratios of these isoforms may explain different functions of KLF4 in cancer development and even in wound healing. Because KLF4 is a transcription factor that regulates gene expression, different isoforms of KLF4 will have different patterns of gene regulation of the downstream targets. In analogy to MDSC dynamics and plasticity, we propose a concept of KLF4 plasticity, which reflects the dynamic nature of KLF4 expression under different conditions. It is likely that under one condition, a major isoform of KLF4 regulates a group of genes that are responsible for one signaling transduction pathway. This pathway may be linked to one functional or phenotypical MDSC group. Under a different condition, another KLF4 isoform dominates and regulates a different group of genes and a different signaling pathway. This kind of differential regulation may cause the plastic change of MDSCs in cancer or wound healing. To confirm our hypothesis, future experiments will be needed to characterize the different KLF4 isoforms during the dynamic change of MDSCs. Validation of our hypothesis will not only reveal novel molecular mechanisms whereby KLF4 regulates MDSC plasticity, but also help design KLF4-based therapeutic strategies to manipulate MDSC plasticity in the treatment of cancer and wound healing.

## 4. Conclusion remarks

Studies of immune cell plasticity have recently gained momentum due to their novel functions in tissue repair and robustness beside their well-known functions in system defense. MDSCs, as a myeloid population with unique functions in tumor and tissue repair, are less studied regarding their phenotypical and functional plasticity, compared to macrophages and neutrophils. Given the ample evidence showing MDSC plasticity in cancer and wound healing, it is essential to elucidate the underlying molecular mechanisms in order to harness MDSCs in tissue repair and cancer treatment. In the meantime, we have shown KLF4 as a key molecule to regulate MDSC plasticity in cancer, wound healing, and allergic asthma. KLF4-controlled FSP-1 expression and possible epigenetic alterations are two possible mechanisms underlying MDSC plasticity. In addition, the existence of different KLF4 isoforms prompts us to hypothesize that KLF4 isoforms control gene expression of different signaling pathways that may contribute to MDSC dynamics and plasticity in both cancer and wound healing. In this regard, future studies to characterize different KLF4 isoforms during MDSC plastic changes and the relevant signaling pathways will pave the way to harness MDSC plasticity in the treatment of cancer and wound healing.

## Acknowledgements

This work was supported by NSF HRD-1436222 and SC INBRE grant (NIH P20GM103499). We also thank Ms. Anna Harper for her proofreading of the manuscript.

## Author details

Daping Fan[1], Samir Raychoudhury[2] and Walden Ai[2]*

1 Department of Cell Biology and Anatomy, University of South Carolina School of Medicine, Columbia, SC, USA

2 Department of Biology, Chemistry and Environmental Health Science, Benedict College, Columbia, SC, USA

*Address all correspondence to: walden.ai@benedict.edu

# References

[1] Bieker JJ. Kruppel-like factors: Three fingers in many pies. The Journal of Biological Chemistry. 2001;**276**(37):34355-34358. DOI: 10.1074/jbc.R100043200

[2] Philipsen S, Suske G. A tale of three fingers: The family of mammalian Sp/XKLF transcription factors. Nucleic Acids Research. 1999;**27**(15):2991-3000

[3] Turner J, Crossley M. Mammalian Kruppel-like transcription factors: More than just a pretty finger. Trends in Biochemical Sciences. 1999;**24**(6):236-240

[4] Kaczynski J, Cook T, Urrutia R. Sp1- and Kruppel-like transcription factors. Genome Biology. 2003;**4**(2):206

[5] Ghaleb AM, Yang VW. Kruppel-like factor 4 (KLF4): What we currently know. Gene. 2017;**611**:27-37. DOI: 10.1016/j.gene.2017.02.025

[6] Li J, Zheng H, Yu F, Yu T, Liu C, Huang S, et al. Deficiency of the Kruppel-like factor KLF4 correlates with increased cell proliferation and enhanced skin tumorigenesis. Carcinogenesis. 2012;**33**(6):1239-1246. DOI: 10.1093/carcin/bgs143

[7] Cui J, Shi M, Quan M, Xie K. Regulation of EMT by KLF4 in gastrointestinal cancer. Current Cancer Drug Targets. 2013;**13**(9):986-995

[8] Shi Y, Ou L, Han S, Li M, Pena MM, Pena EA, et al. Deficiency of Kruppel-like factor KLF4 in myeloid-derived suppressor cells inhibits tumor pulmonary metastasis in mice accompanied by decreased fibrocytes. Oncogene. 2014;**3**:e129. DOI: 10.1038/oncsis.2014.44

[9] Segre JA, Bauer C, Fuchs E. Klf4 is a transcription factor required for establishing the barrier function of the skin. Nature Genetics. 1999;**22**(4):356-360. DOI: 10.1038/11926

[10] Liao X, Sharma N, Kapadia F, Zhou G, Lu Y, Hong H, et al. Kruppel-like factor 4 regulates macrophage polarization. The Journal of Clinical Investigation. 2011;**121**(7):2736-2749. DOI: 10.1172/JCI45444

[11] Ou L, Shi Y, Dong W, Liu C, Schmidt TJ, Nagarkatti P, et al. Kruppel-like factor KLF4 facilitates cutaneous wound healing by promoting fibrocyte generation from myeloid-derived suppressor cells. The Journal of Investigative Dermatology. 2015;**135**(5):1425-1434. DOI: 10.1038/jid.2015.3

[12] Gabrilovich DI, Nagaraj S. Myeloid-derived suppressor cells as regulators of the immune system. Nature Reviews Immunology. 2009;**9**(3):162-174. DOI: 10.1038/nri2506

[13] Manjili MH. Phenotypic plasticity of MDSC in cancers. Immunological Investigations. 2012;**41**(6-7):711-721. DOI: 10.3109/08820139.2012.673670

[14] Tcyganov E, Mastio J, Chen E, Gabrilovich DI. Plasticity of myeloid-derived suppressor cells in cancer. Current Opinion in Immunology. 2018;**51**:76-82. DOI: 10.1016/j.coi.2018.03.009

[15] Mahdipour E, Charnock JC, Mace KA. Hoxa3 promotes the differentiation of hematopoietic progenitor cells into proangiogenic Gr-1+CD11b+ myeloid cells. Blood. 2011;**117**(3):815-826. DOI: 10.1182/blood-2009-12-259549

[16] Laurent P, Jolivel V, Manicki P, Chiu L, Contin-Bordes C, Truchetet ME, et al. Immune-mediated repair: A matter of plasticity. Frontiers in Immunology. 2017;**8**:454. DOI: 10.3389/fimmu.2017.00454

[17] Yang XD, Ai W, Asfaha S, Bhagat G, Friedman RA, Jin G, et al. Histamine deficiency promotes inflammation-associated carcinogenesis through reduced myeloid maturation and accumulation of CD11b+Ly6G+ immature myeloid cells. Nature Medicine. 2011;**17**(1):87-95. DOI: 10.1038/nm.2278

[18] Yu F, Shi Y, Wang J, Li J, Fan D, Ai W. Deficiency of Kruppel-like factor KLF4 in mammary tumor cells inhibits tumor growth and pulmonary metastasis and is accompanied by compromised recruitment of myeloid-derived suppressor cells. International Journal of Cancer. 2013;**133**(12): 2872-2883. DOI: 10.1002/ijc.28302

[19] Reilkoff RA, Bucala R, Herzog EL. Fibrocytes: Emerging effector cells in chronic inflammation. Nature Reviews Immunology. 2011;**11**(6):427-435. DOI: 10.1038/nri2990

[20] Kao HK, Chen B, Murphy GF, Li Q , Orgill DP, Guo L. Peripheral blood fibrocytes: Enhancement of wound healing by cell proliferation, re-epithelialization, contraction, and angiogenesis. Annals of Surgery. 2011;**254**(6):1066-1074. DOI: 10.1097/ SLA.0b013e3182251559

[21] Nimpong JA, Gebregziabher W, Singh UP, Nagarkatti P, Nagarkatti M, Hodge J, et al. Deficiency of KLF4 compromises the lung function in an acute mouse model of allergic asthma. Biochemical and Biophysical Research Communications. 2017;**493**(1):598-603. DOI: 10.1016/j.bbrc.2017.08.146

[22] Das A, Sinha M, Datta S, Abas M, Chaffee S, Sen CK, et al. Monocyte and macrophage plasticity in tissue repair and regeneration. The American Journal of Pathology. 2015;**185**(10):2596-2606. DOI: 10.1016/j.ajpath.2015.06.001

[23] Bronte V, Brandau S, Chen SH, Colombo MP, Frey AB, Greten TF, et al. Recommendations for myeloid-derived suppressor cell nomenclature and characterization standards. Nature Communications. 2016;**7**:12150. DOI: 10.1038/ncomms12150

[24] Viale A, Pettazzoni P, Lyssiotis CA, Ying H, Sanchez N, Marchesini M, et al. Oncogene ablation-resistant pancreatic cancer cells depend on mitochondrial function. Nature. 2014;**514**(7524): 628-632. DOI: 10.1038/nature13611

[25] Ben-Meir K, Twaik N, Baniyash M. Plasticity and biological diversity of myeloid derived suppressor cells. Current Opinion in Immunology. 2018;**51**:154-161. DOI: 10.1016/j. coi.2018.03.015

[26] Condamine T, Ramachandran I, Youn JI, Gabrilovich DI. Regulation of tumor metastasis by myeloid-derived suppressor cells. Annual Review of Medicine. 2015;**66**:97-110. DOI: 10.1146/annurev-med-051013-052304

[27] Ko HJ, Lee JM, Kim YJ, Kim YS, Lee KA, Kang CY. Immunosuppressive myeloid-derived suppressor cells can be converted into immunogenic APCs with the help of activated NKT cells: An alternative cell-based antitumor vaccine. Journal of Immunology. 2009;**182**(4):1818-1828. DOI: 10.4049/ jimmunol.0802430

[28] Corzo CA, Condamine T, Lu L, Cotter MJ, Youn JI, Cheng P, et al. HIF-1alpha regulates function and differentiation of myeloid-derived suppressor cells in the tumor microenvironment. The Journal of Experimental Medicine. 2010;**207**(11): 2439-2453. DOI: 10.1084/jem.20100587

[29] Kumar V, Cheng P, Condamine T, Mony S, Languino LR, McCaffrey JC, et al. CD45 phosphatase inhibits STAT3 transcription factor activity in myeloid cells and promotes tumor-associated macrophage differentiation. Immunity.

2016;**44**(2):303-315. DOI: 10.1016/j. immuni.2016.01.014

[30] Blakaj A, Bucala R. Fibrocytes in health and disease. Fibrogenesis & Tissue Repair. 2012;**5**(Suppl 1):S6. DOI: 10.1186/1755-1536-5-S1-S6

[31] Kisseleva T, von Kockritz-Blickwede M, Reichart D, McGillvray SM, Wingender G, Kronenberg M, et al. Fibrocyte-like cells recruited to the spleen support innate and adaptive immune responses to acute injury or infection. Journal of Molecular Medicine. 2011;**89**(10):997-1013. DOI: 10.1007/s00109-011-0756-0

[32] Ortiz ML, Lu L, Ramachandran I, Gabrilovich DI. Myeloid-derived suppressor cells in the development of lung cancer. Cancer Immunology Research. 2014;**2**(1):50-58. DOI: 10.1158/2326-6066.CIR-13-0129

[33] Kitano H. Biological robustness. Nature Reviews Genetics. 2004; **5**(11):826-837. DOI: 10.1038/nrg1471

[34] Stelling J, Sauer U, Szallasi Z, Doyle FJ 3rd, Doyle J. Robustness of cellular functions. Cell. 2004;**118**(6):675-685. DOI: 10.1016/j. cell.2004.09.008

[35] Jameson J, Ugarte K, Chen N, Yachi P, Fuchs E, Boismenu R, et al. A role for skin gammadelta T cells in wound repair. Science. 2002;**296**(5568):747-749. DOI: 10.1126/science.1069639

[36] Silva-Santos B, Serre K, Norell H. Gammadelta T cells in cancer. Nature Reviews Immunology. 2015;**15**(11): 683-691. DOI: 10.1038/nri3904

[37] Almeida FF, Belz GT. Innate lymphoid cells: Models of plasticity for immune homeostasis and rapid responsiveness in protection. Mucosal Immunology. 2016;**9**(5):1103-1112. DOI: 10.1038/mi.2016.64

[38] Arpaia N, Green JA, Moltedo B, Arvey A, Hemmers S, Yuan S, et al. A distinct function of regulatory T cells in tissue protection. Cell. 2015;**162**(5):1078-1089. DOI: 10.1016/j.cell.2015.08.021

[39] Silverstein SC, Rabadan R. How many neutrophils are enough (redux, redux)? The Journal of Clinical Investigation. 2012;**122**(8):2776-2779. DOI: 10.1172/JCI63939

[40] Yang F, Feng C, Zhang X, Lu J, Zhao Y. The diverse biological functions of neutrophils, beyond the defense against infections. Inflammation. 2017;**40**(1):311-323. DOI: 10.1007/s10753-016-0458-4

[41] Takashima A, Yao Y. Neutrophil plasticity: Acquisition of phenotype and functionality of antigen-presenting cell. Journal of Leukocyte Biology. 2015;**98**(4):489-496. DOI: 10.1189/jlb.1MR1014-502R

[42] Iking-Konert C, Ostendorf B, Sander O, Jost M, Wagner C, Joosten L, et al. Transdifferentiation of polymorphonuclear neutrophils to dendritic-like cells at the site of inflammation in rheumatoid arthritis: Evidence for activation by T cells. Annals of the Rheumatic Diseases. 2005;**64**(10):1436-1442. DOI: 10.1136/ard.2004.034132

[43] Wynn TA, Barron L. Macrophages: Master regulators of inflammation and fibrosis. Seminars in Liver Disease. 2010;**30**(3):245-257. DOI: 10.1055/s-0030-1255354

[44] Brancato SK, Albina JE. Wound macrophages as key regulators of repair: Origin, phenotype, and function. The American Journal of Pathology. 2011;**178**(1):19-25. DOI: 10.1016/j. ajpath.2010.08.003

[45] London A, Itskovich E, Benhar I, Kalchenko V, Mack M, Jung S, et al.

Neuroprotection and progenitor cell renewal in the injured adult murine retina requires healing monocyte-derived macrophages. The Journal of Experimental Medicine. 2011;**208**(1):23-39. DOI: 10.1084/jem.20101202

[46] Mosteiro L, Pantoja C, Alcazar N, Marion RM, Chondronasiou D, Rovira M, et al. Tissue damage and senescence provide critical signals for cellular reprogramming in vivo. Science. 2016;**354**(6315):1-10. Article id: aaf4445. DOI: 10.1126/science.aaf4445

[47] Cash JL, Martin P. Myeloid cells in cutaneous wound repair. Microbiology Spectrum. 2016;**4**(3):1-17. DOI: 10.1128/microbiolspec.MCHD-0017-2015

[48] Bochaton-Piallat ML, Gabbiani G, Hinz B. The myofibroblast in wound healing and fibrosis: Answered and unanswered questions. F1000Res. 2016;**5**:1-8. DOI: 10.12688/f1000research.8190.1

[49] Darby IA, Laverdet B, Bonte F, Desmouliere A. Fibroblasts and myofibroblasts in wound healing. Clinical, Cosmetic and Investigational Dermatology. 2014;**7**:301-311. DOI: 10.2147/CCID.S50046

[50] Gunaydin G, Kesikli SA, Guc D. Cancer associated fibroblasts have phenotypic and functional characteristics similar to the fibrocytes that represent a novel MDSC subset. Oncoimmunology. 2015;**4**(9):e1034918. DOI: 10.1080/2162402X.2015.1034918

[51] Zhang H, Maric I, DiPrima MJ, Khan J, Orentas RJ, Kaplan RN, et al. Fibrocytes represent a novel MDSC subset circulating in patients with metastatic cancer. Blood. 2013;**122**(7):1105-1113. DOI: 10.1182/blood-2012-08-449413

[52] Feinberg MW, Cao Z, Wara AK, Lebedeva MA, Senbanerjee S, Jain MK. Kruppel-like factor 4 is a mediator of proinflammatory signaling in macrophages. The Journal of Biological Chemistry. 2005;**280**(46):38247-38258. DOI: 10.1074/jbc.M509378200

[53] Tetreault MP, Wang ML, Yang Y, Travis J, Yu QC, Klein-Szanto AJ, et al. Klf4 overexpression activates epithelial cytokines and inflammation-mediated esophageal squamous cell cancer in mice. Gastroenterology. 2010;**139**(6):2124-34 e9. DOI: 10.1053/j.gastro.2010.08.048

[54] Alder JK, Georgantas RW 3rd, Hildreth RL, Kaplan IM, Morisot S, Yu X, et al. Kruppel-like factor 4 is essential for inflammatory monocyte differentiation in vivo. Journal of Immunology. 2008;**180**(8):5645-5652

[55] Feinberg MW, Wara AK, Cao Z, Lebedeva MA, Rosenbauer F, Iwasaki H, et al. The Kruppel-like factor KLF4 is a critical regulator of monocyte differentiation. The EMBO Journal. 2007;**26**(18):4138-4148. DOI: 10.1038/sj.emboj.7601824

[56] Yu F, Li J, Chen H, Fu J, Ray S, Huang S, et al. Kruppel-like factor 4 (KLF4) is required for maintenance of breast cancer stem cells and for cell migration and invasion. Oncogene. 2011;**30**(18):2161-2172. DOI: 10.1038/onc.2010.591

[57] Bronte V, Serafini P, De Santo C, Marigo I, Tosello V, Mazzoni A, et al. IL-4-induced arginase 1 suppresses alloreactive T cells in tumor-bearing mice. Journal of Immunology. 2003;**170**(1):270-278

[58] Youn JI, Nagaraj S, Collazo M, Gabrilovich DI. Subsets of myeloid-derived suppressor cells in tumor-bearing mice. Journal of Immunology. 2008;**181**(8):5791-5802

[59] Black JM, Edsberg LE, Baharestani MM, Langemo D, Goldberg M, McNichol L, et al. Pressure ulcers: Avoidable or unavoidable? Results of the National Pressure Ulcer Advisory Panel Consensus Conference. Ostomy/Wound Management. 2011;**57**(2):24-37

[60] Bly D, Schallom M, Sona C, Klinkenberg DA. Model of pressure, oxygenation, and perfusion risk factors for pressure ulcers in the intensive care unit. American Journal of Critical Care. 2016;**25**(2):156-164. DOI: 10.4037/ajcc201684025/2/156 [pii]

[61] Thompson D. A critical review of the literature on pressure ulcer aetiology. Journal of Wound Care. 2005;**14**(2):87-90

[62] Bry KE, Buescher D, Sandrik M.Never say never: A descriptive study of hospital-acquired pressure ulcers in a hospital setting. Journal of Wound, Ostomy, and Continence Nursing. 2012;**39**(3):274-281. DOI: 10.1097/WON.0b013e3182549102

[63] Gorecki C, Brown JM, Nelson EA, Briggs M, Schoonhoven L, Dealey C, et al. Impact of pressure ulcers on quality of life in older patients: A systematic review. Journal of the American Geriatrics Society. 2009;**57**(7):1175-1183. DOI: 10.1111/j.1532-5415.2009.02307.x

[64] Shih B, Garside E, McGrouther DA, Bayat A. Molecular dissection of abnormal wound healing processes resulting in keloid disease. Wound Repair and Regeneration. 2010;**18**(2):139-153. DOI: 10.1111/j.1524-475X.2009.00553.x

[65] Li W, Dasgeb B, Phillips T, Li Y, Chen M, Garner W, et al. Wound-healing perspectives. Dermatologic Clinics. 2005;**23**(2):181-192. DOI: 10.1016/j.det.2004.09.004

[66] Kondo T, Ishida Y. Molecular pathology of wound healing. Forensic Science International. 2010;**203**(1-3):93-98. DOI: 10.1016/j.forsciint.2010.07.004

[67] Gist S, Tio-Matos I, Falzgraf S, Cameron S, Beebe M. Wound care in the geriatric client. Clinical Interventions in Aging. 2009;**4**:269-287

[68] Lumbley JL, Ali SA, Tchokouani LS. Retrospective review of predisposing factors for intraoperative pressure ulcer development. Journal of Clinical Anesthesia. 2014;**26**(5):368-374. DOI: 10.1016/j.jclinane.2014.01.012

[69] Li J, Zheng H, Wang J, Yu F, Morris RJ, Wang TC, et al. Expression of Kruppel-like factor KLF4 in mouse hair follicle stem cells contributes to cutaneous wound healing. PLoS One. 2012;**7**(6):e39663. DOI: 10.1371/journal.pone.0039663

[70] Desmouliere A, Chaponnier C, Gabbiani G. Tissue repair, contraction, and the myofibroblast. Wound Repair and Regeneration. 2005;**13**(1):7-12. DOI: 10.1111/j.1067-1927.2005.130102.x

[71] Hinz B, Phan SH, Thannickal VJ, Prunotto M, Desmouliere A, Varga J, et al. Recent developments in myofibroblast biology: Paradigms for connective tissue remodeling. The American Journal of Pathology. 2012;**180**(4):1340-1355. DOI: 10.1016/j.ajpath.2012.02.004

[72] Stadler I, Zhang RY, Oskoui P, Whittaker MS, Lanzafame RJ. Development of a simple, noninvasive, clinically relevant model of pressure ulcers in the mouse. Journal of Investigative Surgery. 2004;**17**(4):221-227. DOI: 10.1080/08941930490472046

[73] Lanzafame RJ, Stadler I, Cunningham R, Muhlbauer A, Griggs J, Soltz R, et al. Preliminary assessment of photoactivated antimicrobial collagen on bioburden in a murine pressure

ulcer model. Photomedicine and Laser Surgery. 2013;**31**(11):539-546. DOI: 10.1089/pho.2012.3423

[74] Kasuya A, Sakabe J, Tokura Y. Potential application of in vivo imaging of impaired lymphatic duct to evaluate the severity of pressure ulcer in mouse model. Scientific Reports. 2014;**4**:4173. DOI: 10.1038/srep04173

[75] Robbins CS, Swirski FK. The multiple roles of monocyte subsets in steady state and inflammation. Cellular and Molecular Life Sciences. 2010;**67**(16):2685-2693. DOI: 10.1007/s00018-010-0375-x

[76] Schouppe E, De Baetselier P, Van Ginderachter JA, Sarukhan A. Instruction of myeloid cells by the tumor microenvironment: Open questions on the dynamics and plasticity of different tumor-associated myeloid cell populations. Oncoimmunology. 2012;**1**(7):1135-1145. DOI: 10.4161/onci.21566

[77] Boye K, Maelandsmo GM. S100A4 and metastasis: A small actor playing many roles. The American Journal of Pathology. 2010;**176**(2):528-535. DOI: 10.2353/ajpath.2010.090526

[78] Strutz F, Okada H, Lo CW, Danoff T, Carone RL, Tomaszewski JE, et al. Identification and characterization of a fibroblast marker: FSP1. The Journal of Cell Biology. 1995;**130**(2):393-405

[79] Cabezon T, Celis JE, Skibshoj I, Klingelhofer J, Grigorian M, Gromov P, et al. Expression of S100A4 by a variety of cell types present in the tumor microenvironment of human breast cancer. International Journal of Cancer. 2007;**121**(7):1433-1444. DOI: 10.1002/ijc.22850

[80] Abe R, Donnelly SC, Peng T, Bucala R, Metz CN. Peripheral blood fibrocytes: Differentiation pathway and migration to wound sites. Journal of Immunology. 2001;**166**(12):7556-7562

[81] van Deventer HW, Palmieri DA, Wu QP, McCook EC, Serody JS. Circulating fibrocytes prepare the lung for cancer metastasis by recruiting Ly-6C+ monocytes via CCL2. Journal of Immunology. 2013;**190**(9):4861- 4867. DOI: 10.4049/jimmunol.1202857 jimmunol.1202857 [pii]

[82] Niedermeier M, Reich B, Rodriguez Gomez M, Denzel A, Schmidbauer K, Gobel N, et al. CD4+ T cells control the differentiation of Gr1+ monocytes into fibrocytes. Proceedings of the National Academy of Sciences of the United States of America. 2009;**106**(42): 17892-17897. DOI: 10.1073/pnas.0906070106

[83] Crawford JR, Pilling D, Gomer RH. Improved serum-free culture conditions for spleen-derived murine fibrocytes. Journal of Immunological Methods. 2010;**363**(1):9-20. DOI: 10.1016/j.jim.2010.09.025

[84] Lesokhin AM, Hohl TM, Kitano S, Cortez C, Hirschhorn-Cymerman D, Avogadri F, et al. Monocytic CCR2(+) myeloid-derived suppressor cells promote immune escape by limiting activated CD8 T-cell infiltration into the tumor microenvironment. Cancer Research. 2012;**72**(4):876-886. DOI: 10.1158/0008-5472.CAN-11-1792

[85] Movahedi K, Guilliams M, Van den Bossche J, Van den Bergh R, Gysemans C, Beschin A, et al. Identification of discrete tumor-induced myeloid-derived suppressor cell subpopulations with distinct T cell-suppressive activity. Blood. 2008;**111**(8):4233-4244. DOI: 10.1182/blood-2007-07-099226

[86] Stylianou E. Epigenetics of chronic inflammatory diseases. Journal of Inflammation Research. 2019;**12**:1-14. DOI: 10.2147/JIR.S129027

[87] den Dekker A, Davis FM, Kunkel SL, Gallagher KA. Targeting epigenetic mechanisms in diabetic wound healing. Translational Research. 2019;**204**:39-50. DOI: 10.1016/j.trsl.2018.10.001

[88] Ti D, Li M, Fu X, Han W. Causes and consequences of epigenetic regulation in wound healing. Wound Repair and Regeneration. 2014;**22**(3):305-312. DOI: 10.1111/wrr.12160

[89] Lewis CJ, Mardaryev AN, Sharov AA, Fessing MY, Botchkarev VA. The epigenetic regulation of wound healing. Advances in Wound Care. 2014;**3**(7):468-475. DOI: 10.1089/wound.2014.0522

[90] van den Hurk M, Kenis G, Bardy C, van den Hove DL, Gage FH, Steinbusch HW, et al. Transcriptional and epigenetic mechanisms of cellular reprogramming to induced pluripotency. Epigenomics. 2016;**8**(8):1131-1149. DOI: 10.2217/epi-2016-0032

[91] Oyinlade O, Wei S, Kammers K, Liu S, Wang S, Ma D, et al. Analysis of KLF4 regulated genes in cancer cells reveals a role of DNA methylation in promoter-enhancer interactions. Epigenetics. 2018;**13**(7):751-768. DOI: 10.1080/15592294.2018.1504592

[92] Hien TT, Garcia-Vaz E, Stenkula KG, Sjogren J, Nilsson J, Gomez MF, et al. MicroRNA-dependent regulation of KLF4 by glucose in vascular smooth muscle. Journal of Cellular Physiology. 2018;**233**(9):7195-7205. DOI: 10.1002/jcp.26549

[93] Hujie G, Zhou SH, Zhang H, Qu J, Xiong XW, Hujie O, et al. MicroRNA-10b regulates epithelial-mesenchymal transition by modulating KLF4/KLF11/Smads in hepatocellular carcinoma. Cancer Cell International. 2018;**18**(10). DOI: 10.1186/s12935-018-0508-0

[94] Shen L, Gan M, Li Q, Wang J, Li X, Zhang S, et al. MicroRNA-200b regulates preadipocyte proliferation and differentiation by targeting KLF4. Biomedicine & Pharmacotherapy. 2018;**103**:1538-1544. DOI: 10.1016/j.biopha.2018.04.170

[95] Zhu M, Zhang N, He S. Transcription factor KLF4 modulates microRNA-106a that targets Smad7 in gastric cancer. Pathology, Research and Practice. 2019;**215**:1-11. Article id: 152467. DOI: 10.1016/j.prp.2019.152467

[96] Xu Q, Liu M, Zhang J, Xue L, Zhang G, Hu C, et al. Overexpression of KLF4 promotes cell senescence through microRNA-203-survivin-p21 pathway. Oncotarget. 2016;**7**(37):60290-60302. DOI: 10.18632/oncotarget.11200

[97] Yadav SS, Nair RR, Yadava PK. KLF4 signalling in carcinogenesis and epigenetic regulation of hTERT. Medical Hypotheses. 2018;**115**:50-53. DOI: 10.1016/j.mehy.2018.03.012

[98] Li H, Wang J, Xiao W, Xia D, Lang B, Wang T, et al. Epigenetic inactivation of KLF4 is associated with urothelial cancer progression and early recurrence. The Journal of Urology. 2014;**191**(2):493-501. DOI: 10.1016/j.juro.2013.08.087

[99] Lv S, Ji L, Chen B, Liu S, Lei C, Liu X, et al. Histone methyltransferase KMT2D sustains prostate carcinogenesis and metastasis via epigenetically activating LIFR and KLF4. Oncogene. 2018;**37**(10):1354-1368. DOI: 10.1038/s41388-017-0026-x

[100] Shang W, Tang Z, Gao Y, Qi H, Su X, Zhang Y, et al. LncRNA RNCR3 promotes chop expression by sponging miR-185-5p during MDSC differentiation. Oncotarget. 2017;**8**(67):111754-111769. DOI: 10.18632/oncotarget.22906

[101] Lavin Y, Winter D, Blecher-Gonen R, David E, Keren-Shaul H,

Merad M, et al. Tissue-resident macrophage enhancer landscapes are shaped by the local microenvironment. Cell. 2014;**159**(6):1312-1326. DOI: 10.1016/j.cell.2014.11.018

[102] Wei D, Kanai M, Huang S, Xie K. Emerging role of KLF4 in human gastrointestinal cancer. Carcinogenesis. 2006;**27**(1):23-31. DOI: 10.1093/carcin/bgi243

[103] Pandya AY, Talley LI, Frost AR, Fitzgerald TJ, Trivedi V, Chakravarthy M, et al. Nuclear localization of KLF4 is associated with an aggressive phenotype in early-stage breast cancer. Clinical Cancer Research. 2004;**10**(8):2709-2719

[104] Foster KW, Liu Z, Nail CD, Li X, Fitzgerald TJ, Bailey SK, et al. Induction of KLF4 in basal keratinocytes blocks the proliferation-differentiation switch and initiates squamous epithelial dysplasia. Oncogene. 2005;**24**(9): 1491-1500. DOI: 10.1038/sj.onc.1208307

[105] Akaogi K, Nakajima Y, Ito I, Kawasaki S, Oie SH, Murayama A, et al. KLF4 suppresses estrogen-dependent breast cancer growth by inhibiting the transcriptional activity of ERalpha. Oncogene. 2009;**28**(32):2894-2902. DOI: 10.1038/onc.2009.151

[106] Rowland BD, Peeper DS. KLF4, p21 and context-dependent opposing forces in cancer. Nature Reviews Cancer. 2006;**6**(1):11-23. DOI: 10.1038/nrc1780

[107] Godmann M, Kromberg I, Mayer J, Behr R. The mouse Kruppel-like factor 4 (Klf4) gene: Four functional polyadenylation sites which are used in a cell-specific manner as revealed by testicular transcript analysis and multiple processed pseudogenes. Gene. 2005;**361**:149-156. DOI: 10.1016/j. gene.2005.07.025

[108] Wang L, Shen F, Stroehlein JR, Wei D. Context-dependent functions of KLF4 in cancers: Could alternative splicing isoforms be the key? Cancer Letters. 2018;**438**:10-16. DOI: 10.1016/j. canlet.2018.09.005

[109] Wei D, Wang L, Kanai M, Jia Z, Le X, Li Q, et al. KLF4alpha up-regulation promotes cell cycle progression and reduces survival time of patients with pancreatic cancer. Gastroenterology. 2010;**139**(6):2135-2145. DOI: 10.1053/j.gastro.2010.08.022

[110] Ferralli J, Chiquet-Ehrismann R, Degen M. KLF4alpha stimulates breast cancer cell proliferation by acting as a KLF4 antagonist. Oncotarget. 2016;**7**(29):45608-45621. DOI: 10.18632/oncotarget.10058

[111] Ehlermann J, Pfisterer P, Schorle H. Dynamic expression of Kruppel-like factor 4 (Klf4), a target of transcription factor AP-2alpha during murine mid-embryogenesis. The Anatomical Record. Part A, Discoveries in Molecular, Cellular, and Evolutionary Biology. 2003;**273**(2):677-680. DOI: 10.1002/ar.a.10089

[112] Malik D, Kaul D, Chauhan N, Marwaha RK. miR-2909-mediated regulation of KLF4: A novel molecular mechanism for differentiating between B-cell and T-cell pediatric acute lymphoblastic leukemias. Molecular Cancer. 2014;**13**:175. DOI: 10.1186/1476-4598-13-175

[113] Noti JD, Johnson AK, Dillon JD. The leukocyte integrin gene CD11d is repressed by gut-enriched Kruppel-like factor 4 in myeloid cells. The Journal of Biological Chemistry. 2005;**280**(5): 3449-3457. DOI: 10.1074/jbc.M412627200

# 3

# Sorption Detoxification as an Addition to Conventional Therapy of Acute Radiation Sickness and Iatrogenic Leukopenia

*Oksana O. Shevchuk, Elisaveta A. Snezhkova,*
*Anatoliy G. Bilous, Veronika V. Sarnatskaya,*
*Kvitoslava I. Badakhivska, Larysa A. Sakhno,*
*Vasyl F. Chekhun and Volodymyr G. Nikolaev*

**Abstract**

Leukopenia is an essential part of the clinical course of acute radiation sickness and is a side effect of anti-cancer treatment. In both situations, the main factors which determine the survival are the degree of bone marrow suppression and gastrointestinal tract damage due to the presence of a large pool of fast-dividing cells. Leuko- and neutropenia are main limiting factors which may contribute to chemotherapy failure. Hematopoietic cytokines the part of conventional therapy in this field, but their effects require boosting. That is why the use of means and methods of adsorption therapy is considered promising. Sorption therapy creates a basis for sorption detoxification, a doctrine of curative measures directed to the removal of toxic endogenous or exogenous compounds from body fluids. The most widely used types are the purification of blood or its components (hemosorption), oral administration of sorption materials (enterosorption) and application-sorption therapy of wounds and burns. In this chapter, the results of early and recent research and prospects for the use of carbon adsorption therapy for the treatment of acute radiation sickness and cytostatic myelosuppression are discussed.

**Keywords:** leukopenia, ionizing irradiation, anti-cancer chemotherapy, granulocyte colony stimulating factor, hemosorption, enterosorption, application-sorption therapy

## 1. Introduction

The danger of acute and chronic radiation injuries, which provoke leukopenia, is not just a myth today. The explosion at Unit 4 of Chernobyl Nuclear Power Plant (NPP) in 1986 showed how unprepared people were to such a problem. The collective dose of irradiation for liquidators (clean-up workers) was huge; no one knows the exact numbers (all dosimetric equipment measured only gamma irradiation). And until today, about five million people, who live in areas of Belarus, the Russian

Federation and Ukraine, which are contaminated with radionuclides, still experience the consequences of pollution [1–3]. An earthquake and tsunami struck Fukushima Dai-ichi NPP in 2011 contaminated the soil and water with radioactive cesium, iodine, etc. It poses significant risks of exposure to the residents [4, 5]. Terroristic threats or military conflicts with the use of radioactive weapons could be considered as a potential risk of injuries also.

One more source of contact with myelosuppressive factors is radiation therapy, which is routinely used in oncology (up to 70% of patients with malignant tumors are treated with) as well as anti-cancer chemotherapy with cytostatics [6–8]. Medical use of radiation accounts for 98% of the population dose contribution from all artificial sources and represents approximately 20% of the total exposure. Annually worldwide, more than 3600 million diagnostic radiology examinations are performed, 37 million nuclear medicine procedures are carried out and 7.5 million radiotherapy treatments are given [9]. In spite of side effects, the concomitant use of radiotherapy and chemotherapy resulted in significantly improved clinical outcomes [10–12]. Different radiomimetics have effects similar to ionizing irradiation. Among them, a lot of anti-cancer drugs and leukopenia is a common side effect of dose-dense and dose-intense tumoricidal chemotherapy.

The organs and tissues with high speed cell proliferation is the most sensitive for radiation- and radiomimetic damage. Leukopenia, because of aggressive direct ionizing irradiation or anti-cancer chemotherapy with cytostatics, is an important prognostic factor for overall survival [13, 14]. The association between chemotherapy-induced leukopenia and clinical outcome has been reported for several types of cancer. The development of such health impairments gains more and more attention, especially after the success of modern techniques such as stem cell transplantation and cytokine treatment to restore hematopoietic functions. But even now, it is not enough for the treatment of acute radiation sickness.

In last decades, we observe combined injury by ionizing radiation and toxic effects of xenobiotic, thermal burns, mechanical trauma, etc. Despite significant achievements in oncology, precise and targeted irradiation of tumors, the development of effective means for enhancement of bone marrow cell and peripheral blood cells proliferation (granulocyte colony stimulating factors (G-CSF), erythropoietin, interleukin-11 and others), the problems of fighting the negative consequences of ionizing radiation and radiomimetics remain very important.

In this chapter, the results of early and recent research and prospects for the use of carbon adsorption therapy for the treatment of myelosuppression caused by acute radiation sickness and cytostatics use are discussed.

## 2. About radiation injuries

Acute radiation syndrome is a definition to reflect severe damage to specific organs that occurs because of whole-body or significant partial-body irradiation greater than 1 Gy, over a short time period (high dose rate) [15]. The main syndromes are hematopoietic (doses >2–3 Gy), gastrointestinal (doses 5–12 Gy) and cerebrovascular one (doses 10–20 Gy) [16]. Depending on exposed and absorbed doses and its duration, cells exposed to ionizing radiation or radiomimetics present DNA mutations, apoptosis, necrosis, chromosomal aberrations or increased mutation frequency [17, 18]. The most profound injury is to lymphoid organs (lymphatic nodes, spleen and thyroid gland), bone marrow, testicles, ovaries, gastrointestinal mucosa. Parenchymal organs, namely liver, adrenal glands, kidneys, salivary glands and lungs possess quite high radioresistance. According to World Health Organization (WHO), acute radiation sickness (ARS) is composed of the hematopoietic subsyndrome

(HS), gastrointestinal subsyndrome (GIS), neurovascular subsyndrome (NVS) and cutaneous subsyndrome (CS) [19]. The main factors which determine the survival of victims are the degree of bone marrow suppression and gastrointestinal tract damage due to the presence of a large pool of fast-dividing cells [20–22]. Acute radiation sickness (ARS) could be considered as a sequence of immediate radiation injury and long-lasting bystander cross-effects.

Management of patients with ARS includes early use of hematopoietic cyto-kines, antimicrobials and transfusion support; in addition, antiemetic agents and analgesics, and even hematopoietic stem cells transplantation [16, 23]. Since 1997, granulocyte colony-stimulating factor (G-CSF) and granulocyte-macrophage colony-stimulating factor (GM-CSF) are used and their doses are driven by the radiation dose and physiologic responses for ARS [24] and by clinical protocols for leukopenia and neutropenia caused by anti-cancer treatment [25, 26]. However, these drugs still are of high cost, and pharmacoeconomic benefits seem to be questionable [27]. Singh et al. concluded that cytokine therapy has significant but modest effects [28]. All these facts force the researches to search new methods and means for additions to the management of post-aggressive iatrogenic leukopenia and related ARS- and radiomimetic-induced damage.

## 3. Adsorptive hemoperfusion therapy for ARS

Sorption detoxification types, quite widely used today in medicine, are: (1) hemoperfusion (when blood is filtered through the column with activated carbon); (2) enterosorption—enteral use of oral adsorbents of a different type and (3) application-sorption therapy - use of carbon dressing for the healing of the burns and wounds.

The ground for use of direct perfusion of the blood through an adsorbent column for its purification (hemoperfusion) was the Kuzin A.M. Structural-Metabolic Theory in Radiobiology (1970) [29]. Organs and tissues exposed to ionizing radiation and radiomimetic influences are damaged by radiotoxins, which affect radio-sensitive structures, and direct radiation-dependent changes in the macromolecules of the genome. Further investigations demonstrated that "radiotoxins" are reactive oxygen species (ROS) formed by water radiolysis. Oxidative stress causes DNA, protein and lipid oxidation and is responsible for the whole range of signs and syndromes of ARS [29]. Because of excessive lipid peroxidation, a lot of damaged cells appear that deepens the primary radiation injury repeatedly. In summary, ARS is a sum of primary damage due to oxidative stress plus so-called bystander effects [18], when cells exposed to ionizing radiation or radiomimetics can release signals that induce very similar effects on non-targeted neighboring cells.

Our first research of adsorptive therapy effects for acute radiation sickness (ARS) started in 1976 [30]. In this study, 69 inbred dogs were irradiated by external X-ray at the dose of 525 Rad (5.25 Gy). They were randomly assigned to three groups: first control group (n = 31), which received standard antibiotics therapy; second group (n = 19) got antibiotics + hemoperfusion 2 hours after irradiation and third group (n = 19) underwent saline infusion 4–5 hours after irradiation plus furosemide, and hemoperfusion 24 hours later. The results are presented in **Table 1**.

The highest survival rate was in the second group—68.4%, while in the control group, it was only 3.2%. Late hemoperfusion also resulted in a high survival rate—62.4%. Only 16% of an animal with hemoperfusion treatment (three dogs in each group) had critical leukopenia. In the control group, it was 93.5% of animals.

It is noteworthy, that mitotic index (a marker of the rate of cells division) (**Figure 1**) was significantly higher in the second group compared to the control one

| Group | Survival rate, % | Animals with critical hematological indices, % | | |
|---|---|---|---|---|
| | | Bone marrow cellularity $<1.0 \times 10^9/L$ | Leukopenia $<1.0 \times 10^9/L$ | Thrombocytopenia, $<50.0 \times 10^9/L$ |
| 1 (n = 31) | 3.2 | 13.4 ± 1.1 | 93.5 | 70 |
| 2 (n = 19) | 68.4 | 17.0 ± 1.6 | 16.0 | 52.6 |
| 3 (n = 19) | 62.4 | 16.6 ± 1.9 | 16.0 | 38.9 |

**Table 1.**
*Hemoperfusion for ARS treatment [30].*

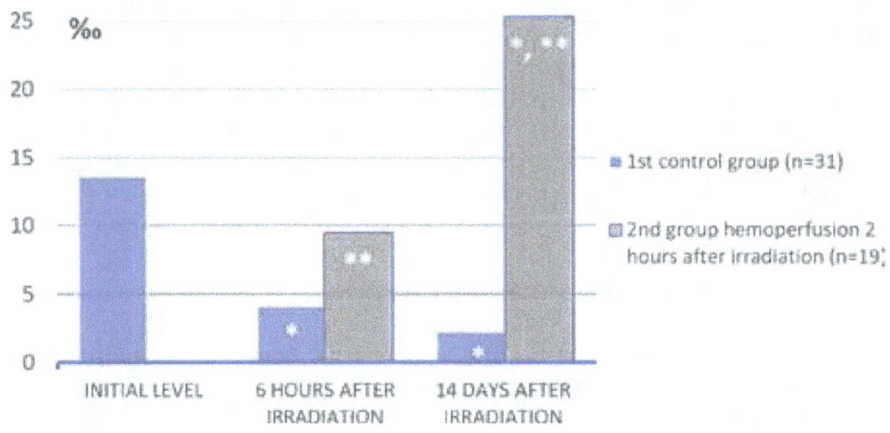

**Figure 1.**
*Mitotic index (‰) in the bone marrow of the dogs, exposed to external ionizing and hemoperfusion. Notes: \**
*$p \leq 0.05$ compared to the initial level; \*\* $p \leq 0.05$ compared to the control group.*

(6 hours after irradiation) and even to the initial level (14th day after exposure to ionizing irradiation) [31].

Hemoperfusion with activated carbon also provided survival of 50% of dogs exposed to ionizing irradiation at the doses of 3.46 and 3.65 Gy [32]. These results were re-tested and developed within a special closed program of Research institutions of the Ministry of Health and the Ministry of Defense of USSR. Hemoperfusion methods were implemented into clinics [33, 34].

A team of researchers who carried out the experiment on dogs by irradiating them at the dose of 5.25 Gy, witnesses that perfusions of the blood through the column with a carbon adsorbent were quite short. Slugging of columns was the main reason for incomplete procedures (only 0.3-0.5 of circulating blood volume was purified) [35]. Despite these factors, the survival rate and other studied parameters were quite successful. We suppose that it could be explained by washout of dust particles from the surface of the adsorbent in the moment of primary contact with the blood, and viscosity changes inside the column after the replacement of rinsing solution to the blood also contributed to it. We think that positive secondary effects could be provided by nano- and microparticles (1–2 μ) of activated carbon, which contact with the blood. Their content is not controlled according to the standards of British (BP) and American (USP) Pharmacopeia.

Today, we have a lot of evidence that positive curative effects of carbon nanoparticles, alone or as a part of a composite, are obliged to their ability to scavenge the ROS and simulate suppose the effects of free oxygen radical scavenging enzymes. Sandhir R. et al. [36] believe that nanoantioxidants (inorganic nanoparticles possessing intrinsic antioxidant properties) would be more effective against

ROS-induced damage because they cross the blood-brain barrier. It is a potential application in treating and preventing neurodegenerative conditions [36]. Arifa R.D. et al. research demonstrated that nanocomposite with fullerol decreases the intensity of irinotecan-induced leukopenia and gastrointestinal damage in mice and do not diminish the tumoricidal effects of the drug [37]. The aftertreatment with the same nanocomposite ameliorates the graft-versus-host disease reactions in mice and reduces intestinal lesions and bacterial translocation; prevents mortality and morbidity [38]. Nano-fullerenes promote osteogenesis of human adipose-derived stem cells and possess a great antioxidant capacity [39].

Encouraging results have been found concerning the amelioration of side effects of one more radiomimetic—anthracycline antibiotic doxorubicin (DOX), which also is known by its ability to cause oxidative stress and leukopenia. Fullerenol $C_{60}(OH)_{24}$ nanoparticles improved the myocardial morphology of DOX-treated animals, but cause a certain degree of parenchymal degeneration by itself [40]. Such and similar cases [41] evidence the need for designing and searching for the nanocomposites with specific features, which will possess antioxidant capacity without notable cytotoxicity. One of the solutions could be the conjugation of carbon nanomaterials with albumin [42]. It was found that $C_{60}(OH)_{24}$ decreases the consequences of DOX-induced excessive oxidation in the tissues of kidneys, testis and lungs in mice [43]. An aqueous solution of fullerenol was quite effective to fight experimental arthritis in rats [44]. Andrievsky G.V. et al. demonstrated significant (but only by 15%) radioprotective properties of hydrate $C_{60}$ fullerene in X-ray irradiation of the mice at the lethal dose of 7 Gy [45]. Water-soluble polyvinilpyrrolidone-wrapped fullerene derivative showed to significantly inhibit UVA-promoted melanogenesis in normal human epidermis melanocytes and human melanoma HMV-II cells within a non-cytotoxicity dose range [46]. Huq R. et al. showed that nontoxic poly(ethylene glycol)-functionalized hydrophilic carbon clusters, known scavengers of the ROS superoxide and hydroxyl radical, are preferentially internalized by T lymphocytes over other splenic immune cells [47]. It was successfully used to reduce T-lymphocyte-mediated inflammation in experimental autoimmune encephalomyelitis (an animal model of multiple sclerosis) [47].

Another type of carbon material—carboxylated nanodiamonds, diminish the biochemical and histological signs of damage of γ-irradiated human erythrocytes [48]. On the other hand, hydrogenated nanodiamonds dramatically increase the sensitivity to radiation effects of human radioresistant cancer cell lines [49]. The same effect was seen considering the radiomimetic neocarcinostatin. Single-walled carbon nanotubes were found to be the efficient nanocarriers for drug delivery in the murine model of breast cancer [50, 51]. The team of researchers [52] synthesized the magnetic particles $Fe_3O_4$ in the shell from partially graphitized carbon and demonstrated their high intrinsic peroxidase-like catalytic activity, which promotes oxidative stress in human prostate cancer PC-3 cells in the presence of ascorbic acid. One more interesting study with a composite system of reduced graphene oxide—iron oxide nanoparticles showed that such a combination can synergistically induce physical and chemical damage to methicillin-resistant *Staphylococcus aureus* (MRSA) [53].

We must notice, that carbon nanoparticles possess great antioxidant properties and could be perspective for designing the nanopharmaceutical means and drugs to treat the disorders, when oxidative stress is an intrinsic part of pathogenesis, for leukopenia also. It means that further studies of carbon micro- and nanoparticles effects at parenteral routes of administration could finalize the discovery of quite a new method of mass treatment of acute radiation sickness.

Recently, several detailed reviews have been published on the pharmacological potential and prospects for the therapeutic use of cerium nanoparticles as traps of highly reactive oxygen (ROS) and nitrogen species (RNS) [54–56]. These reviews are based on a variety of experimental studies both *in vitro* and *in vivo*. Not less interesting results for use of nanocrystal cerium dioxide ($CeO_2$) on the model of DOX-induced cardiomyopathy in rats we got [57]. Cardiomyocytes mostly are damaged because of the radiomimetic impact of the drug, and the violation of blood components was quite similar to the effects of ionizing irradiation. It is known that oxidative stress is an intrinsic part of the cytotoxic effects of DOX, and heart tissues are vulnerable because of a lack of intracellular antioxidant defense factors compared to other organs and systems [58].

In this study, we used 21 female white mongrel rats, which were randomly assigned to the next groups (n = 7): first control groups got weekly intraperitoneal (IP) injection of saline; rats of second (DOX) and third groups got three times a week IP injections of doxorubicin at a dose of 2.5 mg/kg (n = 7); rats of third (DOX + $CeO_2$) group got twice weekly IP injections of nanodisperse $CeO_2$ (0.2 mg/kg) next day after doxorubicin injections additionally. Treatments lasted for 2 weeks (**Figure 2**).

Injections of nanodisperse $CeO_2$ caused positive changes in myocardium structure. We observed improvement of a structure, decreased vacuolization of sarcoplasm, a number of cells with nuclei pathology was much lower (**Figure 4**) compared to the second group (**Figure 3**). A part of myocardium cells still had pyknotic nuclei with karyolysis signs. But mostly, the intensity of dystrophy and necrosis reduced and nuclei acquired oval shape again.

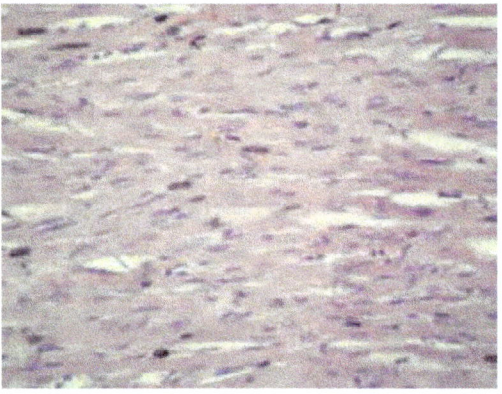

**Figure 2.**
*Myocardium tissue of rat of the control group. H&E. ×600.*

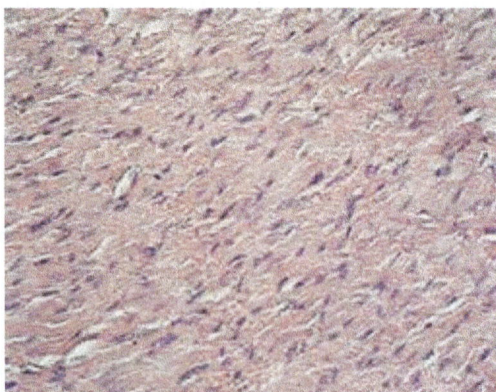

**Figure 3.**
*Myocardium tissue of rat of the DOX group. H&E. ×600.*

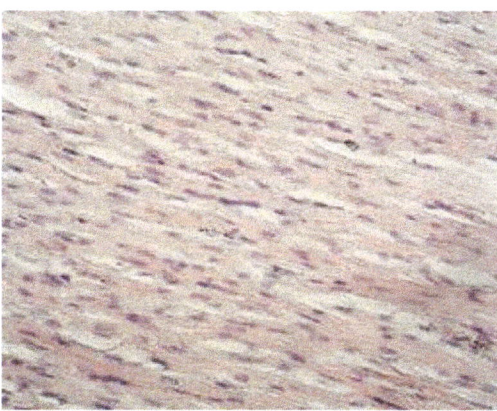

**Figure 4.**
*Myocardium tissue of rat of the DOX + CeO$_2$ group. H&E. ×600.*

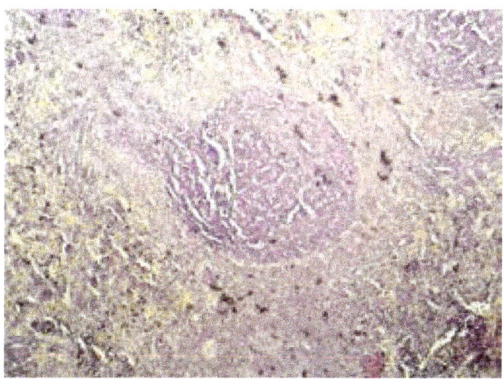

**Figure 5.**
*Spleen structure of rat of the control group. H&E. ×600.*

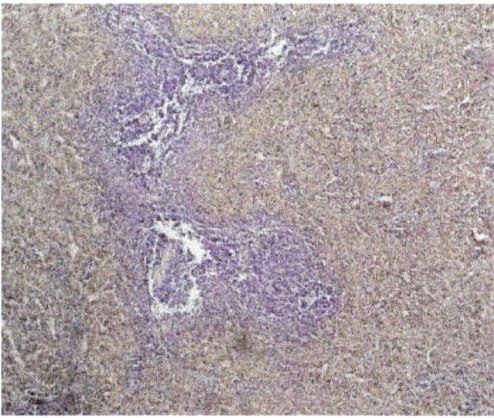

**Figure 6.**
*Spleen structure of rat of the DOX group. H&E. ×600.*

Also, we observed an increased number of lymphoid follicles in the spleen, which restored a circle-like shape (**Figures 5–7**).

There were no significant positive changes in the structure of liver parenchyma. We may just note restoring nuclei sizes and shape and a little bit lighter pale pink

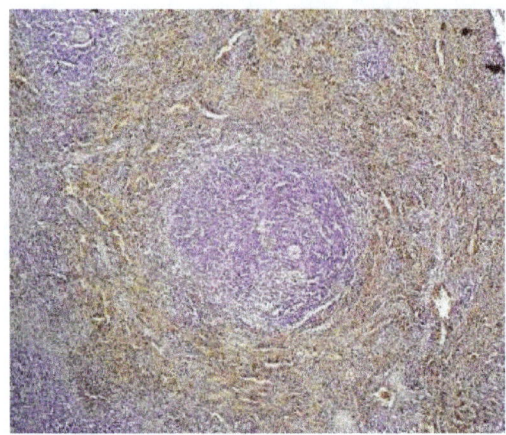

**Figure 7.**
*Spleen structure of rat of the DOX + CeO2 group. H&E. ×600.*

color of cytoplasm. It witnesses that the synthetic function of the liver was partly restored. Concerning the kidneys, no positive changes had been found.

Biochemical indices of lipid and protein peroxidation, antioxidant defense system showed that $CeO_2$ increased the activity of catalase by 24.6%, raised the level of reduced glutathione by 10.9% and decreased the level of oxidative modification of protein and lipids by 28.1 and 23.6%, respectively (compared to the group with untreated DOX-induced cardiomyopathy).

Bakht M.K. et al. proposed to reduce the actual radiation burden in patients exposed to radioisotope studies by arranging radiolabels for cerium oxide [59], and Colon J. et al. could achieve a good prophylactic result for radiation pneumonitis in mice that received nanocrystalline dioxide Ce [60]. One more fact should be mentioned here: because of bone marrow suppression and leukopenia development, lungs are fragile to injury by ionizing irradiation. They have their own host defense system, based on alveolar macrophages. Because of leukocytes toxic damage (by ionizing injury or radiation therapy or as the side effects of anti-cancer chemo-therapy), resting macrophages can no longer be transformed which lead to radiation pneumonitis [24]. Heslet L. et al. showed that systemic administration of myelo stimulative cytokines was not helpful to prevent it because they do not penetrate the alveoli. That is why we suggest that oral adsorbents and/or parenteral use of $CeO_2$ (it penetrated the alveoli and prevents radiation pneumonitis on mice model) will enhance the prophylaxis and treatment of ARS and decrease the intensity of side effects of radiation therapy and cytostatic drugs.

## 4. Local signs of whole-body irradiation and efficacy of application-sorption therapy

External exposure to ionizing irradiation frequently results in radiation burns of the skin. Leukopenia just deepens the injury because of oppressing the regeneration processes. A retrospective report on injuries caused by the atomic bombing of Hiroshima showed that up to 65% of all type of injuries were "radiation-combined injury," when ionizing irradiation was coupled with burns, wounds and infections [61]. Regarding these facts and negative contribution of leukopenia also, we want to demonstrate the efficiency of activated carbon. The remarkable result was observed on the model of the thermal non-full depth burn in Albino rats [62]. The early application (within first

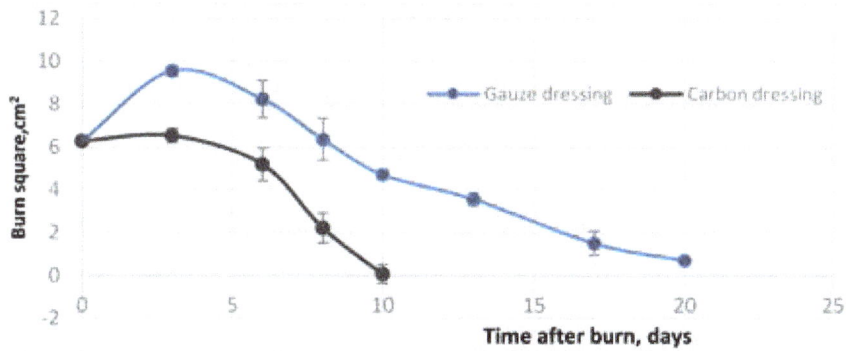

**Figure 8.**
*The dynamics of healing of the non-full depth burn after application of the gauze and carbon dressing.*

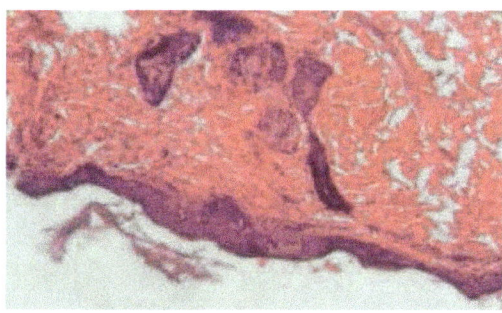

**Figure 9.**
*Morphological structure of normal skin. H&E. ×200.*

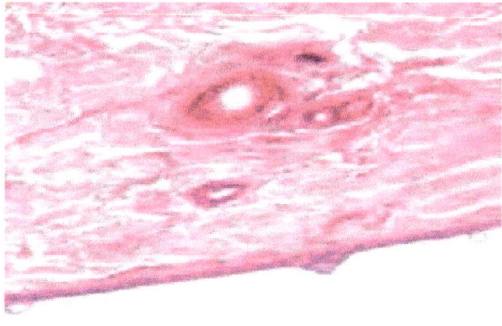

**Figure 10.**
*Morphological structure of burned skin after use of gauze dressing on the 7th day after the thermal non-full depth burn. H&E. ×200.*

60 min) of the highly active carbon fabrics ($S_{BET}$ > 2000 m$^2$/g) twofold reduced the healing time: 10.80 ± 1.27 and 20.60 ± 0.86 days for adsorptive carbon and gauze dress-ings use, respectively (**Figure 8**).

Histological analysis demonstrated that adsoptive carbon dressings' application promoted the restoration of skin structure on the 7th day after injury in rats with the non-full burn (**Figures 9–11**).

Similar results were observed on the burns caused by external irradiation at the dose of 8 Gy. Epithelialization of burn wounds has been completed on 21.1 ± 4.1 versus 27.3 ± 5.7 days after trauma for carbon and gauze dressings use, respectively. One

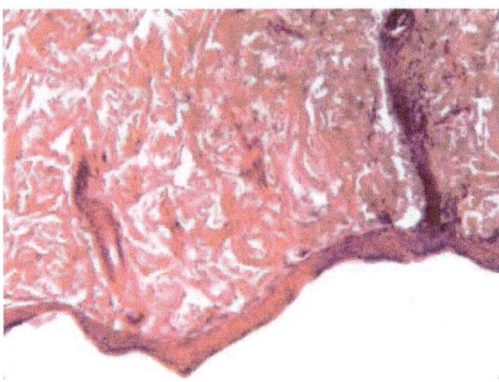

**Figure 11.**
*Morphological structure of the burned skin after use of carbon dressing on the 7th day after the thermal non-full depth burn. H&E. ×200.*

more fact relates to the treatment ultraviolet radiation-induced burns. Application of adsorptive carbon dressings significantly (by 1.5–1.7 times) accelerated the burn-healing time. All these data will be published soon.

These results presented the undoubted perspective for use of high capacity carbon fabrics for the treatment of superficial skin lesions, especially complicated by concomitant leukopenia.


## 5. Enterosorption for leukopenia management

Hemoperfusion as a procedure requires well-trained staff, specific equipment and sterility. It means that such method of sorption detoxification is not adapted to emergency exposure situations, during war-time and large human contingent injury. That is why the use of enteral sorption therapy (ingestion of activated carbon) is a more prospective method for such situations. Among the early studies, the great results were observed in the patients with lymphogranulomatosis undergoing radiotherapy [63], who were treated with fibrous carbon oral adsorbent. Enterosorption treatment allowed to continue planned schemes of radiation therapy and was more efficient than conventional methods for leukopenia healing. In the next study [64], cyclophosphane was given to Guerin tumor-grafted rats at the dose of 100 mg/kg of body weight on 10th and 13th days after tumor transplantation; enterosorption with synthetic SCN carbons (bulk density 0.3–0.4 g/cm$^3$) was administered next day after cyclophosphane injection. These expressed myeloprotective effects we approved and confirmed in the clinic. One more radiomimetic anti-cancer agent cisplatin was used in an experiment on Guerin tumor-grafted rats [65] and highly activated fibrous carbon material Carboline (Ukraine) successfully ameliorated a wide range of its side effects. Carboline is used in clinical practice also and demonstrates promising results [66].

Our latest experiments on rats exposed to X-ray irradiation in a total dose of 6 Gy (63 Rad per min, t = 11 min) demonstrated great results of novel oral carbon adsorbents administration to ameliorate radiation-caused leukopenia. We used two granulated activated carbons (AC) with a diameter of granules (0.25–0.5 mm) and bulk density 0.1 and 0.2 g/cm$^3$ (ES1 and ES2, respectively). Enterosorbents were administrated as radioprotectors, radiomitigators and therapeutic agents (at the dose of 10 ml/kg, admixed to the food, three days before and nine days after ionizing irradiation exposure). Irradiation caused a 10-fold decrease in the white blood

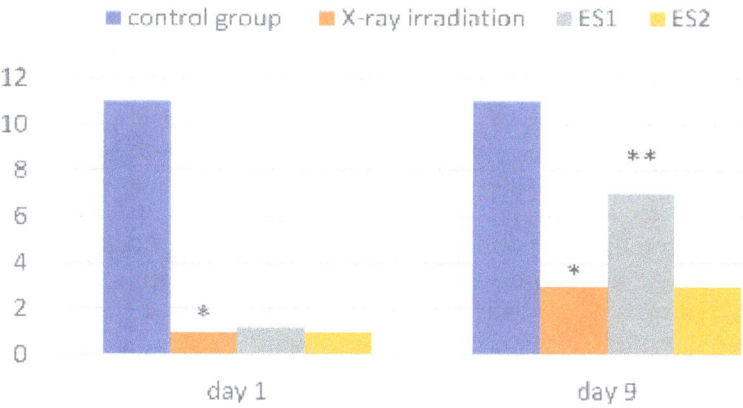

**Figure 12.**
*White blood cells count ($10^9$/L) in X-ray irradiation at the dose of 6 Gy and oral adsorbents administration. Notes: $p < 0.05$ compared to: \*—the control group, \*\*—X-ray irradiation group.*

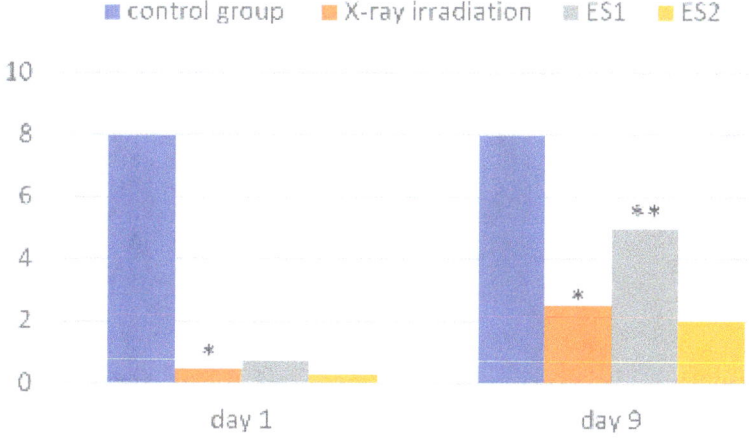

**Figure 13.**
*Lymphocytes count ($10^9$/L) in X-ray irradiation at the dose of 6 Gy and oral adsorbents administration. Notes. $p < 0.05$ compared to: \*—the control group, \*\*—X-ray irradiation group.*

cells count. ES1 administration raised the index twice on the 9th day after X-ray exposure, while ES2 produced fewer results (**Figure 12**).

The same effect was observed concerning the lymphocytes count (**Figure 13**). Structural differences among those two carbon adsorbents are estimated. These results will be published soon in detail.

So, as we observed, specific oral adsorbents with specified porosity and pores distribution are quite successful to fight the iatrogenic leukopenia because of the influence of ARS or anti-cancer treatment.

Oral carbon materials have a high capability to decrease the emesis caused by anti-cancer treatment [66, 67]. Also, it is a unique mean with anti-diarrhea action, which could be implemented in the clinics for the treatment of ARS-induced gastrointestinal subsyndrome as well as for dyspepsia syndrome caused by tumoricidal therapy.

Thus, enterosorption for the results on the animal study and use in clinics do prevent hematotoxicity of anti-cancer treatment and significantly ameliorated leukopenia and its consequences.

## 6. Oral carbon adsorbents as an addition to classical treatment of leukopenia with G-CSF

Abovementioned positive results led us to design of a new improved version of carbon oral adsorbent, which was used in early experiments [64, 68]. An old prototype C1 and his new version C2 were approved on the model of melphalan-induced bone marrow suppression [69–71]. We demonstrated that myeloprotective action of carbon granulated enterosorbent C1 (bulk density of 0.28 g/cm$^3$, specific surface of 1719 m$^2$/g and mesopore area of 239 m$^2$/g) is significantly less compared to effects of adsorbent C2 with bulk density of 0.18 g/cm$^3$, total specific surface of 2162 m$^2$/g and mesopore area of 565 m$^2$/g (**Figure 14**).

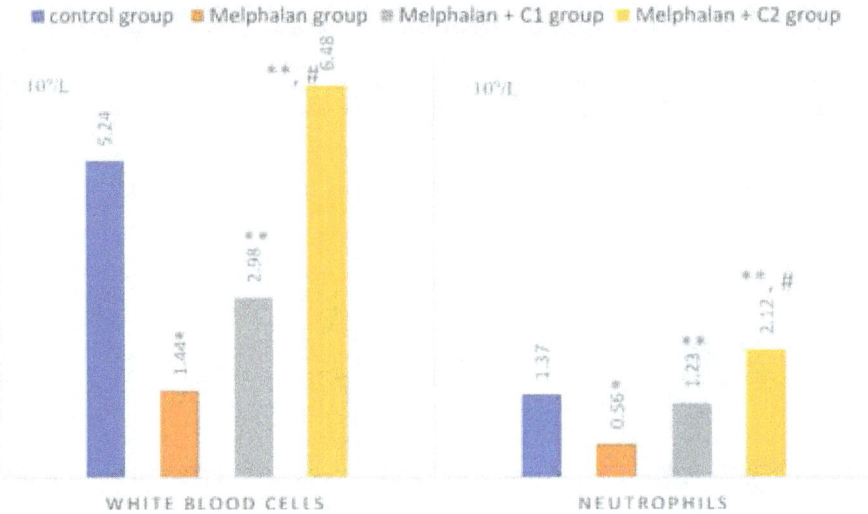

**Figure 14.**
*White blood cells and neutrophils counts ($10^9$/L) on the 8th day after melphalan injection at the dose of 3 mg/kg and administration of oral carbon adsorbents C1 and C2 in a study on rats. Notes. \*—p < 0.05 compared to the control group; \*\*—p < 0.05 compared to the melphalan group; #—p < 0.05 and compared to the Melphalan + C1group.*

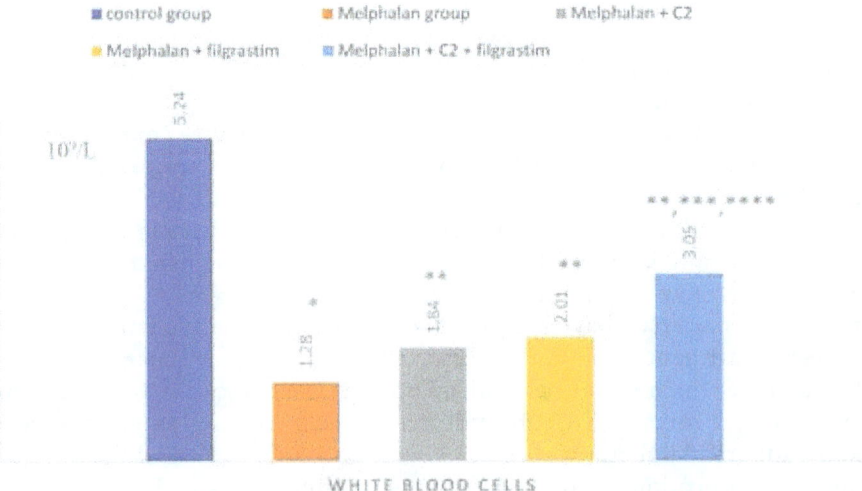

**Figure 15.**
*White blood cells count ($10^9$/L) on the 8th day after melphalan injection at the dose of 4 mg/kg and administration of oral carbon adsorbent and filgrastim in the study on rats. Notes. p < 0.05 compared to: \*—Control group; \*\*—Melphalan group; \*\*\*—Melphalan + C2 group; \*\*\*\*—Melphalan + filgrastim group.*

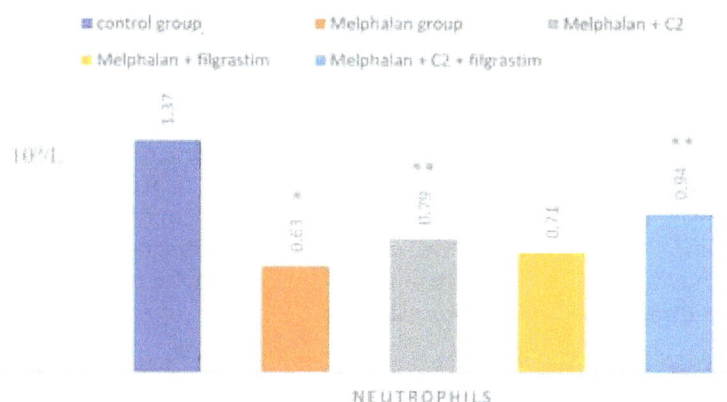

**Figure 16.**
*Neutrophils count ($10^9$/L) on the 8th day after melphalan injection at the dose of 4 mg/kg and administration of oral carbon adsorbent and filgrastim in a study on rats. Notes. p < 0.05 compared to: \*—Control group; \*\* —Melphalan group.*

C2 enterosorbent administration normalized the prooxidant/antioxidant system indices too [71]. Oxidative stress is an intrinsic part of ionizing radiation and radio-mimetic injury, and enteral sorption therapy possesses notable antioxidant effects.

Adding the carbon oral adsorbent to classical scheme for the treatment of leukopenia with G-CSF (caused by single intravenous melphalan injection at the dose of 4 mg/kg) demonstrated significant myeloprotective effect and synergy compared to single-use effects of each agent alone [70] (**Figures 15** and **16**). C2 and filgrastim combination caused increase of white blood cells count by 138.3% compared to the melphalan group; by 65.8% compared to melphalan + C2 group, and by 51.7% compared to use of filgrastim alone.

We must note that in this study, we got an unexpected significant increase of platelets level from (254.60 ± 45.59) to (505.40 ± 70.68) × $10^9$/L in a group of rats that received the combined treatment with oral adsorbent and G-CSF. Isolated administration of enterosorbent C2 tended to raise the level of thrombocytes, we suppose because of general detoxification action.

Use of enterosorbent or combined use of both preparations provided significantly better effects toward the prooxidant/antioxidant balance in rats.

The important issue is that combination of G-CSF and carbon adsorbents [69] as well as enteral sorption therapy use alone [65] does not affect the efficacy of anti-cancer treatment; we proved it by our experiments on Guerin tumor-grafted rats.

## 7. Conclusions

Leukopenia is an essential part of the damage caused by ionizing irradiation and/or radiomimetic influences (as tumoricidal chemotherapy). Leukocytes play an important role in immune defense, tissue regeneration, the functioning of the main organs and systems; and the degree of bone marrow suppression determines the survival of victims in ionizing radiation exposure as well as the efficacy of anti-cancer chemotherapy. All three methods of sorption detoxification with activated carbons such as hemoperfusion (when blood is filtered through the column with activated carbon); enterosorption—peroral use of oral adsorbents and application-sorption therapy (use of carbon dressing for the healing of the burns and wounds), can be successfully used for the leukopenia prophylaxis and treatment in ionizing irradiation exposure, side effects of anti-cancer chemotherapy, as well as for the boosting of healing of associated skin damage.

Enterosorption demonstrates significant synergy with hemopoietic cytokines in the treatment of bone marrow suppression caused by such an aggressive agent as melphalan (a derivative of mustard nitrogen). Nanocrystal cerium dioxide could be useful for oxidative stress modulation caused by such radiomimetic as anti-cancer anthracycline antibiotic doxorubicin. Modification of pathological biochemical processes which provoke bone marrow suppression and leukopenia is a basis of the efficacy of sorption detoxification in acute radiation syndrome as well as to decrease the side effects of anti-cancer chemotherapy. Our findings may contribute to the refinement of current risk stratification algorithms for acute radiation sickness treatment.

## Abbreviations

NPP         nuclear power plants
ARS         acute radiation sickness.
G-CSF       granulocyte colony-stimulating factor.
ROS         reactive oxygen species.
Gy          gray, unit of ionizing radiation dose.

## Author details

Oksana O. Shevchuk[1*], Elisaveta A. Snezhkova[2], Anatoliy G. Bilous[3], Veronika V. Sarnatskaya[2], Kvitoslava I. Badakhivska[2], Larysa A. Sakhno[2], Vasyl F. Chekhun[2] and Volodymyr G. Nikolaev[2]

1 I. Horbachevsky Ternopil State Medical University, Ternopil, Ukraine

2 R.E. Kavetsky Institute of Experimental Pathology, Oncology and Radiobiology of National Academy of Science of Ukraine, Kyiv, Ukraine

3 Institute of General and Inorganic Chemistry of National Academy of Science of Ukraine, Kyiv, Ukraine

*Address all correspondence to: shevchukoo@tdmu.edu.ua

# References

[1] Davis S, Day RW, Kopecky KJ, Mahoney MC, McCarthy PL, Michalek AM, et al. Childhood leukaemia in Belarus, Russia, and Ukraine following the Chernobyl power station accident: Results from an international collaborative population-based case—Control study. International Journal of Epidemiology. 2006;**35**:386-396. DOI: 10.1093/ije/dyi220

[2] Mettler FA, Gus'kova AK, Gusev I. Health effects in those with acute radiation sickness from the Chernobyl accident. Health Physics. 2007;**93**:462-469. DOI: 10.1097/01. HP.0000278843.27969.74

[3] Belyi D, Kovalenko A, Bazyka D, Bebeshko V. Non-cancer effects in acute radiation syndrome survivors in Ukraine. Health Physics. 2010;**98**:876- 884. DOI: 10.1097/HP.0b013e3181d270e4

[4] Hayano RS, Tsubokura M, Miyazaki M, Satou H, Sato K, Masaki S, et al. Internal radiocesium contamination of adults and children in Fukushima 7 to 20 months after the Fukushima NPP accident as measured by extensive whole-body-counter surveys. Proceedings of the Japan Academy. Series B. 2013;**89**:157-163. DOI: 10.2183/pjab.89.157

[5] Kobayashi T, Nagai H, Chino M, Kawamura H. Source term estimation of atmospheric release due to the Fukushima Dai-ichi nuclear power plant accident by atmospheric and oceanic dispersion simulations. Journal of Nuclear Science and Technology. 2013;**50**:255-264. DOI: 10.1080/00223131.2013.772449

[6] Parakkal D, Ehrenpreis ED. Medical management of radiation effects on the intestines. Radiation Therapy for Pelvic Malignancy and its Consequences. New York, NY: Springer New York; 2015. DOI:10.1007/978-1-4939-2217-8_15

[7] Shadad AK, Sullivan FJ, Martin JD, Egan LJ. Gastrointestinal radiation injury: Prevention and treatment. World Journal of Gastroenterology. 2013;**19**:199-208

[8] Teo MTW, Sebag-Montefiore D, Donnellan CF. Prevention and management of radiation-induced late gastrointestinal toxicity. Clinical Oncology. 2015;**27**:656-667. DOI: 10.1016/j.clon.2015.06.010

[9] WHO. Ionizing radiation, health effects and protective measures. Fact Sheet; 2016

[10] Bartelink H, Roelofsen F, Eschwege F, Rougier P, Bosset JF, Gonzalez DG, et al. Concomitant radiotherapy and chemotherapy is superior to radiotherapy alone in the treatment of locally advanced anal cancer: Results of a phase III randomized trial of the European organization for research and treatment of cancer radiotherapy and gastro. Journal of Clinical Oncology. 1997;**15**:2040-2049. DOI: 10.1200/ JCO.1997.15.5.2040

[11] D'Amico AV, Whittington R, Bruce Malkowicz S, Schultz D, Blank K, Broderick GA, et al. Biochemical outcome after radical prostatectomy, external beam radiation therapy, or interstitial radiation therapy for clinically localized prostate cancer. Journal of the American Medical Association. 1998;**280**:969-974. DOI: 10.1001/jama.280.11.969

[12] Nagata Y, Takayama K, Matsuo Y, Norihisa Y, Mizowaki T, Sakamoto T, et al. Clinical outcomes of a phase I/II study of 48 Gy of stereotactic body radiotherapy in 4 fractions for primary lung cancer using a stereotactic body frame. International Journal of Radiation Oncology, Biology, Physics. 2005;**63**:1427-1431. DOI: 10.1016/j. ijrobp.2005.05.034

[13] Liu W, Zhang C-C, Li K. Prognostic value of chemotherapy-induced leukopenia in small-cell lung cancer. Cancer Biology and Medicine. 2013;**10**:92-98. DOI: 10.7497/j.issn.2095-3941.2013.02.005

[14] Xing C, Liang B, Wu J, Yang Q, Hu G, Yan Y, et al. Prognostic significance of leukopenia during the induction phase in adult B cell acute lymphoblastic leukemia. Cancer Management and Research. 2018;**10**: 625-635. DOI: 10.2147/CMAR.S158359

[15] Management of Terrorist Events Involving Radioactive Material. NCRP report No. 138; Bethesda; 2001

[16] López M, Martín M. Medical management of the acute radiation syndrome. Reports of Practical Oncology & Radiotherapy. 2011;**16**:138-146. DOI: 10.1016/j.rpor.2011.05.001

[17] Popov D, Jones J, Maliev V. Radiation toxins—Effects of radiation toxicity, molecular mechanisms of action, radiomimetic properties and possible countermeasures for radiation injury. In: Current Topics in Ionizing Radiation Research. Rijeka, Croatia: InTech; 2012. pp. 215-242. DOI: 10.5772/33806

[18] Rzeszowska-Wolny J, Przybyszewski WM, Widel M. Ionizing radiation-induced bystander effects, potential targets for modulation of radiotherapy. European Journal of Pharmacology. 2009;**625**:156-164. DOI: 10.1016/j.ejphar.2009.07.028

[19] Dainiak N. Medical management of acute radiation syndrome and associated infections in a high-casualty incident. Journal of Radiation Research. 2018;**59**:ii54-ii64. DOI: 10.1093/jrr/rry004

[20] Povirk LF. DNA damage and mutagenesis by radiomimetic DNA-cleaving agents: Bleomycin, neocarzinostatin and other enediynes. Mutation Research. 1996;**355**:71-89

[21] Hauer-Jensen M, Kumar KS, Wang J, Berbee M, Fu Q, Marjan B. Intestinal toxicity in radiation—And combined injury: Significance, mechanisms, and countermeasures. In: Global Terrorism Issues and Developments. Hauppauge (NY): Nova Science Publishers; 2008. pp. 61-100

[22] Levis AG, Spanio L, De Nadai A. Radiomimetic effects of a nitrogen mustard on survival, growth, protein and nucleic acid synthesis of mammalian cells in vitro. Experimental Cell Research. 1963;**31**:19-30. DOI: 10.1016/0014-4827(63)90151-4

[23] Waselenko JK, MacVittie TJ, Blakely WF, Pesik N, Wiley AL, Dickerson WE, et al. Medical management of the acute radiation syndrome: Recommendations of the strategic national stockpile radiation working group. Annals of Internal Medicine. 2004;**140**:1037. DOI: 10.7326/0003-4819-140-12-200406150 - 00015

[24] Heslet L, Bay C, Nepper-Christensen S. Acute radiation syndrome (ARS)—Treatment of the reduced host defense. International Journal of General Medicine. 2012;**5**:105-115. DOI: 10.2147/IJGM.S22177

[25] Aapro MS, Bohlius J, Cameron DA, Lago LD, Donnelly JP, Kearney N, et al. 2010 update of EORTC guidelines for the use of granulocyte-colony stimulating factor to reduce the incidence of chemotherapy-induced febrile neutropenia in adult patients with lymphoproliferative disorders and solid tumours. European Journal of Cancer. 2011;**47**:8-32. DOI: 10.1016/j.ejca.2010.10.013

[26] Schwenkglenks M, Pettengell R, Jackisch C, Paridaens R, Constenla M, Bosly A, et al. Risk factors for chemotherapy-induced neutropenia occurrence in breast cancer patients: Data from the INC-EU prospective

observational European neutropenia study. Support Care Cancer. 2011;**19**:483-490. DOI: 10.1007/ s00520-010-0840-y

[27] Barnes G, Pathak A, Schwartzberg L. Pharmacoeconomics of granulocyte colony-stimulating factor: A critical review. Advances in Therapy. 2014;**31**:683-695. DOI: 10.1007/ s12325-014-0133-9

[28] Singh VK, Newman VL, Seed TM. Colony-stimulating factors for the treatment of the hematopoietic component of the acute radiation syndrome (H-ARS): A review. Cytokine. 2015;**71**:22-37

[29] Kuzin AM. Structural-Metabolic Theory in Radiobiology. Moscow: Nauka; 1970

[30] Nikolaev VG, Pinchuk LB, Umansky MA, Pinchuk VG, Burushkina TN, Petrenko SV, et al. Early experimental studies on hemoperfusion as a treatment modality for acute radiation disease. Artificail Organs. 1993;**17**:362-368

[31] Nikolaev VG. Sorption therapy with the use of activated carbons: Effects on regeneration of organs and tissues, hemoperfusion, plasmaperfusion and other clinical uses of general, biospecific, immuno and leucocyte Adsorbents. Singapore: World Scientific Publishing Co Pte Ltd.; April 2017. p. 221-243. doi:10.1142/9789814749084_0007.

[32] Chertkov KS, Andrianova IY, Andrushchenko VN, Vernigorova LA. Experimental development of combined treatment for acute radiation sickness. In: Horn B, editor. 9th Int. Congr. of Int. Radiat. Prot. Assoc. Vienna, Austria: International Atomic Energy Agency (IAEA); 1996. pp. 129-131

[33] Chertkov KS, Andrianova IE, Andrushchenko VN, Vernigorova LA, Glushkov VA, Davydova SA, et al.

Advances and prospects of a combined therapy of acute radiation injury in experiments. Radiatsionnaia Biologiia, Radioecologiia. 1999;**39**:563-567

[34] Vernigorov LA, Chertkov KS. Methodical Recommendations on the Use of Hemosorption in Clinical Conditions for Treatment of Acute Radiation Sickness. Moscow: Meditsina; 1983

[35] Nikolaev VG, Strelko VV. Method of Hemocarboperfusion in Experiments and in Clinics. Kyiv: Naukova Dumka; 1984

[36] Sandhir R, Yadav A, Sunkaria A, Singhal N. Nano-antioxidants: An emerging strategy for intervention against neurodegenerative conditions. Neurochemistry International. 2015;**89**:209-226. DOI: 10.1016/j. neuint.2015.08.011

[37] Arifa RDN, De Paula TP, Madeira MFM, Lima RL, Garcia ZM, Ávila TV, et al. The reduction of oxidative stress by nanocomposite Fullerol decreases mucositis severity and reverts leukopenia induced by Irinotecan. Pharmacological Research. 2016;**107**:102-110. DOI: 10.1016/j. phrs.2016.03.004

[38] Bernardes PTT, Rezende BM, Resende CB, De Paula TP, Reis AC, Gonçalves WA, et al. Nanocomposite treatment reduces disease and lethality in a murine model of acute graft-versus-host disease and preserves anti-tumor effects. PLoS One. 2015;**10**:e0123004. DOI: 10.1371/ journal.pone.0123004

[39] Yang X, Li C-J, Wan Y, Smith P, Shang G, Cui Q. Antioxidative fullerol promotes osteogenesis of human adipose-derived stem cells. International Journal of Nanomedicine. 2014;**9**: 4023-4031. DOI: 10.2147/IJN.S66785

[40] Borović ML, Ičević I, Kanački Z, Žikić D, Seke M, Injac R, et al. Effects

of Fullerenol $C_{60}(OH)_{24}$ nanoparticles on a single-dose doxorubicin-induced cardiotoxicity in pigs: An ultrastructural study. Ultrastructural Pathology. 2014;**38**:150-163. DOI: 10.3109/01913123.2013.822045

[41] Injac R, Prijatelj M, Strukelj B. Fullerenol nanoparticles: Toxicity and antioxidant activity. In: Methods Molecular Biology Oxidative Stress Nanotechnology. Totowa, NJ: Humana Press; 2013. pp. 75-100. DOI: 10.1007/978-1-62703-475-3_5

[42] Liu Y, Ge Y-S, Jiang F-L, Xu Z-Q, Zhang M-F. Binding of fullerol to human serum albumin: Spectroscopic and electrochemical approach. Journal of Photochemistry and Photobiology B: Biology. 2011;**108**:34-43. DOI: 10.1016/j.jphotobiol.2011.12.006

[43] Srdjenovic B, Milic-Torres V, Grujic N, Stankov K, Djordjevic A, Vasovic V. Antioxidant properties of fullerenol $C_{60}(OH)_{24}$ in rat kidneys, testes, and lungs treated with doxorubicin. Toxicology Mechanisms and Methods. 2010;**20**:298- 305. DOI: 10.3109/15376516.2010.485622

[44] Yudoh K, Karasawa R, Masuko K, Kato T. Water-soluble fullerene (C60) inhibits the development of arthritis in the rat model of arthritis. International Journal of Nanomedicine. 2009;**4**:217-225

[45] Andrievsky GV, Bruskov VI, Tykhomyrov AA, Gudkov SV. Peculiarities of the antioxidant and radioprotective effects of hydrated C60 fullerene nanostuctures in vitro and in vivo. Free Radical Biology & Medicine. 2009;**47**:786-793. DOI: 10.1016/J. FREERADBIOMED.2009.06.016

[46] Xiao L, Matsubayashi K, Miwa N. Inhibitory effect of the water-soluble polymer-wrapped derivative of fullerene on UVA-induced melanogenesis via downregulation of tyrosinase expression in human melanocytes and skin tissues. Archives of Dermatological Research. 2007;**299**:245-257. DOI: 10.1007/s00403-007-0740-2

[47] Huq R, Samuel ELG, Sikkema WKA, Nilewski LG, Lee T, Tanner MR, et al. Preferential uptake of antioxidant carbon nanoparticles by T lymphocytes for immunomodulation. Scientific Reports. 2016;**6**:33808. DOI: 10.1038/srep33808

[48] Santacruz-Gomez K, Silva-Campa E, Melendrez-Amavizca R, Teran Arce F, Mata-Haro V, Landon PB, et al. Carboxylated nanodiamonds inhibit γ-irradiation damage of human red blood cells. Nanoscale. 2016;**8**: 7189-7196. DOI: 10.1039/C5NR06789H

[49] Grall R, Girard H, Saad L, Petit T, Gesset C, Combis-Schlumberger M, et al. Impairing the radioresistance of cancer cells by hydrogenated nanodiamonds. Biomaterials. 2015;**61**:290-298. DOI: 10.1016/J. BIOMATERIALS.2015.05.034

[50] Al Faraj A, Shaik AP, Shaik AS. Magnetic single-walled carbon nanotubes as efficient drug delivery nanocarriers in breast cancer murine model: Noninvasive monitoring using diffusion-weighted magnetic resonance imaging as sensitive imaging biomarker. International Journal of Nanomedicine. 2015;**10**:157-168. DOI: 10.2147/IJN.S75074

[51] Al Faraj A, Shaik AS, Al Sayed B. Preferential magnetic targeting of carbon nanotubes to cancer sites: Noninvasive tracking using MRI in a murine breast cancer model. Nanomedicine. 2015;**10**:931-948. DOI: 10.2217/nnm.14.145

[52] An Q, Sun C, Li D, Xu K, Guo J, Wang C. Peroxidase-like activity of $Fe_3O_4$@carbon nanoparticles enhances ascorbic acid-induced oxidative stress and selective damage to PC-3 prostate cancer cells. ACS Applied Materials &

Interfaces. 2013;**5**:13248-13257. DOI: 10.1021/am4042367

[53] Pan W-Y, Huang C-C, Lin T-T, Hu H-Y, Lin W-C, Li M-J, et al. Synergistic antibacterial effects of localized heat and oxidative stress caused by hydroxyl radicals mediated by graphene/iron oxide-based nanocomposites. Nanomedicine: Nanotechnology, Biology and Medicine. 2016;**12**:431-438. DOI: 10.1016/J.NANO.2015.11.014

[54] Celardo I, Pedersen JZ, Traversa E, Ghibelli L. Pharmacological potential of cerium oxide nanoparticles. Nanoscale. 2011;**3**:1411. DOI: 10.1039/c0nr00875c

[55] Das S, Dowding JM, Klump KE, McGinnis JF, Self W, Seal S. Cerium oxide nanoparticles: Applications and prospects in nanomedicine. Nanomedicine. 2013;**8**:1483-1508. DOI: 10.2217/nnm.13.133

[56] Walkey C, Das S, Seal S, Erlichman J, Heckman K, Ghibelli L, et al. Catalytic properties and biomedical applications of cerium oxide nanoparticles. Environmental Science. Nano. 2015;**2**:33-53. DOI: 10.1039/c4en00138a

[57] Khudenko NV, Sarnatska VV, Paziuk LM, Timashkov IP, Nikolaev VG. Experimental doxorubicin-induced cardiomyopathy: Effects of nanodisperse cerium dioxide. Experimental Oncology. 2019. In press

[58] Golubtsov OU, Tyrenko VV, Lutov VV, Maslyakov VV, Makiev RG. Cardiovascular complications of anticancer therapy. Modern problems of science and education. 2017;(2):1-15. (In Russian)

[59] Bakht MK, Hosseini V, Honarpisheh H. Radiolabeled nanoceria probes may reduce oxidative damages and risk of cancer: A hypothesis for radioisotope-based imaging procedures. Medical Hypotheses. 2013;**81**:1164-1168. DOI: 10.1016/j.mehy.2013.10.008

[60] Colon J, Herrera L, Smith J, Patil S, Komanski C, Kupelian P, et al. Protection from radiation-induced pneumonitis using cerium oxide nanoparticles. Nanomedicine: Nanotechnology, Biology and Medicine. 2009;**5**:225-231. DOI: 10.1016/j.nano.2008.10.003

[61] DiCarlo AL, Ramakrishnan N, Hatchett RJ. Radiation combined injury: Overview of NIAID research. Health Physics. 2010;**98**:863-867. DOI: 10.1097/HP.0b013e3181a6ee32

[62] Sakhno L, Yurchenko O, Sidorenko A, Dvorshchenko O, Maslenny V, Korotich V, et al. Application of adsorptive carbon dressing accelerates skin regeneration after the non-full depth burn. The International Journal of Artificial Organs. 2014;**37**:642

[63] Muravskaya GV, Nikolaev VG, Sergeev VP, Krutilina NI, Bonatskaya LV, Klevtsov VN, et al. Enterosorption in Oncotherapy. Artificial Cells, Blood Substitutes, and Immobilization Biotechnology. 1991;**19**:167-174. DOI: 10.3109/10731199109117823

[64] Bonatskaya LV, Plotnikov VM, Nikolaev VG. Decrease of hematotoxicity of anticancer preparation upon enterosorption. Experimental Oncology. 1989;**23**(11):71-73. (In Russian)

[65] Sakhno LA, Yurchenko OV, Maslenniy VN, Bardakhivskaya KI, Nikolaeva VV, Ivanyuk AA, et al. Enterosorption as a method to decrease the systemic toxicity of cisplatin. Experimental Oncology. 2013;**35**:45-52

[66] Nikolaev VG, Andreychin MA, Bardakhivskaya KI, Sakhno LA, Kopcha VS, Yushko LA, et al. Practical Recommendations on the Use of Granulated Carbon Enterosorbents "Carboline". Kyiv: DIA; 2013

[67] Ponomarova OV, Pivnyuk VM, Nosko MM, Sakhno LO, Dekhtiar TV,

Nikolaev VG, et al. Prophylaxis by coal enterosorbent of acute and extended emethogenic toxicity of cancer patient chemotherapy. Oncology. 2008;**3**: 370-373. (In Ukrainian)

[68] Bonatskaya LV, Zinevich AK. Enterosorption as a method of prophylaxis and treatment of some complication of cancer chemotherapy. In: Proceedings of the Conference Sorption Methods for Detoxification and Immune System Correction. Kharkiv; 1982. p. 4

[69] Shevchuk OO, Posokhova KA, Todor IN, Lukianova NY, Nikolaev VG, Chekhun VF. Prevention of myelosuppression by combined treatment with enterosorbent and granulocyte colony-stimulating factor. Experimental Oncology. 2015;**37**:135-138

[70] Shevchuk OO, Bodnar YY, Bardakhivska KI, Datsko TV, Volska AS, Posokhova KA, et al. Enterosorption combined with granulocyte colony stimulating factor decreases melphalan gonadal toxicity. Experimental Oncology. 2016;**38**:172-175

[71] Shevchuk OO, Posokhova KA, Sidorenko AS, Bardakhivska KI, Maslenny VM, Yushko LA, et al. The influence of enterosorption on some haematological and biochemical indices of the normal rats after single injection of melphalan. Experimental Oncology. 2014;**36**:94-100

# 4

# Mucosal Macrophage Polarization Role in the Immune Modulation

*Tsung-Meng Wu, Shiu-Nan Chen and Yu-Sheng Wu*

## Abstract

Immunotherapy has advantages including few side effects and low probability of abuse by patients. Recently, functional materials with immunomodulatory functions, which act through reduction of free radicals, have been developed for cancer and anti-inflammatory therapy. However, the therapeutic application of natural functional materials involves a complex mechanism along with various organic factors. These substances, including polysaccharides and triterpenoids, have immunomodulatory effects. However, to our knowledge, the mechanism underlying the action of such substances in the physiological immunity of animals remains unclear. Immune cells, particularly macrophages, are crucial in the modulation of immune response. Macrophages polarise into two types, namely, M1 and M2, from the M0 form, based on the physiological microenvironment factors. M1 macrophages have functions in pathogen elimination through phagocytosis, oxidative damage, and complement system activation. M2 macrophages are involved in tissue recovery and tumour tissues containing ample M2 macrophages that release growth factors, which promote angiogenesis. In this study, we focus on the immunomodulation of the macrophage to further understand the effects of the physiological microenvironment factors on macrophage polarisation.

**Keywords:** macrophage, polarisation, immune modulation

## 1. Introduction: immune cells in the mucosal system

The mucosal system is ubiquitous throughout the body; the mucosal tissue is typically present in association with various organ systems, including the gastro-intestinal tract, respiratory tract, and genitourinary tract, as well as the exocrine glands associated with these systems, such as the pancreas, lacrimal glands, salivary glands, and breasts. According to their location and function, mucosal tissues can be divided into nasopharynx-associated lymphoid tissue (NALT) [1], bronchus-associated lymphoid tissue (BALT) [2], and gut-associated lymphoid tissue (GALT) [3]. The surface area of the mucosal system is very broad; its physiological functions include gas exchange, food absorption, and sensory function. The mucus on the mucosal surface acts as a protective barrier inside the body to protect the body from foreign pathogenic infections [4]. Because of the distribution of mucus over a large surface area, the probability of mucosal tissues coming in contact with pathogens is higher than that of other tissues in the body. Nevertheless, these tissues are responsible for the evasion of the pathogens. Adhesion molecules, expressed by tissues and organs, enable the binding of lymphocyte receptors that attract lymphocytes towards the mucosal surface.

GALT, the largest lymphoid organ in the human body, contains 70–80% of the lymphoid tissues of the human body. The main GALT components include lamina propria (LP), Peyer's patches (PP), and mesenteric lymph node (MLN).

A mucosal immune response involves various cells, particularly macrophages. Macrophages are present in almost all tissues and have distinct location-specific phenotypes; their gene expression profiles demonstrate considerable functional diversity in innate immune response, tissue development, and tissue homoeostasis [5, 6]. Resident macrophages in different organ tissues are named differently. For instance, microglia cells have pathogenetic significance regarding perivascular inflammatory phenomena in the brain [7, 8], Kupffer cells have a major role in the homoeostatic function of the liver and are associated with the tissue damage [9], and alveolar macrophages (AMs) are a key determinant of pulmonary immune responses and thus have a role in lung inflammation (e.g. asthma) [10]. Previously, tissue-resident macrophages were considered to be recruited from circulating blood monocytes. However, recent studies have demonstrated that tissue-resident macrophages, such as microglial, Kupffer, and Langerhans cells, are established prenatally; they arise independently from the haematopoietic transcription factor [11, 12], which is required for the development of haematopoietic stem cells (HSCs) and all $CD11b^{high}$ monocytes and macrophages, but is not required for yolk sac (YS) macrophages and for YS-derived $F4/80^{bright}$ macrophages in several tissues, which can all persist in adult mice independently of HSCs [12]. Kupffer cells and other resident macrophages (e.g. microglia) originate from the YS in a colony-stimulating factor-1 receptor (CSF-1R)-dependent and Myb-independent manner and may be maintained through local proliferation, resulting in extensive mitosis after stress or an exchanged tissue microenvironment [13, 14].

## 2. Phenomenon of macrophage and its importance in the immune response

Macrophages are primarily divided into two types based on function and differentiation: classically activated (M1) and alternatively activated (M2) macrophages (**Figure 1**). Both have roles in innate resistance and constitute a link between inflammation and autoimmune disease. In mouse models, macrophages contain CD11b, F4/80, and CSF-1R, where F4/80 is the surface protein for M1 and M2 macrophages [15, 16]; these are circulating monocytes (present in the peripheral blood), which are secreted in response to chemokines produced in response to exposure to an antigen (e.g. pathogens entering the organism from the portal vein of the intestines). When interacting with pattern recognition receptors, antigens may lead to M1- or M2-polarising activities, depending on the secreted Th1 cytokine [interferon (IFN)-γ], Th2 cytokines [interleukin (IL)-4 and IL-13], and other immune factors [17–19]. Macrophage is also role in the antigen presenting, to induce the B cell active and response to the antibody production. The antibody production is from the plasma cell (active B cell), where there is a molecule material expression on its surface. A part of these receptors is named B-cell receptors (BCRs).

B-cell receptor is a B-cell membrane-bound surface protein that acts as a cellular receptor. During B-cell differentiation, differentiated B cells, transferred as plasma cells, secrete immunoglobulins (Igs). Structurally, Igs are similar to the BCRs and are called antibodies [20].

The main functions of antibodies include neutralising the antigen, activating complement reaction, and participating in the adaptive immunity. An antibody comprises two heavy and two light chains, is Y shaped, and is divided into variable and constant regions. The variable region contains the antigen-binding sites [21],

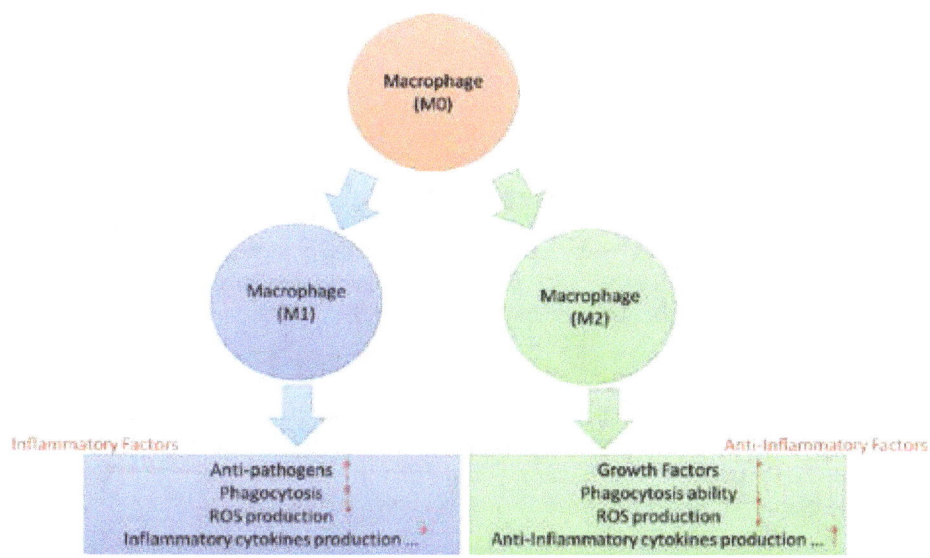

**Figure 1.**
*The inactive macrophage is differentiated into M1 or M2 macrophage by various stress and stimulants in the host microenvironment. M1 macrophage is participating in the inflammatory response, a major function in the pathogen clearance. M2 macrophage is in contrast to the M1 macrophage.*

and each antigen-binding site has three structures complementary to the antigen and a highly recognisable region that determines the antigen-antibody specificity, called the complementarity-determining region (CDR) [22]. By using different combinations of CDRs with heavy and light chains, B cells can be induced to produce various specific antibodies. The antibody immobilisation region has several major functions. First, these regions in different antibody types can bind to Fc receptors (FcRs) on different cells, such as FcRγ on phagocytic cells (e.g. neutrophils and macrophages) [23]. Similarly, the IgG-immobilised region binds to the antigen bound to the antibody; the FcRε on mast cells, neutrophils, and basophils can bind to the IgE-immobilised region [24], inducing the cell to perform a specific antigenic reaction with an inflammatory response modifier. Second, the FcR of the antigen-antibody complex binds to complement, triggering a complement chain reaction. IgG secreted by pregnant women is also transported to the abdomen through their blood flow [25]. Some lymphocytes are called innate-like lymphocytes (ILLs), and the mechanism by which B-1 cells secrete antibodies is different from that used by B cells [26].

## 2.1 B-1 cells

B-1 cells are called natural antibodies and include the IgG, IgA, and IgM isotypes [27, 28]. Natural antibodies are secreted when B-1 cells are not stimulated by foreign pathogens, which can bind to different pathogens but have low affinity.

## 2.2 Ig isotype switching (class switching)

B cells can express different C-region genes during cell maturation and proliferate during the reaction [29]. It simultaneously expresses IgM and IgD through RNA modification [30]. As the immune function continues to respond, antibodies in the same variant region can be expressed as IgG, IgA, and IgE. This process is called homotypic conversion or class switching, which protects all parts of the body at the appropriate time by using specific antibodies produced by the same antigen.

## 2.3 Ig isotype

According to the structural differences of the heavy chain, Igs are divided into five isotypes [25]:

i. IgG, a major Ig in the blood, exists in a monomeric form and thus easily spreads throughout the body through peripheral blood. For instance, in humans, IgG enters the foetus through the placenta, providing passive immunity to the foetus. IgG has a modulating function, which efficiently promotes the phagocytosis of pathogens [31].

ii. IgA, present in serum as a monomer, can diffuse outside blood vessels. In most of the body, IgA is present as a dimer, mainly in mucus and particularly the intestinal and respiratory mucosa. The main function of IgA is antigen neutralisation [32]. Transforming growth factor (TGF)-β and IL-4 can effectively promote IgA isotype switching [33].

iii. IgM is mainly distributed in the blood and less in the lymph. IgM is effective in activating the complement system and is important for controlling infection [34].

iv. IgE is the immunoglobulin that the body mainly produces when the allergens invade. IgE is relatively low in blood and body fluids and strongly binds to the Fc receptors of the mast cells under the blood vessels, submucosa, and connective tissue [35].

v. IgD is the least among other types of immunoglobulins in the body, and there is no clear biological function discovery [36].

Class switching is mainly caused through the influence of cytokines or antigen secretion, which stimulates B cells to express different Igs. For instance, IL-4, IL-5, IL-10, and TGF, present in GALT, enable B cells to secrete IgA after isotype switching [37, 38]. When B cells isolated from mice were exposed to TGF-β in an in vitro culture, the proportion of IgA secreted by the TGF-β-treated B cells was significantly higher than that secreted by the untreated cells [33]. Through homologous switching, B cells secrete antibodies specific for an antigen and supply it to the appropriate body part in a timely manner. The vertebrate intestinal mucosal immune system secretes a large amount of secretory IgA (sIgA) [39]. In mucus, the proportion of sIgA is higher than that of other antibody isotypes. sIgA mainly neutralises pathogens and limits the entry of pathogens into the body. Mcghee et al. found that coculture of B cells of PP with either IL-5 or IL-6 can promote the differentiation of B cells into IgA-secreting plasma cells [40]. Plasma cells release intact J chain-linked IgA dimers, which bind to the endothelial Ig receptors expressed by intestinal epithelial cells and undergo transcytosis [41]. Piskurich et al. cocultured human colonic cell line (HT-29) with IFN-γ and found that IFN-γ stimulated the expression of the poly-Ig receptor gene in a concentration-dependent manner, as detected through immunofluorescence [42]. In other words, IFN-γ can stimulate the expression of poly-Ig receptors. In mice with poly-Ig receptor gene deficiency, IgA expression in serum is significantly higher than that in normal mice, whereas sIgA expression in the mucosal sites is significantly lower than that in normal mice; taken together, poly-Ig receptor gene defects cause IgA to accumulate in the serum of mice. Thus, poly-Ig receptors are crucial for sIgA expression in the mucosal sites [43–45].

## 3. Immunomodulation in the mucosal system

In the mucosal system, the immune response is an important reaction regulating the physiological homoeostasis, including immunomodulation, in the whole body. The major mucosal systems controlling the immune response are as follows:

### 3.1 LP of the intestinal mucosa

The LP of the intestinal mucosa is located below the intestinal epithelial cells and includes various cell types, including Ig-derived plasma cells, T cells, dendritic cells, macrophages, and various cytokines [46]. Under normal conditions, the LP of the intestinal mucosa exhibits high levels of TGF-β [47] and IL-10 [48], which promotes antigen-activated B-cell isoforms. The pathogen enters the LP of the intestinal mucosa from the intestines. The pathogen is recognised by the immune system, and it stimulates B cells to undergo isotype switching to secrete IgA, IgG, and IgM. In a study, rats were administered inactivated *Entamoeba histolytica* through feeding, and IgA, IgG, and IgM were detected in serum and faeces on postfeeding days 2, 4, 6, 8, and 10. IgG and IgM expression in rat serum increased, and IgG and IgA expression in faeces also increased [49].

### 3.2 PP

PP, located below intestinal epithelial cells, is also the induction sites of the intestinal mucosal immune response [50] and has a high number of B and T cells compared with other lymph nodes [51]. PP contains numerous cytokines, including TGF-β, IL-4, IL-6, and IL-10, which stimulate B cells to secrete Igs [52, 53]. The upper part of PP includes specialised epithelial cells called microfold (M) cells [54]. The antigen in the intestine can enter the lymphoid tissue of the subsequent layer through M cells and initiate an immune reaction. However, the proportion of M cells in the intestine is not high; thus, the ability of M cells to deliver antigens is limited [55]. PP is an indispensable immunotolerance-related tissue, particularly in mice [56].

### 3.3 MLN

Lymph nodes are tissues located at the junction of the lymphatic system and higher organs [57]. The vast lymphatic vasculature collects lymph from tissues and returns it to the blood. MLNs are the lymph nodes in the intestinal mucosal immune system [58]. When an antigen enters the body through the intestinal mucosal system, it encounters the lymphatic system and is recognised; the antigen-presenting cells are then activated. These cells carry the antigen to the MLN, perform the antigen presentation reaction, and finally activate appropriate T and B cells [59–61].

### 3.4 Relationship between intestinal immune response and Igs

GALT macrophages have different characteristics from macrophages in other parts of the body; that is, they have good phagocytic and bactericidal abilities [62]. CD4$^+$FOXP3$^+$ regulatory T ($T_{Reg}$) cells are located in the regulatory layer of the intestinal mucosa. T cells differentiate into $T_{Reg}$ cells in the presence of TGF-β. The balance between functional T and $T_{Reg}$ cells highly affects the homoeostasis of intestinal mucosal immune response [63].

## 4. Immunomodulation of macrophages in the immune system

Polysaccharides extracted from mushrooms or algae have immunomodulatory functions, such as increasing macrophage activity, regardless of whether innate or adaptive immunity is activated [64]. For instance, the phagocytic activity of cells, the killing ability of natural killer cells, and the promotion of immune cells to secrete cytokines activate the immune system. In our previous laboratory studies, mushroom polysaccharide administration could enhance the tumour-suppressive and antiallergic ability in mice, along with significant enhancement in the wound-healing ability in rats. Immune cells of the innate immune response, such as macrophages and dendritic cells, or other nonimmune cells, such as epithelial cells, have many nonspecific recognition receptors associated with antigens that evade pathogens. Based on molecular identification and binding, complement receptor type 3 (CR3) on these cells can identify polysaccharides [65]. When polysaccharides bind to CR3, it triggers a series of signalling to activate transcription factors. Cells secrete a cytokine that triggers an inflammatory response, and the antigen exhibits the major histocompatibility complex of the cell, thereby activating other immune cells to achieve immunomodulatory functions [66, 67]. Dectin-1 belongs to the c-type lectin receptor family and is expressed on the cell membranes of macrophages, dendritic cells, neutrophils, and T and B cells [68]. Dectin-1 binds to polysaccharides to promote macrophage phagocytosis and respiratory burst; it also promotes the degranulation of neutrophils and secretion of cytokines and chemokines from immune cells [69–72]. Polysaccharides from *Antrodia camphorata* were cocultured with immature dendritic and T cells isolated from healthy human blood, and the polysaccharides could promote dendritic cell maturation and stimulate T-cell proliferation and IFN-γ performance [73, 74]. Coculture of polysaccharides with macrophages can promote the secretion of immune-related factors and cytokine gene expression, such as nitric oxide (NO), tumour necrosis factor (TNF)-α, IL-1β, and IL-6, to promote macrophage activity [75–78].

Based on our teams' experimental results, the functional polysaccharide can stimulate macrophages and further activate cytokines TNF-α, IL-12, IFN-γ, IL-2, IL-4, IL-10, and IL-17, which are associated with apoptosis and cell cycle. Growth hormone, a multipeptide hormone regulator, promotes growth and cell proliferation [75, 78, 79]. Polysaccharides can reduce $CCl_4$-induced liver damage by regulating related antioxidant enzymes and effectively reducing oxidative damage in liver tissue[80, 81]. In mice, intraperitoneal polysaccharide injection could effectively prevent lipid peroxidation and inhibit the production of reactive oxygen species in the liver [82, 83]. Taken together, the immunomodulation function of polysaccharides may effectively regulate cellular immune response [84].

## 5. Immunomodulation of macrophage differentiation

Immune cells are crucial in immune response modulation. As mentioned, macrophages polarise into M1 and M2 macrophages, which have distinct functions and are affected by the physiological microenvironment factors. M1 macrophages perform pathogen elimination through phagocytosis, inflict oxidative damage, and complement system activation. M2 macrophages have tissue recovery functions. Tumour tissues contain considerable amounts of M2 macrophages that release angiogenesis-promoting growth factors.

Inflammatory reactions can induce chronic diseases; thus, reducing inflammation is important for inhibiting chronic disease. To achieve anti-inflammatory effects, immunotherapy is a novel therapeutic approach without known side effects and drug resistance problems. However, anti-inflammatory processes involve complex reactions; for instance, cellular ROS production for eliminating pathogens can also induce cellular apoptosis [85, 86]. Thus, the balance between inflammatory and anti-inflammatory processes is essential. In case of any imbalance, natural functional materials, such as triterpenoids and polysaccharides, can be applied for immunomodulation.

In summary, polysaccharides can regulate macrophage differentiation to modulate host physiological response through cytokine secretion. Polysaccharides, such as beta-glucan, are known biological response modifiers that can activate leukocytes, monocytes, and macrophages [87, 88]. The activation mechanism involves the polysaccharides binding to the receptors, such as Toll-like receptor, expressed on AMs or Kupffer, Langerhans, mesangial, or microglial cells. After the binding, the immune cells are activated via Toll-like receptor four-mediated signalling pathways to modulate the immune capacity. The activated immune cells then produce IFN-$\gamma$, TNF-$\alpha$, ILs, and other cytokines to modulate the anti-inflammatory process.

In conclusion, the use of the functional materials as alternative medicines in clinical therapy is feasible; however, before implementation, the substance's immunomodulatory mechanism should be clearly realised, particularly in the immune cell signal transduction.

## Acknowledgements

This project was supported by the Ministry of Science and Technology, Taiwan (MOST. 107-2313-B-020-004).

## Author details

Tsung-Meng Wu[1], Shiu-Nan Chen[2] and Yu-Sheng Wu[1]*

1 Department of Aquaculture, National Pingtung University of Science and Technology, Pingtung, Taiwan

2 Department of Life Science, National Taiwan University, Taipei, Taiwan

*Address all correspondence to: wuys0313@mail.npust.edu.tw

# References

[1] Mutoh M, Kimura S, Takahashi-Iwanaga H, Hisamoto M, Iwanaga T, Iida J. RANKL regulates differentiation of microfold cells in mouse nasopharynx-associated lymphoid tissue (NALT). Cell and Tissue Research. 2016;**364**(1):175-184

[2] Hwang JY, Randall TD, Silva-Sanchez A. Inducible bronchus-associated lymphoid tissue: Taming inflammation in the lung. Frontiers in Immunology. 2016;**7**:258

[3] Stanisavljević S, Lukić J, Momčilović M, Miljković M, Jevtić B, Kojić M, et al. Gut-associated lymphoid tissue, gut microbes and susceptibility to experimental autoimmune encephalomyelitis. Beneficial Microbes. 2016;**7**(3):363-373

[4] Peterson LW, Artis D. Intestinal epithelial cells: Regulators of barrier function and immune homeostasis. Nature Reviews Immunology. 2014;**14**(3):141

[5] Wu YS, Ho SY, Nan FH, Chen SN. Ganoderma lucidum beta 1, 3/1, 6 glucan as an immunomodulator in inflammation induced by a high-cholesterol diet. BMC Complementary and Alternative Medicine. 2016;**16**(1):500

[6] Haldar M, Murphy KM. Origin, development, and homeostasis of tissue-resident macrophages. Immunological Reviews. 2014;**262**(1):25-35

[7] Silva-Gomes S, Decout A, Nigou J. Pathogen-associated molecular patterns (PAMPs). Compendium of Inflammatory Diseases. 2016. pp. 1055-1069

[8] Hong S, Beja-Glasser VF, Nfonoyim BM, Frouin A, Li S, Ramakrishnan S, et al. Complement and microglia mediate early synapse loss in Alzheimer mouse models. Science. 2016;**352**(6286):712-716

[9] Sica A, Invernizzi P, Mantovani A. Macrophage plasticity and polarization in liver homeostasis and pathology. Hepatology. 2014;**59**(5):2034-2042

[10] Byrne AJ, Mathie SA, Gregory LG, Lloyd CM. Pulmonary macrophages: Key players in the innate defence of the airways. Thorax. 2015;**70**(12):1189-1196

[11] Palis J. Hematopoietic stem cell-independent hematopoiesis: Emergence of erythroid, megakaryocyte, and myeloid potential in the mammalian embryo. FEBS Letters. 2016;**590**(22):3965-3974

[12] Schulz C, Perdiguero EG, Chorro L, Szabo-Rogers H, Cagnard N, Kierdorf K, et al. A lineage of myeloid cells independent of Myb and hematopoietic stem cells. Science. 2012;**336**(6077):86-90

[13] Widmann JJ, Fahimi HD. Proliferation of mononuclear phagocytes (Kupffer cells) and endothelial cells in regenerating rat liver. A light and electron microscopic cytochemical study. The American Journal of Pathology. 1975;**80**(3):349

[14] Li P, He K, Li J, Liu Z, Gong J. The role of Kupffer cells in hepatic diseases. Molecular Immunology. 2017;**85**:222-229

[15] Hambardzumyan D, Gutmann DH, Kettenmann H. The role of microglia and macrophages in glioma maintenance and progression. Molecular Immunology. 2016;**19**(1):20

[16] Prinz M, Priller J. Microglia and brain macrophages in the molecular age: From origin to neuropsychiatric disease. Nature Reviews Neuroscience. 2014;**15**(5):300

[17] Thirunavukkarasu S, de Silva K, Plain KM, Whittington J. Role of host-and pathogen-associated lipids in directing the immune response in mycobacterial infections, with emphasis on Mycobacterium avium subsp paratuberculosis. Critical Reviews in Microbiology. 2016;**42**(2):262-275

[18] Zhou T, Hu Z, Yang S, Sun L, Yu Z, Wang G. Role of adaptive and innate immunity in type 2 diabetes mellitus. Journal Diabetes Research. 2018;**2018**:7457269. DOI: 10.1155/2018/7457269

[19] Franca RF, Costa RS, Silva JR, Peres RS, Mendonça LR, Colón DF, et al. IL-33 signaling is essential to attenuate viral-induced encephalitis development by downregulating iNOS expression in the central nervous system. Journal of Neuroinflammation. 2016;**13**(1):159

[20] Kurosaki T, Kometani K, Ise W. Memory B cells. Nature Reviews Immunology. 2015;**15**(3):149

[21] Murphy K, Weaver C. Janeway's Immunobiology. 9th ed. New York: Garland Science; 2016

[22] Bowen A, Casadevall A. The role of the constant region in antibody-antigen interactions: Redefining the modular model of immunoglobulin structure. In: Structural Biology in Immunology. Elsevier; 2017. pp. 145-170

[23] Delves PJ, Martin SJ, Burton DR, Roitt IM. Essential Immunology. 13th ed. Hoboken: John Wiley & Sons; 2017

[24] Pober JS, Kluger MS, Schechner JS. Human endothelial cell presentation of antigen and the homing of memory/effector T cells to skin. Annals of the New York Academy of Sciences. 2001;**941**:12-25

[25] Adler R. Janeway's immunobiology. Choice: Current Reviews for Academic Libraries. 2008;**45**(10):1793-1794

[26] Iwasaki A, Medzhitov R. Control of adaptive immunity by the innate immune system. Nature Immunology. 2015;**16**(4):343-353

[27] Stall AM, Wells SM, Lam KP. B-1 cells: Unique origins and functions. Seminars in Immunology. 1996;**8**(1):45-59

[28] Jankovic M, Casellas R, Yannoutsos N, Wardemann H, Nussenzweig MC. RAGs and regulation of autoantibodies. Annual Review of Immunology. 2004;**22**:485-501

[29] Zhang Y, Fear DJ, Willis-Owen SA, Cookson WO, Moffatt MF. Global gene regulation during activation of immunoglobulin class switching in human B cells. Scientific Reports. 2016;**6**:37988

[30] Maki R, Roeder W, Traunecker A, Sidman C, Wabl M, Raschke W, et al. The role of DNA rearrangement and alternative RNA processing in the expression of immunoglobulin delta genes. Cell. 1981;**24**(2):353-365

[31] Von Stebut E. Immunology of cutaneous leishmaniasis: The role of mast cells, phagocytes and dendritic cells for protective immunity. European Journal of Dermatology. 2007;**17**(2):115-122

[32] Pabst O. New concepts in the generation and functions of IgA. Nature Reviews Immunology. 2012;**12**(12):821-832

[33] Li MO, Wan YY, Sanjabi S, Robertson AK, Flavell RA. Transforming growth factor-beta regulation of immune responses. Annual Review of Immunology. 2006;**24**:99-146

[34] Janeway CA Jr. A trip through my life with an immunological theme. Annual Review of Immunology. 2002;**20**:1-28

[35] Gould HJ, Sutton BJ. IgE in allergy and asthma today. Nature Reviews Immunology. 2008;**8**(3):205-217

[36] Girschick HJ, Grammer AC, Nanki T, Vazquez E, Lipsky PE. Expression of recombination activating genes 1 and 2 in peripheral B cells of patients with systemic lupus erythematosus. Arthritis & Rheumatology. 2002;**46**(5):1255-1263

[37] Lamkhioued B, Gounni AS, Aldebert D, Delaporte E, Prin L, Capron A, et al. Synthesis of type 1 (IFN gamma) and type 2 (IL-4, IL-5, and IL-10) cytokines by human eosinophils. Annals of the New York Academy of Sciences. 1996;**796**:203-208

[38] Moqbel R. Synthesis and storage of regulatory cytokines in human eosinophils. Advances in Experimental Medicine and Biology. 1996;**409**:287-294

[39] Tlaskalova-Hogenova H, Stepankova R, Hudcovic T, Tuckova L, Cukrowska B, Lodinova-Zadnikova R, et al. Commensal bacteria (normal microflora), mucosal immunity and chronic inflammatory and autoimmune diseases. Immunology Letters. 2004;**93**(2-3):97-108

[40] Beagley KW, Eldridge JH, Kiyono H, Everson MP, Koopman WJ, Honjo T, et al. Recombinant murine IL-5 induces high rate IgA synthesis in cycling IgA-positive Peyer's patch B cells. The Journal of Immunology. 1988;**141**(6):2035-2042

[41] Chorny A, Puga I, Cerutti A. Innate signaling networks in mucosal IgA class switching. Advances in Immunology. 2010;**107**:31-69

[42] Piskurich JF, France JA, Tamer CM, Willmer CA, Kaetzel CS, Kaetzel DM. Interferon-gamma induces polymeric immunoglobulin receptor mRNA in human intestinal epithelial cells by a protein synthesis dependent mechanism. Molecular Immunology. 1993;**30**(4):413-421

[43] Lee CH, Romain G, Yan W, Watanabe M, Charab W, Todorova B, et al. Corrigendum: IgG fc domains that bind C1q but not effector Fcgamma receptors delineate the importance of complement-mediated effector functions. Nature Immunology. 2017;**18**(10):1173

[44] Mihai S, Nimmerjahn F. The role of Fc receptors and complement in autoimmunity. Autoimmunity Reviews. 2013;**12**(6):657-660

[45] Lycke NY, Bemark M. The regulation of gut mucosal IgA B-cell responses: Recent developments. Mucosal Immunology. 2017;**10**(6):1361-1374

[46] Vicente-Suarez I, Larange A, Reardon C, Matho M, Feau S, Chodaczek G, et al. Unique lamina propria stromal cells imprint the functional phenotype of mucosal dendritic cells. Mucosal Immunology. 2015;**8**(1):141-511

[47] Chen HH, Sun AH, Ojcius DM, Hu WL, Ge YM, Lin X, et al. Eosinophils from murine lamina propria induce differentiation of naive T cells into regulatory T cells via TGF-beta1 and retinoic acid. PLoS One. 2015;**10**(11):e0142881

[48] Wenzel U, Turner JE, Krebs C, Kurts C, Harrison DG, Ehmke H. Immune mechanisms in arterial hypertension. Journal of the American Society of Nephrology. 2016;**27**(3):677-686

[49] Navarro-Garcia F, Pedroso M, Lopez-Revilla R. Immunodulation of rat serum and mucosal antibody responses to entamoeba histolytica trophozoites by beta-1,3-glucan and cholera toxin. Clinical Immunology. 2000;**97**(2):182-188

[50] Cheng X, Ming X, Croyle MA. PEGylated adenoviruses for gene delivery to the intestinal epithelium by the oral route. Pharmaceutical Research. 2003;**20**(9):1444-1451

[51] Klose CSN, Artis D. Innate lymphoid cells as regulators of immunity, inflammation and tissue homeostasis. Nature Immunology. 2016;**17**(7):765-774

[52] Sewell WA, Jolles S. Immunomodulatory action of intravenous immunoglobulin. Immunology. 2002;**107**(4):387-393

[53] Vassilev T, Kazatchkine MD. Mechanisms of immunomodulatory action of intravenous immunoglobulin in autoimmune and systemic inflammatory diseases. Therapeutic Apheresis and Dialysis. 1997;**1**(1):38-41

[54] Roberts CL, Keita AV, Duncan SH, O'Kennedy N, Soderholm JD, Rhodes JM, et al. Translocation of Crohn's disease *Escherichia coli* across M-cells: Contrasting effects of soluble plant fibres and emulsifiers. Gut. 2010;**59**(10):1331-1339

[55] Bron PA, van Baarlen P, Kleerebezem M. Emerging molecular insights into the interaction between probiotics and the host intestinal mucosa. Nature Reviews Microbiology. 2012;**10**(1):66-90

[56] Snyder M, Turrentine JE, Cruz PD Jr. Photocontact dermatitis and its clinical mimics: An overview for the allergist. Clinical Reviews in Allergy and Immunology. 2019;**56**(1):32-40

[57] Bernier-Latmani J, Petrova TV. Intestinal lymphatic vasculature: Structure, mechanisms and functions. Nature Reviews. Gastroenterology & Hepatology. 2017;**14**(9):510-526

[58] Masopust D, Vezys V, Marzo AL, Lefrancois L. Preferential localization of effector memory cells in nonlymphoid tissue. Science. 2001;**291**(5512):2413-2417

[59] Masopust D, Vezys V, Marzo AL, Lefrancois L. Pillars article: Preferential localization of effector memory cells in nonlymphoid tissue. The Journal of Immunology. 2014;**192**(3):845-849

[60] Hodge LM, Bearden MK, Schander A, Huff JB, Williams A Jr, King HH, et al. Lymphatic pump treatment mobilizes leukocytes from the gut associated lymphoid tissue into lymph. Lymphatic Research and Biology. 2010;**8**(2):103-110

[61] Macpherson AJ, Smith K. Mesenteric lymph nodes at the center of immune anatomy. The Journal of Experimental Medicine. 2006;**203**(3):497-500

[62] Platt AM, Mowat AM. Mucosal macrophages and the regulation of immune responses in the intestine. Immunology Letters. 2008;**119**(1-2):22-31

[63] Barnes MJ, Powrie F. Regulatory T cells reinforce intestinal homeostasis. Immunity. 2009;**31**(3):401-411

[64] Kang S, Min H. Ginseng, the 'Immunity Boost': The effects of Panax ginseng on immune system. Journal of Ginseng Research. 2012;**36**(4):354-368

[65] Thornton BP, Vetvicka V, Pitman M, Goldman RC, Ross GD. Analysis of the sugar specificity and molecular location of the beta-glucan-binding lectin site of complement receptor type 3 (CD11b/CD18). The Journal of Immunology. 1996;**156**(3):1235-1246

[66] Frostegard J, Ulfgren AK, Nyberg P, Hedin U, Swedenborg J, Andersson U, et al. Cytokine expression in advanced human atherosclerotic plaques: Dominance of pro-inflammatory (Th1) and macrophage-stimulating cytokines. Atherosclerosis. 1999;**145**(1):33-43

[67] Li X, Xu W, Chen J. Polysaccharide purified from *Polyporus umbellatus* (per) Fr induces the activation and maturation of murine bone-derived dendritic cells via toll-like receptor 4. Cellular Immunology. 2010;**265**(1):50-56

[68] Robinson MJ, Sancho D, Slack EC, LeibundGut-Landmann S, Reis e Sousa C. Myeloid C-type lectins in innate immunity. Nature Immunology. 2006;7(12):1258-1265

[69] Brown GD. Dectin-1: A signalling non-TLR pattern-recognition receptor. Nature Reviews. Immunology. 2006;6(1):33-43

[70] Brown GD, Herre J, Williams DL, Willment JA, Marshall AS, Gordon S. Dectin-1 mediates the biological effects of beta-glucans. The Journal of Experimental Medicine. 2003;197(9):1119-1124

[71] Li X, Utomo A, Cullere X, Choi MM, Milner DA Jr, Venkatesh D, et al. The beta-glucan receptor Dectin-1 activates the integrin mac-1 in neutrophils via Vav protein signaling to promote *Candida albicans* clearance. Cell Host & Microbe. 2011;10(6):603-615

[72] Tsoni SV, Brown GD. Beta-glucans and dectin-1. Annals of the New York Academy of Sciences. 2008;1143:45-60

[73] Liu KJ, Leu SJ, Su CH, Chiang BL, Chen YL, Lee YL. Administration of polysaccharides from Antrodia camphorata modulates dendritic cell function and alleviates allergen-induced T helper type 2 responses in a mouse model of asthma. Immunology. 2010;129(3):351-362

[74] Lu MC, Hwang SL, Chang FR, Chen YH, Chang TT, Hung CS, et al. Immunostimulatory effect of Antrodia camphorata extract on functional maturation of dendritic cells. Food Chemistry. 2009;113(4):1049-1057

[75] Ferreira SS, Passos CP, Madureira P, Vilanova M, Coimbra MA. Structure-function relationships of immunostimulatory polysaccharides: A review. Carbohydrate Polymers. 2015;132:378-396

[76] Ferreira SS, Passos CP, Madureira P, Vilanova M, Coimbra MA. Structure-function relationships of immunostimulatory polysaccharides: A review. Carbohydrate Polymers. 2016;147:557-558

[77] Liu JY, Yang FL, Lu CP, Yang YL, Wen CL, Hua KF, et al. Polysaccharides from Dioscorea batatas induce tumor necrosis factor-alpha secretion via toll-like receptor 4-mediated protein kinase signaling pathways. Journal of Agricultural and Food Chemistry. 2008;56(21):9892-9898

[78] Stout RD, Suttles J. Functional plasticity of macrophages: Reversible adaptation to changing microenvironments. Journal of Leukocyte Biology. 2004;76(3):509-513

[79] Habijanic J, Berovic M, Boh B, Plankl M, Wraber B. Submerged cultivation of Ganoderma lucidum and the effects of its polysaccharides on the production of human cytokines TNF-alpha, IL-12, IFN-gamma, IL-2, IL-4, IL-10 and IL-17. New Biotechnology. 2015;32(1):85-95

[80] Hamid M, Liu D, Abdulrahim Y, Liu Y, Qian G, Khan A, et al. Amelioration of CCl4-induced liver injury in rats by selenizing Astragalus polysaccharides: Role of proinflammatory cytokines, oxidative stress and hepatic stellate cells. Research in Veterinary Science. 2017;114:202-211

[81] Li S, Tan HY, Wang N, Zhang ZJ, Lao L, Wong CW, et al. The role of oxidative stress and antioxidants in liver diseases. International Journal of Molecular Sciences. 2015;16(11):26087-26124

[82] Han B, Gao Y, Wang Y, Wang L, Shang Z, Wang S, et al. Protective effect of a polysaccharide from rhizoma atractylodis macrocephalae on acute liver injury in mice. International

Journal of Biological Macromolecules. 2016;**87**:85-91

[83] Zhou J, Yan J, Bai Z, Li K, Huang K. Hypoglycemic activity and potential mechanism of a polysaccharide from the loach in streptozotocin-induced diabetic mice. Carbohydrate Polymers. 2015;**121**:199-206

[84] Zhao ZK, Yu HL, Liu B, Wang H, Luo Q , Ding XG. Antioxidative mechanism of *Lycium barbarum* polysaccharides promotes repair and regeneration following cavernous nerve injury. Neural Regeneration Research. 2016;**11**(8):1312-1321

[85] Wu YS, Huang SL, Nan FH, Chang CS, Hsiao CM, Lai KC, et al. Over-inhibition of NADPH oxidase reduce the wound healing in liver of finfish. Fish & Shellfish Immunology. 2014;**40**(1):174-181

[86] Wu YS, Nan FH, Huang SL, Hsiao CM, Lai KC, Lu CL, et al. Studies of macrophage cellular response to the extracellular hydrogen peroxide by tilapia model. Fish & Shellfish Immunology. 2014;**36**(2):459-466

[87] Hsiao CM, Wu YS, Nan FH, Huang SL, Chen L, Chen SN. Immunomodulator 'mushroom beta glucan' induces Wnt/ catenin signalling and improves wound recovery in tilapia and rat skin: A histopathological study. International Wound Journal. 2016;**13**(6):1116-1128

[88] Wang WJ, Wu YS, Chen S, Liu CF, Chen SN. Mushroom beta-glucan may immunomodulate the tumor-associated macrophages in the Lewis lung carcinoma. BioMed Research International. 2015. DOI: 10.1155/2015/604385

# 5

# Assessment of Immune Reconstitution Following Hematopoietic Stem Cell Transplantation

*Meenakshi Singh, Selma Z. D'Silva and Abhishweta Saxena*

## Abstract

Allogeneic hematopoietic stem cell transplantation (allo-HSCT) is a potential curative treatment for both congenital and hematological malignancies. Immune reconstitution after allogeneic hematopoietic stem cell transplantation is implicated in successful transplant outcomes such as overall survival and relapse-free survival. The reconstitution of immune cell subsets after HSCT occurs in different phases at different time points encompassing pre-engraftment, engraftment, and post-engraftment. The recovery of innate cellular immunity with the appearance of monocytes, dendritic cells, and natural killer cells in peripheral blood correlates with initiation of cellular engraftment. The cellular adaptive immunity is characterized by both thymic-independent expansion of T cells infused with graft and thymus-dependent expansion of naïve T cells derived from donor stem cells. The humoral immunity consists of B-cell reconstitution, which consists primarily of transitional and naïve subsets with the recovery of memory B cells that occur much later. In this review, we highlight the factors affecting immune reconstitution, the reconstitution of innate and adaptive immunity, techniques to assess immune reconstitution, and ways to enhance it.

**Keywords:** immune reconstitution, hematopoietic stem cell transplantation, innate immunity, adaptive immunity

## 1. Introduction

Hematopoietic stem cell transplantation (HSCT) is a choice of treatment for thousands of leukemic patients. The main outcome expected from HSCT is the life-time engraftment of the donor graft. The preferred donor is a HLA matched-related donor; however, this is available in about 25% of the patients. Other options such as matched unrelated, matched cord blood units, and haploidentical-related donor also do exist. The success of HSCT is marred by conditions such as graft-versus-host disease (GvHD), relapse, treatment-related toxicity, and infection, which lead to higher morbidity and mortality [1]. The effectiveness of HSCT is dependent on the immune reconstitution in the host, which is linked to the number of active T and NK cells present in the graft. Delayed immune reconstitution results in unfavorable transplant outcomes; hence, faster immune reconstitution of donor origin is required for long-term survival of patients.

Soon after HSCT using myeloablative conditioning, the patient experiences a period of pancytopenia. It takes several months or years for immune reconstitution and for patients to regain immunocompetence after transplant. The immune cells start re-appearing in the following order: neutrophils (0.5 months), monocytes (1 month), NK cells (1 month), T cells (2 months), and B cells (3 months); however, the normal levels are reached much later (**Figure 1**) [2].

There are various factors affecting immune reconstitution after transplant such as

1. thymic damage (age-related or pre-transplant conditioning regimens)

2. source of stem cells

3. HLA disparity between donor and host

4. post-transplant immune suppressant

5. occurrence of graft-versus-host disease.

Age or pre transplant chemotherapy or radiation leads to thymic damage. The severity of the damage caused to the thymus depends on the dose of the drugs used and also on the age of the patients, which in turn affect the immune recovery. In younger patients (<18 years), there is faster thymic regeneration after chemotherapy than older patients [3]. The age of the donor also affects the engraftment and reconstitution potential of hematopoietic stem cells as shown in mouse models [4]. Moreover, the thymic recovery is faster and is associated with faster T-cell reconstitution and recovery of normal T-cell repertoire in autologous (9 months) than allo-HSCT (12 months) [5]. This delayed thymic-dependent immune reconstitution is further reduced by the occurrence of aGvHD after allogeneic HSCT [6, 7].

The source of stem cells used as graft could be either bone marrow, peripheral blood, or cord blood. Source of stem cells used predicts the rate of immune reconstitution. It has been observed that platelet (20 × 109/L) reconstitution is faster in peripheral blood (11–18 days) than bone marrow (17–25 days) HSCT. Similarly, neutrophil (>0.5 × 109/L) reconstitution is also faster in peripheral blood (12–19 days) than bone marrow (15–23 days) HSCT. This is because of the presence

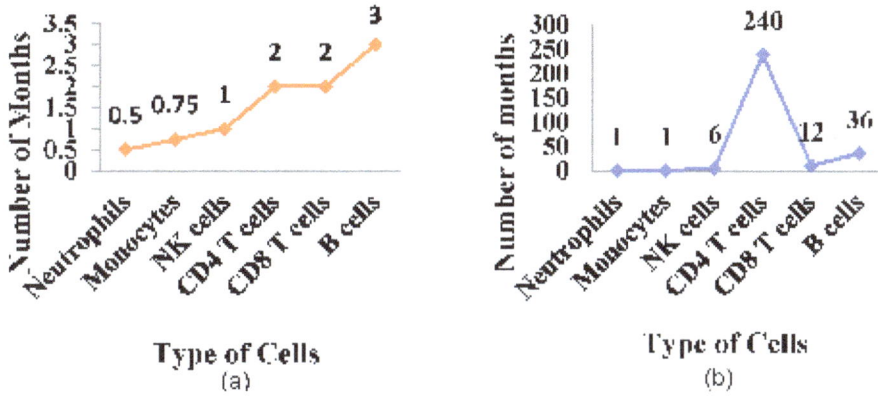

**Figure 1.**
*The time taken for different immune subsets to (A) reappear in circulation and (B) reach normal levels after hematopoietic stem cell transplantation.*

of long-term HSCs and more committed multipotent progenitors in the peripheral blood than bone marrow [8]. Further as compared to transplantation using in vivo or ex vivo T-cell depleted graft, faster immune reconstitution is seen in unmodified graft transplantation [9]. Using peripheral blood graft, faster reconstitution of CMV-specific cytotoxic T cells and CD4+ T cells is observed than stem cells from bone marrow source [10, 11]. The advantages of using umbilical cord blood units are its ready availability and its ability to cross the HLA barrier. The rates of engraftment and post-transplant outcomes are dependent on the number of total nucleated cells (TNCs) and CD34+ cell dose present in the graft source. Martin et al. [12] previously reported high TNC dose in association with positive transplant outcomes such as improved overall survival (OS), lower relapse rate (RR), and increased risk of chronic GvHD. Since there is a higher number of TNCs in the bone marrow and peripheral blood, there is faster engraftment (~14–21 days) after HSCT using this source of graft than umbilical cord blood source (~30 days) [13, 14]. Remberger et al. [15] reported faster engraftment but poor survival and higher relapse after HSCT using high CD34+ cell dose peripheral blood as graft source. Various researchers have reported immune cell reconstitution using different cell sources (**Table 1**).

Graft manipulations such as T-cell depletion (TCD) have resulted in lower chances of GvHD and graft rejection in unrelated and HLA mismatched transplants. However, T-cell depletion results in delayed immune reconstitution and increased morbidity and mortality due to infection [19–21]. An advantage of using T-cell depletion is that in case of malignancies it also leads to better GVL effect depending on the malignant disease being treated. For example, in CML, TCD is related to increased relapse rate [22], whereas in AML and AML cohorts, lower rate of relapse has been observed in TCD transplantation [23–25].

The degree of HLA mismatch is an important factor in immune reconstitution. It has been observed that the outcomes from matched unrelated transplantation are at par with that of matched related transplantation [1]. Chang et al. reported similar reconstitution of T-cell subsets, except for CD4+ cells and CD4+ naïve T cells, in haploidentical and HLA-matched transplantation [16]. Various researchers have reported reconstitution of immune cells following different transplant strategies. It has been observed that the immune reconstitution is best in matched sibling related followed by matched unrelated donor, haploidentical donor, T-cell replete, and T-cell depleted transplants.

Conditioning regimens deplete host immune system, eliminate the leukemic cells, and create space for engraftment of the donor cells. Although this eliminates the patient's leukemic cells, it also reduces the alloreactivity between host and donor cells after HSCT and further results in severe depletion of all immune cells. The use of drugs such as ATG or alemtuzumab depletes the host T cells further and results in

| Cells/L type of transplant | NK cells 1 month | CD4+ T cells 90 days | CD8+ T cells 90 days | B cells 90 days | Reference |
|---|---|---|---|---|---|
| Matched sibling donor | — | 220 | 645 | 33 | [16] |
| Matched unrelated donor | 253 | 198 | 447 | 43 | [17] |
| Haploidentical donor | — | 152 | 672 | 23 | [16] |
| T-cell depleted | 357 | 7 | 7 | 55 | [18] |
| T-cell replete | 183 | 127 | 181 | 64 | [18] |

**Table 1.**
*Reconstitution of various immune subsets in different types of HSCT.*

a delayed recovery of donor-derived T cells. Increase in the severity of the conditioning regimen results in prolonged immune deficiency after transplant [26].

Both thymus-dependent and thymus-independent T-cell reconstitutions are affected by the increase in HLA mismatch between the patient and the donor, probably because of higher risk of GvHD [27]. Clave et al. [28] reported higher reconstitution of both CD4+ and CD8+ T cells in transplants involving unrelated cord blood grafts (190 cells × 103/μL for CD4+ and 280 cells × 103/μL for CD8+) than CD34 selected peripheral blood haploidentical donor grafts (68 cells × 103/μL for CD4+ and 80 cells × 103/μL for CD8+). Mehta et al. [29] showed lower reconstitution of absolute CD4+ and CD8+ T cells at 3 months and higher B-cell counts (6 months) after unrelated cord blood HSCT than HLA matched HSCT (121.53 vs. 261.18 for CD4+, 36.03 vs. 190.56 for CD8+, and 210 vs. 31.2 for B cells). There was similar reconstitution of B cells but lower CD4+ and CD8+ T-cell reconstitution in single unit umbilical cord blood transplantation than HLA mismatched donor HSCT (11 vs. 9 for B cells, 15 vs. 21 for CD4+ cells, and 14 vs. 21 for CD8+ cells) [30].

Acute graft-versus-host disease occurs when donor lymphocytes react against normal host tissue to cause serious complications after allogeneic HSCT. Although there is faster recovery of the innate immune system after allo-HSCT, lymphocyte recovery is delayed due to aGvHD [3, 31]. The recovery of T cells depends on the thymic efficiency as well as the peripheral niche, which provides resources for T-cell survival. As GvHD targets the bone marrow, in patients with graft-versus-host disease, the peripheral resources are reduced because of which there is increased immunosuppression leading to delayed T-cell reconstitution in allogeneic HSCT as compared to autologous HSCT. The options to increase the efficiency of T-cell reconstitution must be selected in a manner so as to not aggravate the already present GvHD [32, 33]. Similarly, the drugs used to treat GvHD can also result in delayed immune reconstitution. Drugs such as cyclosporine A and methotrexate interfere with the T-cell receptor signaling and hence result in alteration of peripheral T-cell survival and B-cell differentiation [34, 35]. Tyrosine kinase inhibitors like imatinib mesylate used for controlling refractory cGvHD also lower T-cell survival by interfering with T-cell receptor (TCR) or IL7 signaling [36, 37]. Reconstitution of dendritic cells is decreased in GvHD [38]. Conversely, it has been suggested that depletion or inactivation of the host dendritic cells before allogeneic HSCT reduces the occurrence of GvHD [39–41].

## 2. Reconstitution of innate immunity

After HSCT, the first cells to engraft are the monocytes, followed by granulocytes, platelets, and NK cells [42]. Monocytes are primarily involved in phagocytosis and release of cytokines. They are classified into classical (CD14++CD16-), intermediate (CD14++CD16+), and nonclassical (CD14+CD16++) based on the expression of CD14 and CD16 [43, 44]. Monocytes remain below the normal levels for up to a year [45, 46].

The conditioning regimen used prior transplant results in a neutropenic phase till the neutrophils reconstitute, which takes approximately 11–12 days in T-cell depleted haploidentical HSCT [47, 48]. Although neutrophil counts rise to normal numbers within 2 weeks after transplant [49], they become functionally competent only after 2 months [50, 51]. The type of graft affects the reconstitution of neutrophils: 2 weeks in case of GCSF mobilized grafts, 3 weeks in case of bone marrow, and around 4 weeks in umbilical cord blood [1]. Use of peripheral blood has decreased the neutrophil recovery time from an average of 16 to 12 days [52].

NK cells recover in both number and function within the first few weeks after transplant [53], and functional reconstitution of NK cells is reached within 2 months [1]. The time taken for NK-cell reconstitution is dependent on the occurrence of GvHD [47, 54] and does not differ if the source of stem cells is peripheral blood or bone marrow [55]. However, the number of functional NK cells is higher when the transplant involves T-cell replete grafts than T-cell depleted grafts [56]. The most prominent functional NK cells after transplant are CD56brightCD16dim [57, 58]. Also, higher overall survival is seen in patients with high CD56bright NK cells at day 14 after unmanipulated haploidentical HSCT. The cytolytic function of NK cells is regulated by the interaction of inhibitory/activating killer immuno-globulin like receptors (KIRs) present on their surface and their specific HLA class I ligands. The reconstitution of the inhibitory and activating KIRs is dependent on factors such as conditioning regimen, T-cell deplete/replete graft, and immunosuppression used after transplant.

In a study evaluating NK-cell reconstitution after matched related/unrelated donor HSCT, it has been reported that the NK-cell counts are lower for longer period (2-3 months) after MUD (156/μL) than MRD (265/μL). The most frequent immature NK cells were CD56bright and NKG2A+CD57-CD56dim NK cells [59]. Russo et al. [60] reported that in haploidentical HSCT using after transplant cyclophosphamide, the immature NK cell starts appearing at 2 weeks; however, the mature NK cells expressing CD16 and CD56 and NKG2A appear at about a year.

Host dendritic cells that escape chemotherapy/radiation activate alloantigenic T cells in the donor and hence play an important role in GvHD. Since host dendritic cells present MHC antigens to donor CD8+ T cells after transplant, depleting these cells could result in lower risk of GvHD [61, 62]. Lower reconstitution of lymphoid dendritic cells has been associated with inferior overall survival [63].

Gamma delta T cells make up ~5% of the T-cell population, and their receptors are composed to gamma and delta chains. These T cells have been reported to enhance engraftment and graft-versus-leukemia effect without an increase in GvHD [64]. Gamma delta T cells reconstitute faster in patients in whom bone marrow (60 days) is used as the graft source than peripheral blood (200 days) [65].

## 3. Reconstitution of adaptive immunity

T-cell reconstitution is faster in transplantation with peripheral blood as graft source than bone marrow due to higher number of T cells present in the graft [55]. Ciurea et al. [18] reported better T-cell reconstitution in recipients of T-cell replete haploidentical HSCT than recipients of T-cell depleted haploidentical HSCT at 6 months after transplant. Use of ATG for T-cell depletion also affects the rate of immune reconstitution. This effect is more prominent in umbilical cord blood transplantation than bone marrow transplantation. T-cell reconstitution in allo-HSCT without the use of ATG is seen in about 7–12 months when using bone marrow and umbilical cord as stem cell source as compared to 6–24 months when using peripheral blood as stem cell source [66]. T cells recover primarily via peripheral expansion of memory T cells or endogenous T-cell development. Hence, functional thymus is required for effective reconstitution of T cells [67]. This is an issue in aging patients where there is thymus atrophy [68]. Due to this, although full immune recovery is possible in middle-aged patients, it is not possible in older patients and is a cause of morbidity and mortality [69]. Reconstitution of T cells is slow probably due to the prolonged depletion and reduced function of naïve T cells [70]. T cells that reconstitute are primarily from the donor origin in case of T-cell replete transplant or host T cells that have escaped the conditioning regimen in case of T-cell depleted transplant. Naïve T cells/T-cell receptor excision circles (TRECs) are lower for approximately 10–30 years after transplant [71, 72]. Reconstitution of functional T cells as observed by their ability to secrete interferon gamma and interleukin-4 to normal levels returns in 30 days after haploidentical HSCT for patients in whom acute GvHD is not observed [73]. Recipients of T-cell depleted haploidentical HSCT show higher CD31+ naïve CD4+ T cells than their donors at approximately 4–6 years [74]. Homeostatic peripheral expansion is induced by various homeostatic cytokines such as IL7 and IL15, inflammatory cytokines, and viral exposure. Peripheral homeostatic expansion leads to an inverse CD4/CD8 ratio in patients for several months after transplant. CD4 counts are considered as the best predictive marker for the recovery of immune competence after HSCT, and its recovery has also been associated with lower risk of infections and improved transplant outcomes [1]. CD4+ T-cell counts are as low as <200 cells/µL in the first 3 months and reach levels of 450 cells/µL at about 5 years after transplant [55, 75]. CD8+ T-cell counts increase rapidly during the first 3 months after transplant possibly due to the expansion of herpesvirus-specific CD8 T cells [55, 76]. GvHD reduces the number of CD4+ T cells by inhibiting the thymic output, whereas CD8+ cells increase in number during GvHD or CMV reactivation [77, 78]. The reconstituting CD4+ T cells have a higher expression of CD11a, CD29, CD45RO, and HLA-DR and a lower expression of CD28, CD45RA, and CD62L than normal individuals [79, 80]. The early reconstituting CD8+ T cells are mostly memory or effector cells. Naïve or TREC+CD8+ T cells recover at a slower rate [77, 81]. The number of regulatory T cells (Tregs) is much higher after transplant than normal individuals and may contribute to remission [82, 83]. A Treg:CD4+ T cell ratio of less than 9% has been associated with higher risk of aGvHD [84]. Chang et al. [16] reported lower CD4+ T cells, dendritic cells, and higher CD28 expression on CD4+ and CD8+ T cells in patients receiving haploidentical HSCT than patients receiving HLA matched HSCT.

B-cell reconstitution is also delayed after HSCT: ~6 months for autologous and ~9 months after allogeneic transplantation and is mainly due to GvHD or its treatment. In the first 2 months after transplant, B-cell counts are low but rise higher than the normal levels in approximately 1–2 years [55, 85]. Since restoration of full humoral immune functioning requires both naïve and memory B cells, all patients who have undergone HSCT remain susceptible to infections for at least a year after transplant [1]. The reconstituted B cells express higher levels of CD1c, CD38, CD5, membrane IgM, and membrane IgD and lower levels of CD25 and CD26L than normal individuals [86].

A number of studies have reported comparisons between reconstitution of different immune cells depending on the graft source. Faster reconstitution of

| Cell type and numbers | Bone marrow | Peripheral blood | Unrelated cord blood | Reference |
|---|---|---|---|---|
| Neutrophils (>0.5 × 109/L) | 16 days | 15 days | 19 days | [87] |
| Natural killer cells (>0.1 × 109/L) | 1.5 months | 4 months | 4 months | [16, 87] |
| T cells (>0.5 × 109/L) CD4 | 2–3 months | 6 months | 3 months | [28, 88] |
| Naïve T cells (>0.5 × 109/L) | 9 months | 24 months | 12 months | [87, 89] |
| Cytotoxic T cells (>0.25 × 109/L | 3 months | 9 months | 8 months | [65, 90] |
| T helper cells (>0.2 × 109/L) | 4 months | 10 months | 1 months | [65, 90] |

Table 2.
*Reconstitution of different immune cells depending on the graft source.*

different immune cells was observed when bone marrow was used as graft source as compared to peripheral blood or cord blood (**Table 2**).

## 4. Assessment of post-transplant immune recovery

There are different methods to assess the immune recovery after transplant, such as estimation of absolute lymphocyte count (ALC), levels of immune cell subsets (NK cells, B cells, and T cells), and antibody titers to assays for T- and B-cell repertoires [91].

ALC levels have been reported in association with overall survival and rate of relapse. ALC >500 cells/µL on day 15 is linked with better OS and lower relapse after autologous as well as allogeneic transplantation [92, 93]. An increase in the levels of CD16+ monocytes has been associated with aGvhD [94].

Early recovery of CD4+ T cells is associated with overall survival, nonrelapse mortality, and risk of infections [95, 96]. Admiral et al. [97] reported the time taken by circulating CD4+ T cells to reach 0.5× 109/L as a strong marker for probability of relapse. In myeloablative allogeneic HSCT, higher levels of CD3+, CD8+ T cells, regulatory T cells, and myeloid dendritic cells are correlated with relapse-free survival [98].

Recently, flow cytometric analysis has been used to differentiate between the T, B, and NK-cell subpopulations. Low levels of NK cells within the first few weeks after transplant have been associated with poor transplant outcomes like lower overall survival and higher risk of infection [99, 100]. Surface markers such as CD45RA, CD28, CD27, CD62L, and CCR7 can be used to differentiate naïve, effector, effector memory, and central memory CD4+ and CD8+ subsets [101, 102]. The surface markers expressed by naïve T cells are CD45RA+CCR7+; central memory T cells are CD45RA-CCR7+; effector memory T cells are CD45RA-CCR7–; and effector T cells are CD45RA+CCR7– [91]. CD4+ T cells also include regulatory T cells (CD25+FoxP3+) and Th17 cells [103, 104]. The expression of CD27, IgM, and IgD helps in distinguishing between naïve B cells (CD27-IgD+), memory B cells (CD27+IgD+), and isotype switched memory B cells (CD27+IgD-) [105]. Myeloid and plasmacytoid dendritic cells can be distinguished based on the expression of CD123 and CD11c: CD123low CD11c+(myeloid) and CD123bright CD11c- (plasma-cytoid) [106].

TRECs have been suggested as a marker for reconstitution of naïve T cells (CD4+CD45RA+) derived from the thymus. TRECs, however, remain low up to 6 months after HSCT [107]. Due to thymic atrophy with age, older patients have T cells with low TCR repertoire, which leads to higher risk of infections leading to lower transplant outcomes [108, 109]. Thymopoiesis can also be evaluated by measuring the number of TRECs by real-time quantitative in purified CD4+ and CD8+ T cells [110]. Lewin et al. [111] reported faster recovery of TRECs in younger patients and patients who received conventional grafts as compared to T-cell depleted grafts. Lower levels of TRECs are associated with GvHD and opportunistic infections [77, 112].

Certain cytokines can also be used as predictive markers for transplant outcomes. One such marker is IL7, which can be used to evaluate successful T-cell recovery. Increased IL7 is associated with delayed reconstitution and increased mortality and aGvHD [113]. High levels of IL6, GCSF, and IL2α have also been indicated in association with risk of aGvHD [96, 114]. For assessing chronic GvHD, high levels of IL8 and low levels of IL17A have been suggested [103, 115]. Min et al. [104] have also correlated high levels of IL6 and IL10 with poor transplant-related outcomes.

Further, T- and B-cell receptor repertoire gene arrangements can be evaluated by molecular techniques such as next generation sequencing [116, 117]. Michalek et al. [118] have demonstrated β chain sequencing of the T-cell receptor in order to identify the T-cell clones that could mediate either graft-versus-host disease or graft-versus-leukemia effect. Brink et al. [9] reported higher diversity in CD4+ T cells than CD8+ T cells following allogeneic HSCT. Greater diversity was observed in cord blood grafts, followed by unmanipulated grafts and T-cell depleted grafts.

## 5. Strategies to improve immune reconstitution

Many strategies, such as administration of recombinant cytokines, adoptive cell therapy, and hormone-based therapies, have recently been used to improve immune reconstitution after transplantation.

IL7 cytokine has been shown to effectively enhance reconstitution of T and B lymphoid cells by enabling thymopoiesis [105, 119]. It has been demonstrated that IL7 increased the CD3+, CD4+, and CD8+ T-cell levels to more than four folds and also leads to increase in functional and diverse T cells [120]. Administering IL-7 predominantly increases the naïve CD8+ T cells. The timing of administering is, however, important, as administering early after transplant aggravates GvHD [116, 121], whereas administering it at a later stage after HSCT results in lower risk of GvHD. This is contributed by the activation of alloreactive T cells that express lower IL-7Rα levels [32, 38]. Other cytokines that enable immune reconstitution are insulin-like growth factor 1(IGF-1), IL22, IL15, and IL12 [122–124]. IL15 has been shown to significantly increase the reconstitution of CD8+ T cells and NK cells and improve the GvL effect in haploidentical murine models [125]. Sauter et al. [126] reported better lymphocyte reconstitution after IL-15 administration in T-cell depleted allogeneic HSCT; however, it has been shown to worsen GvHD.

Recently, it has been suggested that modulating the function of dendritic cells could reduce GvHD while maximizing GvL [127]. Studies on reconstitution of dendritic cells after HSCT have been contradictory. Maraskovsky et al. [128] have shown that treatment with Flt3-L can expand DC subsets; however, when administered after HSCT, it can worsen GvHD [38]. Gauthier et al. [38] have demonstrated that SDF-1α therapy can expand the DC1 subsets and lower the severity of GvHD. Because of their immunosuppressive properties, mesenchymal stem cells have recently been used for suppressing GvHD [129–131]. Mesenchymal stem cells release cytokines such as IL-7, which improve T-cell survival and promote reconstitution of dendritic cells by secreting SDF-1α [132].

NK-cell immunotherapy is one of the novel strategies underway to reduce GvHD and enhance graft-versus-leukemia effect in a KIR-HLA mismatched haploidentical HSCT [133–135].

## 6. Future directions

Recently, few studies have identified the association of reconstitution of certain immune subsets with predicting post-HSCT outcomes. However, these studies are often limited by small sample size, lack of detailed immune reconstitution, and secretome profile, which could be used as biomarkers to predict immune reconstitution. Prospective studies involving a large number of patients should be conducted to determine which immune factors and tests to detect the same could have prognostic value and understand the impact of such predictive risk factors on transplant outcomes. This is most beneficial, especially for recipients of haploidentical HSCT, in which a routine strategy could be adopted to result in faster immune reconstitution and hence lower probability of poor transplant outcomes, such as TRM, relapse, and GvHD.

## Author details

Meenakshi Singh[1*], Selma Z. D'Silva[1] and Abhishweta Saxena[2]

1 HLA and Immunogenetics Laboratory, Tata Memorial Hospital, Mumbai, India

2 Department of Transfusion Medicine, Homi Bhabha Cancer Hospital, Varanasi, India

*Address all correspondence to: meenakshisingha@gmail.com

†Meenakshi Singh and Selma Z. D'Silva share the first authorship.

# References

[1] Mackall C, Fry T, Gress R, Peggs K, Storek J, Toubert A. Background to hematopoietic cell transplantation, including post transplant immune recovery. Bone Marrow Transplantation. 2009;**44**:457-462. DOI: 10.1038/bmt. 2009.255

[2] Storek J. Immunological reconstitution after hematopoietic cell transplantation – Its relation to the contents of the graft. Expert Opinion on Biological Therapy. 2008;**8**(5):583-597. DOI: 10.1517/14712598.8.5.583

[3] Mackall CL, Fleisher TA, Brown MR, Andrich MP, Chen CC, Feuerstein IM, et al. Age, thymopoiesis, and CD4+ T-lymphocyte regeneration after intensive chemotherapy. The New England Journal of Medicine. 1995;**332**:143-149. DOI: 10.1056/NEJM199501193320303

[4] Liang Y, Van Zant G, Szilvassy SJ. Effects of aging on the homing and engraftment of murine hematopoietic stem and progenitor cells. Blood 2005; 106: 1479-1487. DOI: 10.1182/blood-2004-11-4282

[5] Olkinuora H, Talvensaari K, Kaartinen T, Siitonen S, Saarinen-Pihkala U, Partanen J, et al. T cell regeneration in pediatric allogeneic stem cell transplantation. Bone Marrow Transplantation. 2007;**39**(3):149-156. DOI: 10.1038/sj. bmt.1705557

[6] Muller-Hermelink HK, Sale GE, Borisch B, Storb R. Pathology of the thymus after allogeneic bone marrow transplantation in man. A histologic immu-nohistochemical study of 36 patients. The American Journal of Pathology. 1987;**129**(2):242-256

[7] Lum LG. The kinetics of immune reconstitution after human marrow transplantation. Blood. 1987;**69**(2):369-380

[8] Korbling M, Anderlini P. Peripheral blood stem cell versus bone marrow allotransplantation: Does the source of hematopoietic stem cells matter? Blood. 2001;**98**:2900-2908. DOI: 10.1182/blood. v98.10.2900

[9] van den Brink MRM, Velardi E, Perales MA. Immune reconstitution following stem cell transplantation. Hematology. 2015;**2015**(1):215-219. DOI: 10.1182/asheducation-2015.1.215

[10] Hakki M, Riddell SR, Storek J, Carter RA, Stevens-Ayers T, Sudour P, et al. Immune reconstitution to cytomegalovirus after allogeneic hematopoietic stem cell transplantation: Impact of host factors, drug therapy, and sub-clinical reactivation. Blood. 2003;**102**(8):3060-3067. DOI: 10.1182/blood-2002- 11-3472

[11] Cwynarski K, Ainsworth J, Cobbold M, Wagner S, Mahendra P, Apperley J, et al. Direct visualization of cytomegalovirus-specific T-cell reconstitution after allogeneic stem cell transplantation. Blood. 2001;**97**(5):1232-1240. DOI: 10.1182/blood.V97.5.1232

[12] Martin PS, Li S, Nikiforow S, Alyea EP, Antin JH, Armand P, et al. Infused total nucleated cell dose is a better predictor of transplant outcomes than CD34(+) cell number in reduced-intensity mobilized peripheral blood allogeneic hematopoietic cell transplantation. Haematologica. 2016;**101**(4):499-505. DOI: 10.3324/haematol.2015.134841

[13] Seggewiss R, Einsele H. Immune reconstitution after allogeneic transplanta-tion and expanding options for immunomodulation: An update. Blood. 2010;**115**(19):3861-3868. DOI: 10.1182/blood-2009-12-234096

[14] Danby R, Rocha V. Improving engraftment and immune reconstitution

in umbilical cord blood transplantation. Frontiers in Immunology. 2014;5:68. DOI: 10.3389/fimmu.2014.00068

[15] Remberger M, Törlén J, Ringdén O, Engström M, Watz E, Uhlin M, et al. Effect of total nucleated and CD34+ cell dose on outcome after allogeneic hematopoietic stem cell transplantation. Biology of Blood and Marrow Transplantation. 2015;21(5):889-893. DOI: 10.1016/j.bbmt.2015.01.025

[16] Chang YJ, Zhao XY, Huo MR, Xu LP, Liu DH, Liu KY, et al. Immune reconstitution following Unmanipulated HLAMismatched/ Haploidentical transplantation compared with HLA-identical sibling transplantation. Journal of Clinical Immunology. 2012;32:268- 280. DOI: 10.1007/s10875-011-9630-7

[17] Pérez-Martínez A, González-Vicent M, Valentín J, Aleo E, Lassaletta A, Sevilla J, et al. Early evaluation of immune reconstitution following allogeneic CD3/CD19-depleted grafts from alternative donors in childhood acute leukemia. Bone Marrow Transplantation. 2012;47:1419- 1427. DOI: 10.1038/bmt.2012.43

[18] Ciurea SO, Mulanovich V, Saliba RM, Bayraktar UD, Jiang Y, Bassett R, et al. Improved early outcomes using a T cell replete graft compared with T cell depleted Haploidentical hematopoietic stem cell transplantation. Biology of Blood and Marrow Transplantation. 2012;18(12):1835-1844. DOI: 10.1016/j. bbmt.2012.07.003

[19] Cavazzana-Calvo M, Carlier F, Le Deist F, Morillon E, Taupin P, Gautier D, et al. Long-term T-cell reconstitution after hematopoietic stem-cell transplantation in primary T-cell-immunodeficient patients is associated with myeloid chimerism and possibly the primary disease phenotype. Blood. 2007;109:4575-4581. DOI: 10.1182/blood-2006-07-029090

[20] Müller SM, Kohn T, Schulz AS, Debatin KM, Friedrich W. Similar pattern of thymic-dependent T-cell reconstitution in infants with severe combined immunodeficiency after human leukocyte antigen (HLA)-identical and HLA-nonidentical stem cell transplantation. Blood. 2000;96:4344-4349

[21] Neven B, Leroy S, Decaluwe H, Le Deist F, Picard C, Moshous D, et al. Long-term outcome after hematopoietic stem cell transplantation of a single-center cohort of 90 patients with severe combined immunodeficiency. Blood. 2009;113:4114-4124. DOI: 10.1182/ blood-2008-09-177923

[22] Sehn LH, Alyea EP, Weller E, Canning C, Lee S, Ritz J, et al. Comparative outcomes of T-cell-depleted and non-T-cell-depleted allogeneic bone marrow transplantation for chronic myelogenous leukemia: Impact of donor lymphocyte infusion. Journal of Clinical Oncology. 1999;17:561-568

[23] Papadopoulos EB, Carabasi MH, Castro-Malaspina H, Childs BH, Mackinnon S, Boulad F, et al. T-cell-depleted allogeneic bone marrow transplantation as postremission therapy for acute myelogenous leukemia: Freedom from relapse in the absence of graft-versus-host disease. Blood. 1998;91:1083-1090

[24] Jakubowski AA, Small TN, Kernan NA, Castro-Malaspina H, Collins N, Koehne G, et al. T cell-depleted unrelated donor stem cell transplantation provides favorable disease-free survival for adults with hematologic malignancies. Biology of Blood and Marrow Transplantation. 2011;17:1335-1342. DOI: 10.1016/j. bbmt.2011.01.005

[25] Devine SM, Carter S, Soiffer RJ, Pasquini MC, Hari PN, Stein A, et al. Low risk of chronic graft-versus-host

disease and relapse associated with T cell-depleted peripheral blood stem cell transplantation for acute myelogenous leukemia in first remission: Results of the blood and marrow transplant clinical trials network protocol 0303. Biology of Blood and Marrow Transplantation. 2011;**17**:1343-1351. DOI: 10.1016/j.bbmt.2011.02.002

[26] Soderling CC, Song CW, Blazar BR, Vallera DA. A correlation between conditioning and engraftment in recipients of MHC-mismatched T cell-depleted murine bone marrow transplants. Journal of Immunology. 1985;**135**:941-946

[27] Politikos I, Boussiotis VA. The role of the thymus in T-cell immune reconstitution after umbilical cord blood transplantation. Blood. 2014;**124**:3201-3211. DOI: 10.1182/blood-2014-07-589176

[28] Clave E, Lisini D, Douay C, Giorgiani G, Busson M, Zecca M, et al. Thymic function recovery after unrelated donor cord blood or T-cell depleted HLA-haploidentical stem cell transplantation correlates with leukemia relapse. Frontiers in Immunology. 2013;**4**:54. DOI: 10.3389/fimmu.2013.00054

[29] Mehta RS, Bejanyan N, Cao Q, Luo X, Brunstein C, Cooley S, et al. Immune reconstitution after umbilical cord blood versus peripheral blood progenitor cell transplantation in adults following myeloablative conditioning. Blood. 2016;**22**:2246

[30] Servais S, Lengline E, Porcher R, Carmagnat M, Peffault de Latour R, Robin M, et al. Long-term immune reconstitution and infection burden after mismatched hematopoietic stem cell transplantation. Biology of Blood and Marrow Transplantation. 2014;**20**:507-517. DOI: 10.1016/j.bbmt.2014.01.001

[31] Fry TJ, Mackall CL. Immune reconstitution following hematopoietic pro-genitor cell transplantation: Challenges for the future. Bone Marrow Transplantation. 2005;**35**:S53-S57. DOI: 10.1038/sj.bmt.1704848

[32] Sinha ML, Fry TJ, Fowler DH, Miller G, Mackall CL. Interleukin 7 worsens graft-versus-host disease. Blood. 2002;**100**(7):2642-2649. DOI: 10.1182/blood- 2002-04-1082

[33] Blaser BW, Roychowdhury S, Kim DJ, Schwind NR, Bhatt D, Yuan W, et al. Donor-derived IL-15 is critical for acute allogeneic graft-versus-host disease. Blood. 2005;**105**(2):894-901. DOI: 10.1182/blood-2004-05-1687

[34] Hannam-Harris AC, Taylor DS, Nowell PC. Cyclosporin a directly inhibits human B-cell proliferation by more than a single mechanism. Journal of Leukocyte Biology. 1985;**38**(2):231-239. DOI: 10.1002/jlb.38.2.231

[35] Gratama JW, Würsch AM, Nissen C, Gratwohl A, D'Amaro J, de Gast GC, et al. Influence of graft-versus-host disease prophylaxis on early T-lymphocyte regeneration following allogeneic bone marrow transplantation. British Journal of Haematology. 1986;**62**(2):355-365. DOI: 10.1111/j.1365-2141.1986.tb02939.x

[36] Legros L, Ebran N, Stebe E, Rousselot P, Rea D, Cassuto JP, et al. Imatinib sensitizes T-cell lymphocytes from chronic myeloid leukemia patients to FasL-induced cell death: A brief communication. Journal of Immunotherapy. 2012;**35**(2):154-158. DOI: 10.1097/CJI.0b013e318243f238

[37] Thiant S, Moutuou MM, Laflamme P, Sidi Boumedine R, Leboeuf DM, Busque L, et al. Imatinib mesylate inhibits STAT5 phosphorylation in response to IL-7 and promotes T cell lymphopenia in chronic myelogenous leukemia patients. Blood Cancer

Journal. 2017;**7**(4):e551. DOI: 10.1038/bcj. 2017.29

[38] Gauthier SD, Leboeuf D, Manuguerra-Gagne R, Gaboury L, Guimond M. Stromal-derived factor-1alpha and interleukin-7 treatment improves homeostatic proliferation of naive CD4(+) T cells after allogeneic stem cell transplantation. Biology of Blood and Marrow Transplantation. 2015;**21**(10):1721-1731. DOI: 10.1016/j.bbmt.2015.06.019

[39] Chan GW, Gorgun G, Miller KB, Foss FM. Persistence of host dendritic cells after transplantation is associated with graft-versus-host disease. Biology of Blood and Marrow Transplantation. 2003;**9**(3):170-176. DOI: 10.1016/S1083-8791(03)70006-8

[40] Arpinati M, Chirumbolo G, Urbini B, Bonifazi F, Bandini G, Saunthararajah Y, et al. Acute graft-versus-host disease and steroid treatment impair CD11c+ and CD123+ dendritic cell reconstitution after allogeneic peripheral blood stem cell transplantation. Biology of Blood and Marrow Transplantation. 2004;**10**(2):106-115. DOI: 10.1016/j.bbmt.2003.09.005

[41] Vakkila J, Thomson AW, Hovi L, Vettenranta K, Saarinen-Pihkala UM. Circulating dendritic cell subset levels after allogeneic stem cell transplantation in children correlate with time post transplant and severity of acute graft-versus-host disease. Bone Marrow Transplantation. 2005;**35**(5):501-507. DOI: 10.1038/sj.bmt.1704827

[42] Storek J, Geddes M, Khan F, Huard B, Helg C, Chalandon Y, et al. Reconstitution of the immune system after hematopoietic stem cell transplantation in humans. Seminars in Immunopathology. 2008;**30**:425-437. DOI: 10.1007/s00281-008-0132-5

[43] Ziegler-Heitbrock L, Ancuta P, Crowe S, Dalod M, Grau V, Hart DN, et al. Nomenclature of monocytes and dendritic cells in blood. Blood. 2010;**116**:e74-e80. DOI: 10.1182/blood-2010-02-258558

[44] Passlick B, Flieger D, Ziegler-Heitbrock HW. Identification and characterization of a novel monocyte subpopulation in human peripheral blood. Blood. 1989;**74**:2527-2534

[45] Cayeux S, Meuer S, Pezzutto A, Körbling M, Haas R, Schulz R, et al. Allogeneic mixed lymphocyte reactions during a second round of ontogeny: Normal accessory cells did not restore defective interleukin-2 (IL-2) synthesis in T cells but induced responsiveness to exogenous IL-2. Blood. 1989;**74**:2278-2284

[46] Sahdev I, O'Reilly R, Black P, Heller G, Hoffmann M. Interleukin-1 production following T-cell-depleted and unmodified marrow grafts. Pediatric Hematology and Oncology. 1996;**13**:55-67

[47] van Rood JJ, Loberiza Jr FR, Zhang MJ, Oudshoorn M, Claas F, Cairo MS, Champlin RE, Gale RP, Ringdén O, Hows JM, Horowitz MH. Effect of tolerance to noninherited maternal antigens on the occurrence of graft versus- host disease after bone marrow transplantation from a parent or an HLA-haploidentical sibling. Blood 2002;**99**:1572-1577. DOI: 10.1182/blood.v99.5.1572

[48] Passweg JR, Tichelli A, Meyer-Monard S, Heim D, Stern M, Kühne T, et al. Purified donor NK-lymphocyte infusion to consolidate engraftment after haploidentical stem cell transplantation. Leukemia. 2004;**18**:1835-1838. DOI: 10.1038/sj.leu.2403524

[49] Zimmerli W, Zarth A, Gratwohl A, Speck B. Neutrophil function and

pyogenic infections in bone marrow transplant recipients. Blood. 1991;77:393-399

[50] Atkinson K, Biggs JC, Downs K, Juttner C, Bradstock K, Lowenthal RM, et al. GM-CSF after allogeneic BMT: Accelerated recovery of neutrophils, monocytes and lymphocytes. Australian and New Zealand Journal of Medicine. 1991;21:686-692

[51] Bensinger WI, Clift R, Martin P, Appelbaum FR, Demirer T, Gooley T, et al. Allogeneic peripheral blood stem cell transplantation in patients with advanced hematologic malignancies: A retrospective comparison with marrow transplantation. Blood. 1996;88:2794-2800

[52] Przepiorka D, Smith TL, Folloder J, Anderlini P, Chan KW, Körbling M, et al. Controlled trial of filgrastim for acceleration of neutrophil recovery after allogeneic blood stem cell transplantation from human leukocyte antigen-matched related donors. Blood. 2001;97(11):3405-3410. DOI: 10.1182/blood.v97.11.3405

[53] Jacobs R, Stoll M, Stratmann G, Leo R, Link H, Schmidt RE, et al. Natural killer cells after bone marrow transplantation. Blood. 1992;79:3239-3244

[54] Chen H, Liu KY, Xu LP, Liu DH, Chen YH, Zhao XS, et al. Application of real time polymerase chain reaction to the diagnosis and treatment of cytomegalovirus infection after allogeneic hematopoietic stem cell transplantation. Zhonghua Xue Ye Xue Za Zhi. 2009;30:77-81

[55] Storek J, Dawson MA, Storer B, Stevens-Ayers T, Maloney DG, Marr KA, et al. Immune reconstitution after allogeneic marrow transplantation compared with blood stem cell transplantation. Blood.

2001;97(11):3380-3389. DOI: 10.1182/blood.v97.11.3380

[56] Gallez-Hawkins GM, Franck AE, Li X, Thao L, Oki A, Gendzekhadze K, et al. Expression of activating KIR2DS2 and KIR2DS4 genes after hematopoietic cell transplantation: Relevance to cytomegalovirus infection. Biology of Blood and Marrow Transplantation. 2011;17:1662-1672. DOI: 10.1016/j.bbmt.2011.04.008

[57] De Angelis C, Mancusi A, Ruggeri L, Capanni M, Urbani E, Velardi A, et al. Expansion of CD56-negative, CD16-positive, KIR-expressing natural killer cells after T cell-depleted haploidentical hematopoietic stem cell transplantation. Acta Haematologica. 2011;126:13-20. DOI: 10.1159/000323661

[58] Hokland M, Jacobsen N, Ellegaard J, Hokland P. Natural killer function following allogeneic bone marow transplantation. Transplantation. 1988;45:1080-1084. DOI: 10.1097/00007890-198806000-00016

[59] Pical-Izard C, Crocchiolo R, Granjeaud S, Kochbati E, Just-Landi S, Chabannon C, et al. Reconstitution of natural killer cells in HLA-matched HSCT after reduced-intensity conditioning: Impact on clinical outcome. Biology of Blood and Marrow Transplantation. 2015;21:429-439. DOI: 10.1016/j.bbmt.2014.11.681

[60] Russo A, Oliveira G, Berglund S, Greco R, Gambacorta V, Cieri N, et al. NK cell recovery after Haploidentical HSCT with post-TransplantCyclophosphamide: Dynamics and clinical implications. Blood. 2018;131:247-262. DOI: 10.1182/blood-2017-05-780668

[61] Shlomchik WD. Antigen presentation in graft-vs-host

disease. Experimental Hematology. 2003;**31**:1187-1197

[62] Hashimoto D, Merad M. Harnessing dendritic cells to improve allogeneic hematopoietic cell transplantation outcome. Seminars in Immunology. 2011;**23**:50-57. DOI: 10.1016/j.smim.2011.01.005

[63] Koehl U, Bochennek K, Zimmermann SY, Lehrnbecher T, Sörensen J, Esser R, et al. Immune recovery in children undergoing allogeneic stem cell transplantation: Absolute CD8+CD3+ count reconstitution is associated with survival. Bone Marrow Transplantation. 2007;**39**(5):269-278. DOI: 10.1038/sj.bmt.1705584

[64] Booth C, Lawson S, Veys P. The current role of T cell depletion in paediatric stem cell transplantation. British Journal of Haematology. 2013;**162**:177-190. DOI: 10.1111/bjh.12400

[65] Eyrich M, Leiler C, Lang P, Schilbach K, Schumm M, Bader P, et al. A prospective comparison of immune reconstitution in pediatric recipients of positively selected CD34þ peripheral blood stem cells from unrelated donors vs recipients of unmanipulated bone marrow from related donors. Bone Marrow Transplantation. 2003;**32**:379-390. DOI: 10.1038/sj.bmt.1704158

[66] de Koning C, Plantinga M, Besseling P, Boelens JJ, Nierkens S. Immune reconstitution after allogeneic hematopoietic cell transplantation in children. Biology of Blood and Marrow Transplantation. 2016;**22**:195-206. DOI: 10.1016/j.bbmt.2015.08.028

[67] Hakim FT, Memon SA, Cepeda R, Jones EC, Chow CK, Kasten-Sportes C, et al. Age-dependent incidence, time course, and consequences of thymic renewal in adults. The Journal of Clinical Investigation. 2005;**115**:930-939. DOI: 10.1172/JCI22492

[68] Rodewald HR. The thymus in the age of retirement. Nature. 1998;**396**:630-631. DOI: 10.1038/25251

[69] Storek J, Gooley T, Witherspoon RP, Sullivan KM, Storb R. Infectious morbidity in long-term survivors of allogeneic marrow transplantation is associated with low CD4 T cell counts. American Journal of Hematology. 1997;**54**:131-138

[70] Roux E, Dumont-Girard F, Starobinski M, Siegrist CA, Helg C, Chapuis B, et al. Recovery of immune reactivity after T-cell-depleted bone marrow transplantation depends on thymic activity. Blood. 2000;**96**:2299-2303

[71] Storek J, Joseph A, Espino G, Dawson MA, Douek DC, Sullivan KM, et al. Immunity of patients surviving 20 to 30 years after allogeneic or syngeneic bone marrow transplantation. Blood. 2001;**98**:3505-3512. DOI: 10.1182/blood.v98.13.3505

[72] Le RQ, Melenhorst JJ, Battiwalla M, Hill B, Memon S, Savani BN, et al. Evolution of the donor T-cell repertoire in recipients in the second decade after allogeneic stem cell transplantation. Blood. 2011;**117**:5250-5256. DOI: 10.1182/blood-2011-01-329706

[73] Fu YW, Wu DP, Cen JN, Feng YF, Chang WR, Zhu ZL, et al. Patterns of T-cell reconstitution by assessment of T-cell receptor excision circle and T-cell receptor clonal repertoire after allogeneic hematopoietic stem cell transplantation in leukemia patients – A study in Chinese patients. European Journal of Haematology. 2007;**79**(2):138-145. DOI: 10.1111/j.1600-0609.2007.00885.x

[74] Azevedo RI, Soares MV, Albuquerque AS, Tendeiro R, Soares RS,

Martins M, et al. Long-term immune reconstitution of naive and memory T cell pools after haploidentical hematopoietic stem cell transplantation. Biology of Blood and Marrow Transplantation. 2013;**19**(5):703-712. DOI: 10.1016/j.bbmt.2013.01.017

[75] Atkinson K, Hansen JA, Storb R, Goehle S, Goldstein G, Thomas ED. T-cell subpopulations identified by monoclonal antibodies after human marrow transplantation. I. Helper-inducer and cytotoxic-suppressor subsets. Blood. 1982;**59**(6):1292-1298

[76] Marshall NA, Howe JG, Formica R, Krause D, Wagner JE, Berliner N, et al. Rapid reconstitution of Epstein-Barr virus-specific T lymphocytes following allogeneic stem cell transplantation. Blood. 2000;**96**(8):2814-2821

[77] Weinberg K, Blazar BR, Wagner JE, Agura E, Hill BJ, Smogorzewska M, et al. Factors affecting thymic function after allogeneic hematopoietic stem cell transplantation. Blood. 2001;**97**(5):1458e1466. DOI: 10.1182/blood.v97.5.1458

[78] Storek J, Zhao Z, Lin E, Berger T, McSweeney PA, Nash RA, et al. Recovery from and consequences of severe iatrogenic lymphopenia (induced to treat autoimmune diseases). Clinical Immunology. 2004;**113**(3):285-298. DOI: 10.1016/j.clim.2004.07.006

[79] Storek J, Witherspoon RP, Storb R. T cell reconstitution after bone marrow transplantation into adult patients does not resemble T cell development in early life. Bone Marrow Transplantation. 1995;**16**(3):413-425

[80] Weinberg K, Annett G, Kashyap A, Lenarsky C, Forman SJ, Parkman R. The effect of thymic function on immunocompetence following bone marrow transplantation. Biology of Blood and Marrow Transplantation. 1995;**1**(1):18-23

[81] Storek J, Joseph A, Dawson MA, Douek DC, Storer B, Maloney DG. Factors influencing T-lymphopoiesis after allogeneic hematopoietic cell transplantation. Transplantation. 2002;**73**(7):1154-1158. DOI: 10.1097/00007890-200204150-00026

[82] Roord ST, de Jager W, Boon L, Wulffraat N, Martens A, Prakken B, et al. Autologous bone marrow transplantation in autoimmune arthritis restores immune homeostasis through CD4þCD25þFoxp3þ regulatory T cells. Blood. 2008;**111**:5233-5241. DOI: 10.1182/blood-2007-12-128488

[83] Zhang L, Bertucci AM, Ramsey-Goldman R, Burt RK, Datta SK. Regulatory T cell (Treg) subsets return in patients with refractory lupus following stem cell transplantation, and TGF-beta-producing CD8þ Treg cells are associated with immunological remission of lupus. Journal of Immunology. 2009;**183**:6346-6358. DOI: 10.4049/jimmunol.0901773

[84] Federmann B, Bornhauser M, Meisner C, Kordelas L, Beelen DW, Stuhler G, et al. Haploidentical allogeneic hematopoietic cell transplantation In adults using CD3/CD19 depletion and reduced intensity conditioning: A phase II study. Haematologica. 2012;**97**(10):1523-1531. DOI: 10.3324/haematol.2011.059378

[85] Kook H, Goldman F, Padley D, Giller R, Rumelhart S, Holida M, et al. Reconstruction of the immune system after unrelated or partially matched T-cell-depleted bone marrow transplantation in children: Immunophenotypic analysis and factors affecting the speed of recovery. Blood. 1996;**88**(3):1089-1097

[86] Storek J, Ferrara S, Ku N, Giorgi JV, Champlin RE, Saxon A. B cell reconstitution after human bone marrow transplantation: Recapitulation

of ontogeny? Bone Marrow Transplantation. 1993;**12**(4):387e398

[87] Oshrine BR, Li Y, Teachey DT, Heimall J, Barrett DM, Bunin N. Immunologic recovery in children after alternative donor allogeneic transplantation for hematologic malignancies: Comparison of recipients of partially T cell-depleted peripheral blood stem cells and umbilical cord blood. Biology of Blood and Marrow Transplantation. 2013;**19**:1581-1589. DOI: 10.1016/j.bbmt.2013.08.003

[88] Moretta A, Maccario R, Fagioli F, Giraldi E, Busca A, Montagna D, et al. Analysis of immune reconstitution in children undergoing cord blood transplantation. Experimental Hematology. 2001;**29**:371-379

[89] Olkinuora H, von Willebrand E, Kantele JM, Vainio O, Talvensaari K, Saarinen-Pihkala U, et al. The impact of early viral infections and graft-versus-host disease on immune reconstitution following paediatric stem cell transplantation. Scandinavian Journal of Immunology. 2011;**73**:586-593. DOI: 10.1111/j.1365-3083.2011.02530.x

[90] Chiesa R, Gilmour K, Qasim W, Adams S, Worth AJ, Zhan H, et al. Omission of in vivo T cell depletion promotes rapid expansion of naïve CD4þ cord blood lymphocytes and restores adaptive immunity within 2 months after unrelated cord blood transplant. British Journal of Haematology. 2012;**156**:656-666. DOI: 10.1111/j.1365-2141.2011.08994.x

[91] Dudakov JA, Perales MA, van den Brink MRM. Immune reconstitution following hematopoietic cell transplantation. In: Thomas' Hematopoietic Cell Transplantation. 5th ed. Wiley & Sons Publishers; 2015. pp. 160-169. DOI: 10.1002/9781118416426.ch15

[92] Porrata LF, Markovic SN. Timely reconstitution of immune competence affects clinical outcome following autologous stem cell transplantation. Clinical and Experimental Medicine. 2004;**4**:78-85

[93] Kim DH, Kim JG, Sohn SK, Sung WJ, Suh JS, Lee KS, et al. Clinical impact of early absolute lymphocyte count after allogeneic stem cell transplantation. British Journal of Haematology. 2004;**125**:217-224. DOI: 10.1111/j.1365-2141.2004.04891.x

[94] Döring M, Cabanillas Stanchi KM, Haufe S, Erbacher A, Bader P, Handgretinger R, et al. Patterns of monocyte subpopulations and their surface expression of HLA-DR during adverse events after hematopoietic stem cell transplantation. Annals of Hematology. 2014;**94**:825-836. DOI: 10.1007/s00277-014-2287-6

[95] Kim DH, Sohn SK, Won DI, Lee NY, Suh JS, Lee KB. Rapid helper T-cell recovery above 200 × 106/l at 3 months correlates to successful transplant outcomes after allogeneic stem cell transplantation. Bone Marrow Transplantation. 2006;**37**:1119-1128. DOI: 10.1038/sj.bmt.1705381

[96] Berger M, Figari O, Bruno B, Raiola A, Dominietto A, Fiorone M, et al. Lymphocyte subsets recovery following allogeneic bone marrow transplantation (BMT): CD4+ cell count and transplant-related mortality. Bone Marrow Transplantation. 2008;**41**:55-62. DOI: 10.1038/sj.bmt.1705870

[97] Admiraal R, van Kesteren C, Jol-van der Zijde CM, Lankester AC, Bierings MB, Egberts TC, van Tol MJ, Knibbe CA, Bredius RG, Boelens JJ. Association between anti-thymocyte globulin (ATG) exposure and CD4þ immune reconstitution predicting overall survival in paediatric haematopoietic cell transplantation: A multicentre retrospective pharmacodynamic cohort analysis. The

Lancet Haematology 2015;2: e194-e203. DOI: 10.1016/S2352-3026(15)00045-9

[98] Kanda J, Chiou LW, Szabolcs P, Sempowski GD, Rizzieri DA, Long GD, et al. Immune recovery in adult patients after myeloablative dual umbilical cord blood, matched sibling, and matched unrelated donor hematopoietic cell transplantation. Biology of Blood and Marrow Transplantation. 2012;**18**:1664-1676.e1. DOI: 10.1016/j. bbmt.2012.06.005

[99] Bartelink IH, Belitser SV, Knibbe CA, Danhof M, de Pagter AJ, Egberts TC, et al. Immune reconstitution kinetics as an early predictor for mortality using various hematopoietic stem cell sources in children. Biology of Blood and Marrow Transplantation. 2013;**19**:305-313. DOI: 10.1016/j.bbmt.2012.10.010

[100] Thomson BG, Roberston KA, Gowan D, Heilman D, Broxmeyer HE, Emanuel D, et al. Analysis of engraftment, graft-versus-host disease, and immune recovery following unrelated donor cord blood transplantation. Blood. 2000;**96**:2703-2711

[101] Campbell JJ, Murphy KE, Kunkel EJ, Brightling CE, Soler D, Shen Z, et al. CCR7 expression and memory T cell diversity in humans. Journal of Immunology. 2001;**166**:877- 884. DOI: 10.4049/jimmunol.166.2.877

[102] Hamann D, Baars PA, Rep MH, Hooibrink B, Kerkhof-Garde SR, Klein MR, et al. Phenotypic and functional separation of memory and effector human CD8+ T cells. The Journal of Experimental Medicine. 1997;**186**:1407-1418. DOI: 10.1084/ jem.186.9.1407

[103] Resende RG, de Correia-Silva J, Silva TA, Salomão UE, Marques-Silva L, Vieira ÉL, et al. IL-17 genetic and immunophenotypic evaluation in

chronic graft-versus-host disease. Mediators of Inflammation. 2014;**2014**:571231. DOI: 10.1155/2014/571231

[104] Min CK, Lee WY, Min DJ, Lee DG, Kim YJ, Park YH, et al. The kinetics of circulating cytokines including IL-6, TNF-, IL-8 and IL-10 following allogeneic hematopoietic stem cell transplantation. Bone Marrow Transplantation. 2001;**28**:935-940. DOI: 10.1038/sj.bmt.1703258

[105] Kang J, Der SD. Cytokine functions in the formative stages of a lymphocyte's life. Current Opinion in Immunology. 2004;**16**:180-190. DOI: 10.1016/j.coi.2004.02.002

[106] Kim JM, Rudensky A. The role of the transcription factor Foxp3 in the development of regulatory T cells. Immunological Reviews. 2006;**212**:86-98. DOI: 10.1111/ j.0105-2896.2006.00426.x

[107] Harrington LE, Hatton RD, Mangan PR, Turner H, Murphy TL, Murphy KM, et al. Interleukin 17-producing CD4+ effector T cells develop via a lineage distinct from the T helper type 1 and 2 lineages. Nature Immunology. 2005;**6**:1123-1132. DOI: 10.1038/ni1254

[108] Small TN, Robinson WH, Miklos DB. B cells and transplantation: An educational resource. Biology of Blood and Marrow Transplantation. 2009;**15**(1 Suppl):104-113. DOI: 10.1016/ j.bbmt.2008.10.016

[109] Rossi M, Young JW. Human dendritic cells: Potent antigen-presenting cells at the crossroads of innate and adaptive immunity. Journal of Immunology. 2005;**175**:1373-1381. DOI: 10.4049/jimmunol.175.3.1373

[110] Douek DC, Vescio RA, Betts MR, Brenchley JM, Hill BJ, Zhang L, et al. Assessment of thymic output in

adults after haematopoietic stem-cell transplantation and prediction of T-cell reconstitution. Lancet. 2000;355:1875-1881. DOI: 10.1016/S0140-6736(00)02293-5

[111] Lewin SR, Heller G, Zhang L, Rodrigues E, Skulsky E, van den Brink MR, Small TN, Kernan NA, O'Reilly RJ, Ho DD, Young JW. Direct evidence for new T-cell generation by patients after either T-cell-depleted or unmodified allogeneic hematopoietic stem cell transplantations. Blood 2002; 100: 2235-2242

[112] Wils EJ, van der Holt B, Broers AE, Posthumus-van Sluijs SJ, Gratama JW, Braakman E, et al. Insufficient recovery of thymopoiesis predicts for opportunistic infections in allogeneic hematopoietic stem cell transplant recipients. Haematologica. 2011;96:1846-1854. DOI: 10.3324/haematol.2011.047696

[113] Kielsen K, Jordan KK, Uhlving HH, Pontoppidan PL, Shamim Z, Ifversen M, et al. T cell reconstitution in allogeneic haematopoietic stem cell transplantation: Prognostic significance of plasma interleukin-7. Scandinavian Journal of Immunology. 2015;81:72-80. DOI: 10.1111/sji.12244

[114] Paczesny S, Krijanovski OI, Braun TM, Choi SW, Clouthier SG, Kuick R, et al. A biomarker panel for acute graft-versus-host disease. Blood. 2009;113:273-278. DOI: 10.1182/blood-2008-07-167098

[115] Berger M, Signorino E, Muraro M, Quarello P, Biasin E, Nesi F, et al. Monitoring of TNFR1, IL-2Ra, HGF, CCL8, IL-8 and IL-12p70 following HSCT and their role as GVHD biomarkers in paediatric patients. Bone Marrow Transplantation. 2013;48:1230-1236. DOI: 10.1038/bmt.2013.41

[116] Perales MA, Goldberg JD, Yuan J, Koehne G, Lechner L, Papadopoulos EB,

et al. Recombinant human interleukin- 7 (CYT107) promotes T-cell recovery after allogeneic stem cell transplantation. Blood. 2012;120:4882-4891. DOI: 10.1182/blood-2012-06-437236

[117] Keller T, Weber S, Gombert M, Schuster FR, Asang C, Stepensky P, et al. Next-generation-sequencing spectratyping reveals public T-cell receptor repertoires in pediatric very severe aplastic anemia and identifies a beta chain CDR3 sequence associated with hepatitis-induced pathogenesis. Haematologica. 2013;98:1388-1396. DOI: 10.3324/haematol.2012.069708

[118] Michalek J, Collins RH, Hill BJ, Brenchley JM, Douek DC. Identification and monitoring of graft-versus-host specific T-cell clone in stem cell transplantation. The Lancet. 2003;361:1183-1185. DOI: 10.1016/S0140-6736(03)12917-0

[119] van Heijst JW, Ceberio I, Lipuma LB, Samilo DW, Wasilewski GD, Gonzales AM, et al. Quantitative assessment of T cell repertoire recovery after hematopoietic stem cell transplantation. Nature Medicine. 2013;19:372-377. DOI: 10.1038/nm.3100

[120] Sudo T, Nishikawa S, Ohno N, Akiyama N, Tamakoshi M, Yoshida H, et al. Expression and function of the interleukin 7 receptor in murine lymphocytes. Proceedings of the National Academy of Sciences of the United States of America. 1993;90:9125-9129. DOI: 10.1073/pnas.90.19.9125

[121] Hennion-Tscheltzoff O, Leboeuf D, Gauthier SD, Dupuis M, Assouline B, Gregoire A, et al. TCR triggering modulates the responsiveness and homeostatic proliferation of CD4+ thymic emigrants to IL-7 therapy. Blood. 2013;121(23):4684-4693. DOI: 10.1182/blood-2012-09-458174

[122] Alpdogan O, Muriglan SJ, Eng JM, Willis LM, Greenberg AS,

Kappel BJ, et al. IL-7 enhances peripheral T cell reconstitution after allogeneic hematopoietic stem cell transplantation. The Journal of Clinical Investigation. 2003;**112**(7):1095-1107. DOI: 10.1172/JCI200317865

[123] Dudakov JA, Hanash AM, Jenq RR, Young LF, Ghosh A, Singer NV, et al. Interleukin-22 drives endogenous thymic regeneration in mice. Science. 2012;**336**:91-95. DOI: 10.1126/science.1218004

[124] Eisenring M, vom Berg J, Kristiansen G, Saller E, Becher B. IL-12 initiates tumor rejection via lymphoid tissue-inducer cells bearing the natural cytotoxicity receptor NKp46. Nature Immunology. 2010;**11**:1030-1038. DOI: 10.1038/ni.1947

[125] Satoh-Takayama N, Lesjean-Pottier S, Vieira P, Sawa S, Eberl G, Vosshenrich CA, et al. IL-7 and IL-15 independently program the differentiation of intestinal CD3– NKp46+ cell subsets from Id2-dependent precursors. The Journal of Experimental Medicine. 2010;**207**: 273-280. DOI: 10.1084/jem.20092029

[126] Sauter CT, Bailey CP, Panis MM, Biswas CS, Budak-Alpdogan T, Durham A, et al. Interleukin-15 administration increases graft-versus-tumor activity in recipients of haploidentical hematopoietic SCT. Bone Marrow Transplantation. 2013;**48**(9):1237-1242. DOI: 10.1038/bmt.2013.47

[127] Thiant S, Moutuou MM, Leboeuf D, Guimond M. Homeostatic cytokines in immune reconstitution and graft-versus-host disease. Cytokine. 2016;**82**:24-32. DOI: 10.1016/j.cyto.2016.01.003

[128] Maraskovsky E, Brasel K, Teepe M, Roux ER, Lyman SD, Shortman K, et al. Dramatic increase in the numbers of functionally mature dendritic cells in Flt3 ligand-treated mice: Multiple dendritic cell subpopulations identified. The Journal of Experimental Medicine. 1996;**184**(5):1953-1962. DOI: 10.1084/jem.184.5.1953

[129] Spaggiari GM, Capobianco A, Becchetti S, Mingari MC, Moretta L. Mesen-chymal stem cell-natural killer cell interactions: Evidence that activated NK cells are capable of killing MSCs, whereas MSCs can inhibit IL-2-induced NK-cell proliferation. Blood. 2006;**107**(4):1484-1490. DOI: 10.1182/blood-2005-07-2775

[130] Nemeth K, Leelahavanichkul A, Yuen PS, Mayer B, Parmelee A, Doi K, et al. Bone marrow stromal cells attenuate sepsis via prostaglandin E(2)-dependent reprogramming of host macrophages to increase their inter-leukin-10 production. Nature Medicine. 2009;**15**(1):42-49. DOI: 10.1038/nm.1905

[131] Bouchlaka MN, Moffitt AB, Kim J, Kink JA, Bloom DD, Love C, et al. Human mesenchymal stem cell-educated macrophages are a distinct high IL-6- producing subset that confer protection in graft-versus-host-disease and radiation injury models. Biology of Blood and Marrow Transplantation. 2017;**23**(6):897-905. DOI: 10.1016/j.bbmt.2017.02.018

[132] Fujii S, Miura Y, Fujishiro A, Shindo T, Shimazu Y, Hirai H, et al. Graft- versus-host disease amelioration by human bone marrow mesenchymal stromal/stem cell-derived extracellular vesicles is associated with peripheral preservation of naive T cell populations. Stem Cells. 2018;**36**(3):434-445. DOI: 10.1002/stem.2759

[133] Laport GG, Sheehan K, Baker J, Armstrong R, Wong RM, Lowsky R, et al. Adoptive immunotherapy with cytokineinduced killer cells for patients with relapsed hematologic malignancies after allogeneic hematopoietic cell transplantation. Biology of Blood and

Marrow Transplantation. 2011;**17**: 1679-1687. DOI: 10.1016/j. bbmt.2011.05.012

[134] Miller JS, Soignier Y, Panoskaltsis-Mortari A, McNearney SA, Yun GH, Fautsch SK, et al. Successful adoptive transfer and in vivo expansion of human haploidentical NK cells in patients with cancer. Blood. 2005;**105**:3051-3057. DOI: 10.1182/blood-2004-07-2974

[135] Rubnitz JE, Inaba H, Ribeiro RC, Pounds S, Rooney B, Bell T, et al. NKAML: A pilot study to determine the safety and feasibility of haploidentical natural killer cell transplantation in childhood acute myeloid leukemia. Journal of Clinical Oncology. 2010;**28**:955-959. DOI: 10.1200/JCO.2009.24.4590

# 6

# Neutrophil Function Impairment is a Host Susceptibility Factor to Bacterial Infection in Diabetes

*Daniella Insuela, Diego Coutinho, Marco Martins, Maximiliano Ferrero and Vinicius Carvalho*

## Abstract

*Diabetes mellitus* is a highly prevalent noncommunicable disease globally. One of the main complications of diabetes is the increased susceptibility to bacterial infection. Neutrophils play a crucial role in inflammatory response against bacterial infections, once they are the first cells recruited to the sites of injury. In diabetes, there is a failure in the neutrophil functions, including migration, ROS production, phagocytosis, and bacterial killing, which are associated with the high incidence of bacterial infections. Herein, we point out pieces of evidence revealing the primary molecular mechanisms involved with impairment of neutrophil functions in diabetes, with relationship with high susceptibility to bacterial infections.

**Keywords:** diabetes, bacterial infection, neutrophils, inflammation, chemotaxis

## 1. Introduction

*Diabetes mellitus* (DM) is a chronic metabolic disorder characterized by a hyperglycemic condition that results in several complications, such as neuropathy, nephropathy, retinopathy, and increased risk of cardiovascular disease [1]. DM can be classified into type 1 (T1DM) and type 2 (T2DM). T1DM is common in childhood or young adulthood and is a result of autoimmune destruction of beta-cells in pancreatic islets mediated by T cells, leading to defect in insulin synthesis [2, 3]. The T2DM appears mainly in adulthood, affecting people with the most productive age. This type of diabetes is associated with insulin resistance and inadequate compensation by beta-cells, leading to a relative insulin deficiency [1, 4]. Currently, it is known that there are over 425 million people with DM globally. Worryingly, it is estimated that in 2045, this number will grow to over 600 million [5].

Hyperglycemia, a hallmark of DM, is associated with patient vulnerability to bacterial infections, such as tuberculosis and pneumonia, besides more severe sepsis of bacterial origin [5]. In fact, diabetic patients generally present microbial persistence, greater susceptibility to new infections, recurrences, and an increase in the risk of mortality if compared to nondiabetic individuals [5, 6]. This is due to the compromised immune response presented by diabetic patients, which leads to failure in leukocytes protective effects. Cyclically, infection profile in these patients can worsen glycemic control [5]. Neutrophils present an important role in host immune response to bacterial infection, once they are one of the first leukocytes that arrive in the infected area [7]. In normal conditions, these cells act by different manners against microorganism, leading to infection control and resolution of the inflammatory process. However, the immune response in diabetic patients is characterized by impairment in neutrophil function [7, 8]. Here, we revised the mechanisms involved with the failure of neutrophil functions noted in DM and its relationship with the high susceptibility to bacterial infections.

## 2. Role of neutrophils in bacterial infections

### 2.1 Migration of neutrophils to infected sites

Neutrophils are polymorphonuclear (PMN) versatile innate effector cells essential for immune defense, which arise from hematopoietic stem cells (HSCs) in bone marrow [9]. Under normal conditions, about $5 \times 10^{10}$–$10 \times 10^{10}$ new neutrophils are produced in the bone marrow daily [10, 11]. Chemokine gradients and adhesion molecules are central players that regulate neutrophil release from the bone marrow [11]. Neutrophils express CXC receptors (CXCR)-1 and CXCR2 that interact with CXC chemokines (CXCL1/KC, CXCL2/MIP-2, and CXCL8/IL-8) and result in neutrophil migration from bone marrow into the bloodstream. Neutrophils also express CXCR4, which interacts with CXCL12/SDF-1 produced by osteoblasts and other stromal cells to mediate neutrophil maintenance in the bone marrow [10, 12]. Thereby, only a small fraction of mature neutrophils is released into the blood. However, after a bacterial invasion, the host defense activates strong neutrophil release from bone marrow and migration toward infected sites [11, 12].

Under bacterial infection, sentinel cells detect the microorganisms via pattern recognition receptors (PRRs), such as Toll-like receptors (TLRs) and NOD-like receptors (NLRs). These receptors identify highly conserved pathogen-associated molecular patterns (PAMPs), including peptidoglycan (PGN) and lipopolysaccharide (LPS) expressed in the cell membrane surface of bacteria. They can also recognize danger-associated molecular patterns (DAMPs), such as high mobility group protein B1 (HMGB1), ATP, and uric acid, released from damaged and necrotic cells after tissue injury. Then, sentinel cells release mediators such as granulocyte colony-stimulating factor (G-CSF), which leads to neutrophil production and release from bone marrow via upregulation of CXCR2 and its ligands, and reduces expression of CXCL12/SDF-1 and CXCR4. After this event, neutrophils can be mobilized to sites of infection and combat microorganism [13–15].

Correct leukocyte recruitment requires the adhesive interactions between P-selectin glycoprotein ligand-1 (PSGL-1), E-selectin ligand-1 (ESL-1), and CD44 expressed on the neutrophil membrane surface to the P- and E-selectin which are upregulated in endothelial cells of inflamed tissue. These processes will lead to neutrophil capture and fast rolling [16, 17]. Rolling event exposes neutrophils to chemokines that are arrested on the glycocalyx of endothelial cells, such as CXCL8/IL-8. Then occurs the activation of integrin molecules such as VLA-4 (CD49D/CD29), macrophage-1 antigen (MAC-1 or CD11b/CD18), and lymphocyte function-associated antigen-1 (LFA-1 or CD11a/CD18) on neutrophils [10, 18]. The integrin binds to their ligands such as intercellular adhesion molecule (ICAM)-1, ICAM-2, and platelet endothelial cell adhesion molecule-1 (PECAM-1) on endothelial cells, resulting in slow rolling and firm adhesion of the neutrophil to endothelial cells [17]. Thence, the neutrophils perform diapedesis toward the tissue and migrate along a chemokine gradient until they arrive in the infected site. The long-distance recruitment is mediated by chemoattractants, including leukotriene B4 and CXCL8/IL-8, while near chemoattractants are peptides and C5a [17].

Despite the canonical neutrophil migration during infections, in sepsis occurs an inadequate migration of neutrophils even with high levels of chemokines at the infection site [12]. The decrease of CXCR2 expression on the cell surface of neutrophils is among the mechanisms leading to this failure. The prolonged exposure to CXCR2 agonists, which leads to phosphorylation of G protein-coupled receptors (GPCRs) by GPCR kinases (GRKs) and induces the desensitization and internalization of CXCR2, can explain the down-regulation of this receptor [16]. In addition, the activation of lectin-like oxidized low-density lipoprotein receptor-1 (LOX-1) by inflammatory products, such as C-reactive protein (CRP), bacterial products, apoptotic cells, or activated platelets, can also account for CXCR2 neutrophil endocytosis [12, 19].

## 2.2 Actions of neutrophils in infected sites

At the sites of infection, neutrophils can combat pathogenic microorganisms and clear infections by different ways including phagocytosis, degranulation of microbicidal molecules, production and secretion of reactive oxygen species (ROS), and release of neutrophil extracellular traps (NETs) [20]. For efficient bacterial phagocytosis, the microorganism needs to be covered with opsonins, such as immunoglobulins (Igs) and components of the complement system, which are recognized by neutrophil specific surface receptors. After phagocytosis of an opsonized pathogen by neutrophils, there is a mobilization of intracellular granules or lysosomes, leading to the killing of the ingested bacteria [21].

Neutrophil activation can induce the production of ROS to combat infection. It happens mainly due to the action of NADPH oxidase complex (NOX), but can also be generated by mitochondria. After neutrophil activation, NOX acts converting molecular oxygen ($O_2$) into superoxide anion ($O_2^{\cdot-}$) which suffers dismutation, spontaneously or catalyzed by myeloperoxidase (MPO), generating hydrogen peroxide ($H_2O_2$) [22, 23]. In addition to ROS, neutrophils can also enhance the inducible nitric oxide synthase (NOS2) expression, which will convert $O_2$ to nitric oxide (NO), resulting in reactive nitrogen species (RNS). Both ROS and RNS contribute to microbicide activity and are crucial for the defense against intracellular microorganisms [22]. Curiously, NO is supposed to be involved in the failure of neutrophil migration during sepsis, once it stimulates the internalization of CXCR2 on the neutrophil surface and reduces expression of adhesion molecules, leading to diminished leucocyte rolling and adhesion to the endothelium [12]. After neutrophil migration, degranulation occurs, which is the process mediated by microbial or inflammatory stimuli in which neutrophils release the granule contents, such as MPO, defensins, cathepsin G, neutrophil elastase, and collagenase. These granule contents are released by exocytosis or into the phagosome to kill microorganisms [24].

Neutrophils may also perform the antimicrobial activity directly attacking and restraining microorganisms by releasing NETs (NETosis) [25, 26]. NETs are extracellular fibrous structures composed by a network of extracellular chro-matin fibers, histones, antimicrobial peptides, and enzymes, including MPO, α-defensins, cathepsin G, elastase, and lactoferrin, to capture and kill microorganisms [12, 20, 26]. NETosis occurs after neutrophil exposure to bacteria or stimulation with mediators such as interleukin CXCL8/IL-8. This neutrophil stimulation will result in activation of intracellular pro-inflammatory kinases, such as Akt, p38 MAPK, or MEK/ERK, a release of neutrophil elastase, oxidative burst, and actin polymerization [20, 26, 27]. This mechanism will result in microorganism destruction and neutrophil death [25]. NETs also limit the microorganism growth and dissemination; however, excessive formation of NETs in association with the uncontrolled inflammatory response that occurs in sepsis can result in multiple organ damage to the host [12, 20].

## 2.3 Resolution of neutrophilic inflammation

Resolution phase is an essential process to interrupt the inflammatory response after the danger signal or when microorganism has been eliminated, preventing the development of chronic inflammation and fibrosis [28]. Resolution of inflammation was previously considered a passive response, associated with clearance of inflammatory stimulus, reduction of pro-inflammatory mediators, and prevention of leukocyte recruitment. Currently, it is known that resolution is an active and tightly controlled process, carried out by specialized pro-resolving mediators (SPM) such as resolvins, lipoxins, maresins, and protectins, which are produced locally from polyunsaturated fatty acids and act orchestrating the end of inflammation, but do not evoke unwanted immunosuppression [29, 30]. For a correct resolution of inflammation, the neutrophil reverse migration, lymphatic drainage, exudation to the external environment, apoptosis of activated neutrophils followed by efferocytosis, and autophagic clearance of intracellular inflammatory signals are necessary [31, 32].

The reduction in neutrophil recruitment is regulated by a class-switch from the production of pro-inflammatory to pro-resolving mediators, resulting in down-regulation of CXCR2 on neutrophils [28]. Pro-resolving lipid mediators also resolve inflammation by promoting neutrophil apoptosis [28, 32]. Apoptotic neutrophils or cell bodies are phagocytosed by professional phagocytes, mainly macrophages, in a process known as efferocytosis. This event is mediated by an interaction between phosphatidylserine expressed on the neutrophil surface and macrophage receptors, such as TIM1 and TIM4 [32, 33]. During resolution, macrophages change their profile decreasing the pro-inflammatory feature and acquiring anti-inflammatory and pro-resolving functions, acting in apoptotic cell clearance, and producing immune regulatory intracellular messengers, including cyclic adenosine monophosphate (cAMP) [28, 34]. Macrophage phagocytosis allows the complete elimination of dead neutrophils and tissue debris of the infected and inflamed area. Generally, this process is followed by macrophage autophagy [35, 36]. Together, all these processes contribute to the resolution of neutrophil inflammation and tissue homeostasis [31].

## 3. Impaired neutrophil migration in diabetes

The causes of increase in susceptibility to infections in DM are not yet fully known, but one of the possible and well-established explanations is that diabetics present an impairment in defense mechanisms of innate immunity, including neutrophil migration to the site of inflammation, phagocytosis, ROS production, and bactericidal activity [37].

The number of neutrophils in the circulation is also altered in DM. Older studies have shown that in T1DM patients, there is an increase in neutrophil counts compared to healthy individuals [38, 39]. Recent researches described a decrease in circulating neutrophil numbers in T1DM patients in comparison with nondiabetics [40, 41]. Impairment in neutrophil yield and maturation in bone marrow, increase in peripheral neutrophil consumption, and/or tissue sequestration could explain this reduction in blood neutrophil counts observed in T1DM [42]. This divergence between studies can be attributed to differences between ethnic groups and the discovery of the existence of various stages of DM [43]. While in T1DM, the data about circulating neutrophil counts are still controversial, most of the studies described that in T2DM patients, there is an increase in the number of neutrophils in circulation in comparison to healthy individuals [40, 44]. This neutrophilia was related to elevation in the circulation levels of inflammatory cytokines, including TNF-α, IL-1β, and IL-6, and CRP, a known marker of inflammation [45].

Regarding migration, *in vitro* studies described a reduction in CXCL8/IL-8, platelet-activating factor (PAF), or N-formyl-methionyl-leucyl-phenylalanine (fMLP)-induced chemotaxis of neutrophils from T1DM or T2DM patients compared to cells from healthy subjects [40, 46]. *In situ* evaluation of chemotaxis toward fMLP using T1DM rat neutrophils also revealed a deficiency in migration. This impairment in neutrophil chemotaxis was positively related to DM severity which was characterized by glycaemia values greater than 400 mg/dL [47]. In addition, blood neutrophils of diabetic animals presented a decreased migratory response to CXCL2/MIP-2 *in vitro* and *in vivo* compared to nondiabetic animals. Despite the deficiency in CXCL2/MIP-2 induced-neutrophil migration, there was no difference between the expression of CXCR-2, a CXCL2/MIP-2 receptor, on neutrophils from diabetic animals [48, 49]. Similarity in CXCR-2 mRNA levels was also found among bone marrow neutrophils obtained from NOD mice (a strain that spontaneously develops T1DM), NOR mice (a strain that is resistant to diabetes), and control mice strain. However, CXCR-1 mRNA levels were reduced in neutrophils isolated from NOD mice in comparison to neutrophils from NOR and control mice [50]. Then, it is possible to consider that alterations in CXCR-1 expression and activity may also contribute to the impairment of neutrophil migratory activity in diabetics.

A feature well described in DM is the increase in oxidative stress which may also be related with impairment of neutrophil migration. Oxidative stress can induce glutathionylation (S-thiolation) of several proteins, including L-plastin (LPL) [51] that is expressed exclusively in leucocytes and controls polarization and migration of neutrophils through bundling of β-actin filaments [52]. Neutrophils from diabetic patients and from T2DM mice showed enhanced S-thiolation of LPL in comparison to neutrophils from nondiabetic subjects, which culminate with impaired fMLP-chemotaxis of neutrophils from diabetics. S-thiolation of LPL reduces its interaction with β-actin and this may be another mechanism involved in defective migration of neutrophils in DM [51].

In addition, T1DM rats administered with LPS by intra-tracheal route exhibited a reduction in neutrophil accumulation in the bronchoalveolar fluid (BAL), which occurred in association with a decrease in TNF-α and IL-1β levels, when compared with nondiabetic rats provoked with LPS. However, no difference was observed in relation to the expression of ICAM-1 and E-selectin in lung vascular endothelium and cytokine-induced neutrophil chemoattractant-1 (CINC-1) amount in BAL [53]. A deficiency in neutrophil migration to airways after LPS intra-tracheal injection was also observed in a spontaneous rat model of T2DM, using Goto-Kakizaki (GK) rats. This reduction in neutrophil migration to the airways in GK rats stimulated with LPS occurred despite an increase in the number of neutrophils in the blood. These data showed that there was no failure in the production of these cells by the bone marrow, but impairment in the recruitment mechanisms of these leukocytes to the lungs. Indeed, GK rats exhibited a decrease in IL1-β, IL-6, and TNF-α concentration in BAL and also a reduction in the expression of adhesion molecules, such as LFA-1 and ICAM-2, on neutrophils. All these alterations were associated with a reduction in the TLR4 expression and activation in neutrophils [54].

## 3.1 Failure in neutrophil migration associated with hyperglycemia

Hyperglycemia can influence various components of the immune response, including activities of inflammatory cells [55]. Incubation of human neutrophils with supraphysiological levels of glucose decreased both chemotaxis in response to zymosan and phagocytosis/killing of the intracellular bacteria *Staphylococci in vitro*. In addition, high glucose concentrations increased neutrophil adherence *in vitro*, and this also can limit neutrophil locomotion from blood vessels toward infected tissues *in vivo* [56].

It is debated which mechanisms are involved in the benefit of insulin treatment on the immune response of diabetics. While some authors argue that the beneficial effects are dependent on the correction of hyperglycemia by insulin, others believe that the insulin may have direct actions on immune system independently of glycemic control [55]. Indeed, it has been shown that insulin *in vitro* increases human neutrophil chemotaxis induced by fMLP, calcium ionophore, or phorbol-myristyl acetate (PMA) [57, 58]. Besides, insulin presents a chemokinesis effect which required activation of tyrosine kinase and phosphatidylinositol 3-kinase (PI3K), but did not depend on protein kinase C (PKC) stimulation [59, 60]. Interestingly, in a hyperglycemic medium, the chemokinetic action of insulin in neutrophils is blocked through a mechanism that involved activation of PKC [60]. These data suggest that insulin is able to exert direct effects on neutrophils, but the maintenance of glucose levels is also important for actions of this hormone on these leukocytes. In addition to acting on neutrophils, insulin can increase expression of the PECAM-1 in endothelial HUVEC cells and thus enhance transmigration of neutrophils across these cells in response to fMLP *in vitro* [61]. Finally, *in vivo* studies showed that insulin restored neutrophil migration to the lungs in T1DM rats subjected to LPS provocation. This effect of insulin occurred in parallel to a reduction of 50% glycemia; however, the glycemic levels continued to be high in these animals compared to nondiabetic rats [53]. These data suggest that the action of insulin on LPS-induced inflammatory response was not totally dependent on its effect on blood glucose.

It is well known that chronic hyperglycemia upregulates the generation of advanced glycation end-products (AGE). AGEs are produced by a nonenzymatic reaction between reducing sugars, such as glucose, and amino acids of proteins. AGEs can induce cross-link between proteins and also can bind cellular receptors; among them, the best described is the receptor for AGE (RAGE) [62]. AGE accumulation has been associated with the development of several diabetic complications, including retinopathy, nephropathy, and neuropathy [63]. RAGE is expressed on neutrophils and its activation by AGEs, like glycated albumin, induces a transient rise in intracellular free-calcium levels and actin polymerization. Nevertheless, the dimension of increase in calcium levels induced by glycated-albumin is smaller than that induced by fMLP. In addition, glycated-albumin pre-treatment in neutrophils inhibited elevation of intracellular calcium levels promoted by fMLP, causing a defective signal processing and, consequently, a reduction in fMLP-induced-transendothelial migration *in vitro* [64]. Furthermore, glycated collagen also inhibited chemotaxis in response to fMLP, and this effect was associated with the capacity of glycated collagen to increase adhesion strength of neutrophils *in vitro* [62]. In addition, the blockade of AGE formation in diabetic animals restored leucocyte rolling, adhesion, and migration in response to zymosan *in vitro* [65], and also restored neutrophil accumulation toward traumatic skin tissue induced by hot water [66]. Therefore, it is possible that in DM, AGEs promote sustained stimulation of neutrophils which decreases the responses of these cells to chemotactic stimulus.

A positive relation between hyperglycemia and serum NO levels was also described in rats [67], and some studies have reported an increase in serum or plasma NO concentrations in T1DM and T2DM patients [67, 68]. Human neutrophils treated with L-Arginine, a NO precursor, have decreased chemotaxis toward CXCL8/IL-8 *in vitro*, while treatment with NOS inhibitor increased CXCL8/

IL-8-induced-chemotaxis of neutrophils *in vitro* [69]. In addition, a NO donor inhibited human chemotaxis promoted by fMLP *in vitro* and incubation with a guanylate cyclase inhibitor did not interfere with the effect of NO donor. These data suggested that the inhibitory action of NO on neutrophil chemotaxis is independent of cGMP [51]. The NO-induced impairment of neutrophil migration was confirmed using bone marrow neutrophils isolated from $NOS2^{-/-}$ mice stimulated with fMLP *in vitro,* which showed increased chemotaxis in comparison to that isolated from $NOS2^{+/+}$ mice [51]. Furthermore, the pre-treatment with NOS inhibitor prevented impairment of neutrophil recruitment toward peritoneal cavity observed in severe sepsis [70]. Therefore, it is possible to hypothesize that deficiency on migration activity of neutrophils may be associated with increased serum levels of NO in diabetics.

## 3.2 Failure in neutrophil migration independent of hyperglycemia

DM has altered levels of several molecules in serum that are not directly related to hyperglycemia, some of which can interfere with components of immune response, including neutrophils. Alpha-1-acid glycoprotein (AGP) is one of the main acute-phase proteins in organisms; its synthesis depends mainly on liver, and during an inflammatory response, the concentration in serum increases. [71]. AGP can bind to hormones and interfere with functions of endothelial cells, platelets, and leukocytes, and in fact, it inhibits human neutrophil chemotaxis in response to fMLP *in vitro* [72]. In addition, intravenous administration of AGP in rats prevented migration of neutrophils to peritoneal cavity, reducing rolling and adhesion of these leukocytes on endothelium of mesenteric microcirculation induced by carrageenan [73]. DM patients present high serum levels of AGP [48], so it is feasible that AGP can mediate the impairment of neutrophil locomotion described in DM.

Furthermore, AGP-mediated neutrophil dysfunction was also demonstrated in diabetic animals upon sepsis induction by cecal ligation and perforation (CLP). Neutrophils from septic T1DM mice showed impaired rolling, adhesion, and migration from mesenteric tissue toward the peritoneal cavity, while accumulated in lung tissue. These observations were associated with an altered expression of adhesion molecules (CD62L-CD11b) and a clear reduction in CXCR2 in neutrophils from diabetic animals compared to nondiabetic, after CLP. Accordingly, neutrophils from diabetic mice presented an increased expression of GRK2, a key modulator of CXCR2 receptor desensitization, upon sepsis induction compared to control septic mice. AGP administration in septic nondiabetic mice impaired neutrophil migration to peritoneal cavity, augmenting GRK2 expression, and reducing CXCR2, which reproduced the diabetic condition. On the other hand, insulin treatment reduced GKR2 and augmented CXCR2 on neutrophils obtained from diabetic mice, while decreased AGP serum concentrations. Thus, AGP increased production is involved in neutrophil impaired migration to infection during diabetes, possibly by enhancing GRK2 expression and/or augmenting NO production in these cells [48]. Notably, CXCR2 downregulation in diabetic animals seems to depend on the presence of comorbidity since several studies showed no difference in CXCR2 expression between normal and diabetic mice.

Histamine for a long time was considered as a pro-inflammatory mediator whose main role is played in allergic inflammation. However, some evidence has shown that histamine can modulate other immunological events. Neutrophils express both histamine receptors, H1 and H2 [74] and activation of H2 inhibited human neutrophil chemotaxis *in vitro* [75]. Furthermore, blood neutrophils obtained after systemic or inhalatory administration of histamine in normal volunteers showed a reduction in chemotactic response to zymosan *in vitro* [75].

After septic stimuli, T1DM mice exhibited mast cell accumulation in the peritoneal cavity and higher plasma levels of histamine than nondiabetic mice. In addition, the augmented activation of H2 receptor promoted an increase in intracellular expression of GRK2 and cAMP levels in diabetic septic mice neutrophils, favoring CXCR2 desensitization [74].

Resistin is a cysteine-rich protein that belongs to the resistin-like molecule (RELM) family that, in humans, is released mainly by macrophages but can be also produced by adipose tissue [76]. Resistin impairs glucose tolerance and insulin action and therefore has been related to obesity-induced insulin resistance and T2DM [77]. Beyond metabolic effects, resistin can act directly in immune cells, including neutrophils. Resistin decreased fMLP-induced neutrophil chemotaxis *in vitro* through inhibition of PI3K pathway activation. Resistin also decreased oxidative burst in neutrophils after stimulation with PMA and *Escherichia coli* [78]. Since resistin directly affects neutrophil function and T2DM patients present higher serum levels of this hormone [79], it can be suggested that resistin is also involved with the deficiency of neutrophil responses in DM independently of hyperglycemia.

## 4. Neutrophil response to bacterial infections in diabetes

It is now generally accepted that high glucose concentrations impaired several functions of neutrophils beyond their migratory capacity, including phagocytosis and bacterial killing. Hyperglycemia hinders neutrophil activity by inducing higher concentrations of intracellular calcium and thereby reducing ATP levels, which in turn leads to reduced phagocytic ability of PMN cells. Nevertheless, under glycemic control, diabetic patients restored intracellular calcium levels and increased cellular ATP content in neutrophils, which consequently improved phagocytosis. In addition, hyperglycemia was shown to affect other immune and hemostatic responses during experimental human endotoxemia. Healthy patients submitted to high blood glucose levels presented a reduction of *E. coli* endotoxin-induced neutrophil degranulation and exaggerated coagulation. A reversal of these effects was observed when glucose was controlled with insulin therapy [55].

Neutrophils from diabetic patients showed increased production of inflammatory cytokines [80] and ROS without any stimulation, although neutrophil oxidative responses to certain pathogens appear to be predominantly suppressed in diabetes [64, 81, 82]. Furthermore, hyperglycemia led to decreased mRNA synthesis of different pro-inflammatory cytokines in neutrophils after LPS stimulation, compared with the euglycemic state [55]. In addition, T1DM mice showed a hyperglycemia-induced pre-activation of NOX, resulting in a significantly higher release of superoxide. Sustained hyperglycemic condition may, therefore, induce oxidative damage and the onset of diabetic complications, particularly at sites with neutrophilia [83, 84].

In DM, neutrophils increased basal ROS generation in a close-relationship to sustained hyperglycemia and the generation of AGEs [64]. On the other hand, decreased pathogen-stimulated ROS production is thought to be related to impaired glucose metabolism by the pentose-phosphate pathway, which produces NADPH that is a requirement for optimal superoxide generation by NOX [6]. Off noted, phagocytosis and NETosis were shown to depend on oxidative burst in neutrophils. Nevertheless, the relevance of the ROS production misbalance noted in neutrophils obtained from diabetics is not clear, since not all the diabetic patients with diminished ROS production presented recurrent bacterial infections [82].

## 4.1 Neutrophil dysfunction and sepsis

According to The Third International Consensus Definitions for Sepsis and Septic Shock, "sepsis is a life-threatening organ dysfunction secondary to a deregulated host response to an infection" [85]. During septic processes, serum inflammatory marker concentration increases in patients although innate immune response appears to be impaired. Particularly, defective neutrophil recruitment to the sites of infection was reported in animal models of sepsis [86, 87]. Clinical studies reported that the incidence of sepsis is increased in diabetic patients [5]. Accordingly, DM is associated with high severity of sepsis, likely due to compromised immune responses, such as adhesion, chemotaxis, phagocytosis, and bacterial killing by immune cells [88]. Few studies reproducing septic inflammations in the context of diabetes had been performed in animals. T1DM or T2DM animals have worse prognosis upon CLP-induced sepsis even though plasma levels of systemic pro-inflammatory cytokines, like TNF-α, CXCL2/MIP-2, and IL-6, are increased in diabetic animals compared with control animals upon sepsis induction. This situation is normally attributed to neutrophil dampened activity [48, 74, 89, 90].

On the other hand, results obtained upon CLP-induced sepsis in a mouse model of T2DM showed an increased neutrophil infiltration in the peritoneal cavity in diabetic animals compared to nondiabetic upon sepsis induction. Nevertheless, neutrophils from diabetic animals presented reduced phagocytic activity and ROS generation after sepsis induction compared to control animals in the same condition. This impairment in neutrophil functions was related to a downregulation of TAM family of receptor tyrosine kinases. The lack of an appropriated innate immune response results in deficient bacterial elimination and augmented death rate in diabetic septic animals compared to control septic animals [90].

Similar results were observed in T1DM NOD mice intraperitoneally challenged with *Staphylococcus aureus*. The augmented neutrophil presence in the peritoneum of diabetic mice was associated with a sustained TNF-α production which prevents apoptosis in these leukocytes. Despite it, diabetic mice were more susceptible to *S. aureus* infection possibly associated to neutrophil decreased oxidative burst [91]. In addition, administration of GM-CSF, a cytokine known to activate PMNs, in diabetic animals submitted to CLP was able to restore neutrophilic activity and prevent the increased mortality of the animals. These effects of GM-CSF were associated with an increased neutrophil phagocytic activity and ROS generation, which controlled bacterial proliferation in the peritoneal cavity [90].

## 4.2 Neutrophil counts and function in tuberculosis

Several clinical and epidemiological studies have identified DM as a risk factor for the development of pulmonary tuberculosis (TB). T2DM and TB are two of the most common co-morbid conditions in many parts of the world. In addition, DM has been associated with a greater severity of TB disease among the infected population and worse outcome in response to treatment [92]. TB-DM co-morbidity is characterized by heightened levels of bacterial loads in sputum accompanied by increased neutrophil counts in peripheral blood [93]. Neutrophilic inflammation is a central feature of TB-DM, accompanied by elevated levels of biomarkers associated with macrovascular complications.

Whole blood gene expression and plasma analyses showed that several inflammatory markers, including IL-1β, CXCL8/IL-8, IL-17A, CCL3/MIP-1, TNF-α, and VEGF, associated with neutrophilic activity and absolute neutrophil counts were highly increased in TB-DM patients compared to TB or DM patients. A higher frequency of participants with high molecular degree of perturbation (MDP) was also noted in the TB-DM subgroup. MDP is a parameter that reflects the "distance to health," based on molecular expression scores in comparison with a healthy population. Consequently, they suggest that epigenetic reprogramming and neutrophilic inflammation determine the pattern of plasma cytokines and growth factors in TB-DM co-morbidity, highlighting neutrophilic inflammation as the main cause of susceptibility to develop TB by DM patients. Thereby, neutrophilic inflammation may be a useful target to improve TB treatment outcomes in this growing TB-DM patient population [94]. In addition, increased levels of three of the most prominent antimicrobial peptides, cathelicidin (LL37), human β-defensin 2 (HBD2), and human neutrophil peptide 1–3 (HNP1–3), principally secreted by neutrophils were found in individuals with TB-DM and TB compared with individuals with latent TB or non-TB-infected [7]. However, neutrophils isolated from T2DM patients showed a decreased capacity to phagocyte *Mycobacterium tuberculosis* or other *M. tuberculosis*-related molecules compared to control donors [95].

There are few studies using animal models of TB-DM co-morbidity focusing on neutrophil activity. Even though it is frequently observed that diabetic animals have an increased accumulation of neutrophils within lung tissue upon infection [96, 97], T2DM animals were more vulnerable to *M. tuberculosis* showing a decreased survival rate compared to control infected animals. Also, diabetic animals recruited more neutrophils and express higher levels of CXCL8/IL-8 in lung tissue than control infected animals [96]. In T1DM mice, infection with *M. tuberculosis* led to a decreased survival rate associated with an impaired bacterial control compared to nondiabetic infected mice. This high mortality of T1DM mice was accompanied by a lung neutrophilia and IL-6 overexpression. The treatment of TB-DM animals with neutralizing anti-IL-6 antibodies reduced neutrophil numbers and controlled bacterial burden in lung tissue, improving the survival rate [97].

## 4.3 Neutrophil counts and function in pneumonia

DM increases the risk of patients acquiring a pneumococcal disease, and besides, adversely affects the severity and outcome of this infectious illness [98]. In fact, DM has been shown to be a significant predictor of hospitalization in patients with community-acquired pneumonia (CAP) and also, a risk factor for the development of bacteremia in patients with pneumococcal pneumonia. T2DM is frequently associated with increased mortality rate from pneumonia, which appeared to be highest in the early phase of infection where neutrophilic inflammation is more important [99]. *Streptococcus pneumoniae* is the most frequent cause of CAP irrespective of age and comorbidity. The phagocytosis of *S. pneumonia* was reduced in neutrophils recovered from eight patients with poorly controlled DM, but this defect improved with insulin treatment. Notably, control neutrophils incubated with serum taken from patients with diabetes also demonstrated a defective phagocytosis, suggesting that the inefficient bacterial opsonization might be occurring in the diabetic patient's serum [100].

Once phagocytosed, bacterial killing by neutrophils depends on the generation of ROS. *Ex-vivo* studies using neutrophils from T2DM patients have demonstrated a defect in the intracellular killing of *S. pneumoniae* together with a reduced $O_2$ production, reduced MPO activity, and $H_2O_2$ generation. In addition, chronic hyperglycemia induces inactivation of the source of leukocyte ROS, which results in high prevalence of oral abscesses, progressive interstitial inflammation, and fibrosis in the lung of mice in the absence of an inflammatory stimulus, leading to cachexia and death. These data suggested that ROS generated by NOX is not only beneficial but also essential to oral and respiratory health in DM, particularly when the glycemia is uncontrolled [84].

*Klebsiella pneumoniae* is emerging as an agent which induces severe CAP. DM is associated with increased susceptibility to *K. pneumoniae* and poor prognosis of infection. Streptozotocin-induced diabetic mice are more susceptible to oropharyngeal infection with *K. pneumoniae*, presenting increased mortality rate and less bacterial control. There was no difference in the antibacterial activity of neutrophils recovered from nondiabetic and diabetic mice, indicating that the higher bacterial burden in hyperglycemia is probably related to a defective inflammatory signaling and late neutrophil recruitment. In fact, *K. pneumoniae* LPS induced a fewer recruitment of neutrophils to the alveolar airspace in diabetic mice compared to nondiabetic mice. Also, diabetic mice reduced neutrophil accumulation and early production of CXCL1/KC, CXCL2/MIP-2, IL-1β, and TNF-α in lung. Additionally, TLR2 and TIRAP, a Toll receptor and adaptor protein, were under-expressed in lungs of diabetic mice following *K. pneumoniae*-LPS provocation compared to nondiabetic infected mice, while no differences were observed for TLR-4 expression. These observations suggested that the failure in neutrophil recruitment and activation during the first hours of infection with *K. pneumoniae* is a most probable mechanism for high susceptibility to pneumonia in diabetics [101].

Commonly, *K. pneumoniae* infections cause pneumonia or urinary tract infections; however, during the past two decades, a distinct invasive syndrome that causes liver abscesses (KLA) has been increasingly reported in Asia, and this syndrome is emerging as a global disease [102]. DM is the most common comorbidity in KLA patients. It was shown that DNA and MPO levels were elevated in the plasma of KLA patients compared to uninfected individuals, indicating neutrophil activation independently of diabetic status. In addition, clinical *K. pneumoniae* isolates induced phagocytosis, bacterial killing, and NETosis comparable by neutrophils from diabetic and nondiabetic patients. Notably, the IL-12-IFNγ axis and its downstream chemokines CXCL9/MIG, CXCL10/IP-10, and CCL5/RANTES were produced at lower levels by peripheral blood mononuclear cells (PBMCs) from T2DM compared to PBMCs from healthy individuals in response to *K. pneumoniae* strains. These observations indicated that although T2DM does not overtly impact on neutrophil intra- and extra-cellular killing of *K. pneumoniae*, it may influence cytokine/chemokine production and intracellular killing by PBMCs.

### 4.4 Neutrophil function in bacterial infection-induced deficiency in wound healing

Delayed wound healing is one of the main diabetes-related morbidities. Neutrophil inefficient activity has been pointed as one of the major responsible factors for the impaired wound healing in diabetes, since neutrophil depletion accelerates wound resolution independently of the presence of an infection [103]. Furthermore, increased serum elastase levels, a marker of neutrophilic inflammation, predicted delayed wound healing in diabetic patients. In addition, proteomic analyses of the diabetic patient's foot ulcers (DFUs) showed elevated expression of NET components, including elastase, histones, neutrophil gelatinase-associated lipocalin, and proteinase-3, in nonhealing wounds as also in circulating blood. Consistently, neutrophils isolated from blood of DFU patients showed an increase of spontaneous NETosis but an impaired inducible NETosis [104]. Isolated neutrophils from T2DM patients presented higher NETosis rate than neutrophils from healthy patients in the absence of stimulation, which was associated with elevated intracellular calcium levels. Hyperglycemia is strongly related to these effects since neutrophils derived from healthy patients produced more NETosis after pre-incubation with high glucose medium *in vitro*. In addition, large amounts of NETs were found in excisional skin sterile-wounds of streptozotocin-induced diabetic mice. Although the role of NETosis in wounds remains elusive, it has been confirmed that the inhibition of NETosis or degrading NETs improved sterile-wound healing and reduced NET-driven chronic inflammation in diabetic mice [105].

Gram-positive bacteria cause more than half of cases of diabetes-related wound infections. Especially, *Staphylococcus aureus* is a major pathogen in these infections, and its presence correlates with significant delays in wound healing [106]. Wounds induced by *S. aureus* in T2DM mice showed delayed resolution compared to nondiabetic mice. Seven days after infection, the lesions of diabetic mice presented exacerbated NETosis, while nondiabetic mice had their inflammatory process already resolved and healing was nearly completed. Although neutrophils derived from both T1DM and T2DM patients produced greater amounts of NETs compared to healthy volunteer's neutrophils, the induction of NETosis cannot be explained just by hyperglycemia. In fact, some works showed that high glucose exposure reduced LPS- or IL-6-induced NETosis *in vitro* [105, 107, 108].

Some mechanisms that could also explain the increased neutrophil NETosis in diabetic patients are the elevated levels of zonulin and the overexpression of PAD4. Zonulin is a protein that modulates the permeability of tight junctions between cells of the digestive tract. Interestingly, the increased zonulin levels in diabetic patients revealed a strong correlation with neutrophil elastase concentration and NET formation in a glucose-independent way [109]. PAD4 is a calcium-dependent enzyme that mediates NETosis. In diabetes, PAD4 was upregulated in neutrophils from individuals with diabetes and was responsible for the unbalanced NET production by these leukocytes.

In T2DM mice, although neutrophil infiltration toward the lesion was augmented, the impaired wound healing upon surgical site infection with *S. aureus* was related to a significant reduction in phagocytic activity and bacterial killing by neutrophils. Consistently, *S. aureus*-induced phagolysosome maturation was abolished and PMA-stimulated superoxide production was decreased in neutrophils recovered from diabetic mice. In addition, treatment of neutrophils with insulin significantly restored neutrophil killing activities and increased phagocytosis. Interestingly, phagosome maturation and superoxide production restoring were dependent on glycemic control and not on a direct effect of insulin. These abnormalities in neutrophil functions were closely related with impaired wound healing in DM, once treatment with insulin restored normal wound healing in diabetic mice [110].

## 5. Conclusion

The increased susceptibility to bacterial infections is one of the hallmarks of diabetic complications. Under comorbidity with diabetes, the high prevalence and severity of bacterial infections, as observed in tuberculosis, pneumonia, and sepsis, is closely associated to impairment in neutrophil functions, such as migration, phagocytosis, ROS production, and NET formation. The alterations in neutrophil functions noted in diabetics occur both dependently and independently of the glycemic control. Among the mechanisms that lead to neutrophil dysfunction in diabetic conditions not related to glycemic control, some targets have been highlighted, such as AGP, H2 receptor, IL-6, PAD4, resistin, and zonulin. These potential targets should be better explored in clinical studies concerning their putative benefits to diabetic patients.

## Acknowledgements

The authors thank Conselho Nacional de Desenvolvimento Científico e Tecnológico (CNPq), Instituto Nacional de Ciência e Tecnologia-NIM, and Fundação Carlos Chagas de Amparo à Pesquisa do Estado do Rio de Janeiro (FAPERJ) for financial support.

## Author details

Daniella Insuela[1], Diego Coutinho[1], Marco Martins[1], Maximiliano Ferrero[1] and Vinicius Carvalho[1,2]*

1 Laboratory of Inflammation, Oswaldo Cruz Institute, Oswaldo Cruz Foundation (FIOCRUZ), Rio de Janeiro, Brazil

2 National Institute of Science and Technology on Neuroimmunomodulation (INCT-NIM), Brazil

*Address all correspondence to: viniciusfrias@hotmail.com

# References

[1] Al-Awar A, Kupai K, Veszelka M, Szűcs G, Attieh Z, Murlasits Z, et al. Experimental diabetes mellitus in different animal models. Journal Diabetes Research. 2016;**2016**:1-12. DOI: 10.1155/2016/9051426

[2] Saberzadeh-Ardestani B, Karamzadeh R, Basiri M, Hajizadeh-Saffar E, Farhadi A, Shapiro AMJ, et al. Type 1 diabetes mellitus: Cellular and molecular pathophysiology at a glance. Cell Journal. 2018;**20**(3):294-301. DOI: 10.22074/cellj.2018.5513

[3] Yi B, Huang G, Zhou Z. Different role of zinc transporter 8 between type 1 diabetes mellitus and type 2 diabetes mellitus. Journal of Diabetes Investigation. 2016;**7**(4):459-465. DOI: 10.1111/jdi.12441

[4] Pedron S, Emmert-Fees K, Laxy M, Schwettmann L. The impact of diabetes on labour market participation: A systematic review of results and methods. BMC Public Health. 2019;**19**(1):19-25. DOI: 10.1186/s12889-018-6324-6

[5] Toniolo A, Cassani G, Puggioni A, Rossi A, Colombo A, Onodera T, et al. The diabetes pandemic and associated infections: Suggestions for clinical microbiology. Reviews in Medical Microbiology: A Journal of the Pathological Society of Great Britain and Ireland. 2019;**30**(1):1-17. DOI: 10.1097/mrm.0000000000000155

[6] Hodgson K, Morris J, Bridson T, Govan B, Rush C, Ketheesan N. Immunological mechanisms contributing to the double burden of diabetes and intracellular bacterial infections. Immunology. 2015;**144**(2):171-185. DOI: 10.1111/imm.12394

[7] Kumar Nathella P, Babu S. Influence of diabetes mellitus on immunity to human tuberculosis. Immunology. 2017;**152**(1):13-24. DOI: 10.1111/imm.12762

[8] Chiang CY, Bai KJ, Lin HH, Chien ST, Lee JJ, Enarson DA, et al. The influence of diabetes, glycemic control, and diabetes-related comorbidities on pulmonary tuberculosis. PLoS One. 2015;**10**(3):1-15. DOI: 10.1371/journal.pone.0121698

[9] Grieshaber-Bouyer R, Nigrovic PA. Neutrophil heterogeneity as therapeutic opportunity in immune-mediated disease. Frontiers in Immunology. 2019;**10**:1-13. DOI: 10.3389/fimmu.2019.00346

[10] Alvarenga DM, Mattos MS, Araujo AM, Antunes MM, Menezes GB. Neutrophil biology within hepatic environment. Cell and Tissue Research. 2018;**371**(3):589-598. DOI: 10.1007/s00441-017-2722-9

[11] Lerman YV, Kim M. Neutrophil migration under normal and sepsis conditions. Cardiovascular & Hematological Disorders Drug Targets. 2015;**15**(1):19-28. DOI: 10.2174/1871529X15666150108113236

[12] Shen XF, Cao K, Jiang JP, Guan WX, Du JF. Neutrophil dysregulation during sepsis: An overview and update. Journal of Cellular and Molecular Medicine. 2017;**21**(9):1687-1697. DOI: 10.1111/jcmm.13112

[13] Liu L, Sun B. Neutrophil pyroptosis: New perspectives on sepsis. Cellular and Molecular Life Sciences. 2019;**76**:1-10. DOI: 10.1007/s00018-019-03060-1

[14] de Oliveira S, Rosowski EE, Huttenlocher A. Neutrophil migration in infection and wound repair: Going forward in reverse. Nature Reviews. Immunology. 2016;**16**(6):378-391. DOI: 10.1038/nri.2016.49

[15] Rosales C. Neutrophil: A cell with many roles in inflammation or several cell types? Frontiers in Physiology. 2018;9:1-17. DOI: 10.3389/fphys.2018.00113

[16] Maas SL, Soehnlein O, Viola JR. Organ-specific mechanisms of transendothelial neutrophil migration in the lung, liver, kidney, and aorta. Frontiers in Immunology. 2018;9(2739):1-24. DOI: 10.3389/fimmu.2018.02739

[17] Caster DJ, Powell DW, Miralda I, Ward RA, McLeish KR. Re-examining neutrophil participation in GN. Journal of the American Society of Nephrology. 2017;28(8):2275-2289. DOI: 10.1681/ASN.2016121271

[18] Mortaz E, Alipoor SD, Adcock IM, Mumby S, Koenderman L. Update on neutrophil function in severe inflammation. Frontiers in Immunology. 2018;9:1-14. DOI: 10.3389/fimmu.2018.02171

[19] Rios-Santos F, Alves-Filho JC, Souto FO, Spiller F, Freitas A, Lotufo CM, et al. Down-regulation of CXCR2 on neutrophils in severe sepsis is mediated by inducible nitric oxide synthase-derived nitric oxide. American Journal of Respiratory and Critical Care Medicine. 2007;175(5):490-497. DOI: 10.1164/rccm.200601-103OC

[20] Li RHL, Tablin F. A comparative review of neutrophil extracellular traps in sepsis. Frontiers in Veterinary Science. 2018;5:1-11. DOI: 10.3389/fvets.2018.00291

[21] van Kessel KPM, Bestebroer J, van Strijp JAG. Neutrophil-mediated phagocytosis of Staphylococcus aureus. Frontiers in Immunology. 2014;5:1-12. DOI: 10.3389/fimmu.2014.00467

[22] Phan QT, Sipka T, Gonzalez C, Levraud J-P, Lutfalla G, Nguyen-Chi M. Neutrophils use superoxide to control bacterial infection at a distance. PLoS Pathogens. 2018;14(7):1-29. DOI: 10.1371/journal.ppat.1007157

[23] Witter AR, Okunnu BM, Berg RE. The essential role of neutrophils during infection with the intracellular bacterial pathogen Listeria monocytogenes. Journal of Immunology. 2016;197(5):1557-1565. DOI: 10.4049/jimmunol.1600599

[24] Taheri N, Fahlgren A, Fällman M. Yersinia pseudotuberculosis blocks neutrophil degranulation. Infection and Immunity. 2016;84(12):3369-3378. DOI: 10.1128/iai.00760-16

[25] van Dam LS, Rabelink TJ, van Kooten C, Teng YKO. Clinical implications of excessive neutrophil extracellular trap formation in renal autoimmune diseases. Kidney International Reports. 2018;4(2):196-211. DOI: 10.1016/j.ekir.2018.11.005

[26] Gray RD, Hardisty G, Regan KH, Smith M, Robb CT, Duffin R, et al. Delayed neutrophil apoptosis enhances NET formation in cystic fibrosis. Thorax. 2018;73(2):134-144. DOI: 10.1136/thoraxjnl-2017-210134

[27] Behnen M, Möller S, Brozek A, Klinger M, Laskay T. Extracellular acidification inhibits the ROS-dependent formation of neutrophil extracellular traps. Frontiers in Immunology. 2017;8:1-22. DOI: 10.3389/fimmu.2017.00184

[28] Schett G, Neurath MF. Resolution of chronic inflammatory disease: Universal and tissue-specific concepts. Nature Communications. 2018;9(1):1-8. DOI: 10.1038/s41467-018-05800-6

[29] Philippe R, Urbach V. Specialized pro-resolving lipid mediators in cystic fibrosis. International Journal of Molecular Sciences. 2018;19(10):1-11. DOI: 10.3390/ijms19102865

[30] Galvão I, Queiroz-Junior CM, de Oliveira VLS, Pinho V, Hirsch E, Teixeira MM. The inhibition of phosphoinositide-3 kinases induce resolution of inflammation in a gout model. Frontiers in Pharmacology. 2019;**9**:1-10. DOI: 10.3389/fphar.2018.01505

[31] Rahtes A, Geng S, Lee C, Li L. Cellular and molecular mechanisms involved in the resolution of innate leukocyte inflammation. Journal of Leukocyte Biology. 2018;**104**(3):535-541. DOI: 10.1002/jlb.3ma0218-070r

[32] Cartwright JA, Lucas CD, Rossi AG. Inflammation resolution and the induction of granulocyte apoptosis by cyclin-dependent kinase inhibitor drugs. Frontiers in Pharmacology. 2019;**10**:1-18. DOI: 10.3389/fphar.2019.00055

[33] Rossaint J, Margraf A, Zarbock A. Role of platelets in leukocyte recruitment and resolution of inflammation. Frontiers in Immunology. 2018;**9**:1-13. DOI: 10.3389/fimmu.2018.02712

[34] Bang S, Xie Y-K, Zhang Z-J, Wang Z, Xu Z-Z, Ji R-R. GPR37 regulates macrophage phagocytosis and resolution of inflammatory pain. Journal of Clinical Investigation. 2018;**128**(8):3568-3582. DOI: 10.1172/jci99888

[35] Skendros P, Mitroulis I, Ritis K. Autophagy in neutrophils: From granulopoiesis to neutrophil extracellular traps. Frontiers in Cell and Development Biology. 2018;**6**:1-12. DOI: 10.3389/fcell.2018.00109

[36] Prieto P, Rosales-Mendoza CE, Terrón V, Toledano V, Cuadrado A, López-Collazo E, et al. Activation of autophagy in macrophages by pro-resolving lipid mediators. Autophagy. 2015;**11**(10):1729-1744. DOI: 10.1080/15548627.2015.1078958

[37] Knapp S. Diabetes and infection: Is there a link?—A mini-review. Gerontology. 2013;**59**(2):99-104. DOI: 10.1159/000345107

[38] Collier A, Jackson M, Bell D, Patrick AW, Matthews DM, Young RJ, et al. Neutrophil activation detected by increased neutrophil elastase activity in type 1 (insulin-dependent) diabetes mellitus. Diabetes Research. 1989;**10**(3):135-138

[39] Jackson MH, Collier A, Nicoll JJ, Muir AL, Dawes J, Clarke BF, et al. Neutrophil count and activation in vascular disease. Scottish Medical Journal. 1992;**37**(2):41-43. DOI: 10.1177/003693309203700205

[40] Huang J, Xiao Y, Zheng P, Zhou W, Wang Y, Huang G, et al. Distinct neutrophil counts and functions in newly diagnosed type 1 diabetes, latent autoimmune diabetes in adults, and type 2 diabetes. Diabetes/Metabolism Research and Reviews. 2019;**35**(1):1-10. DOI: 10.1002/dmrr.3064

[41] Valle A, Giamporcaro GM, Scavini M, Stabilini A, Grogan P, Bianconi E, et al. Reduction of circulating neutrophils precedes and accompanies type 1 diabetes. Diabetes. 2013;**62**(6):2072-2077. DOI: 10.2337/db12-1345

[42] Battaglia M. Neutrophils and type 1 autoimmune diabetes. Current Opinion in Hematology. 2014;**21**(1):8-15. DOI: 10.1097/MOH.0000000000000008

[43] Huang J, Xiao Y, Xu A, Zhou Z. Neutrophils in type 1 diabetes. Journal of Diabetes Investigation. 2016;**7**(5):652-663. DOI: 10.1111/jdi.12469

[44] Zhang H, Yang Z, Zhang W, Niu Y, Li X, Qin L, et al. White blood cell subtypes and risk of type 2 diabetes. Journal of Diabetes and its

Complications. 2017;**31**(1):31-37. DOI: 10.1016/j.jdiacomp.2016.10.029

[45] Yang M, Liu J, Xu J, Sun T, Sheng L, Chen Z, et al. Elevated systemic neutrophil count is associated with diabetic macroalbuminuria among elderly Chinese. International Journal of Endocrinology. 2015;**2015**:1-6. DOI: 10.1155/2015/348757

[46] Trevelin SC, Carlos D, Beretta M, da Silva JS, Cunha FQ. Diabetes mellitus and sepsis: A challenging association. Shock. 2017;**47**(3):276-287. DOI: 10.1097/SHK.0000000000000778

[47] Ozsoy N, Bostanci H, Ayvali C. The investigation of the ultrastructural neutrophil changes in alloxan-induced diabetes in rats: Response to a chemotactic challenge. Cell Biochemistry and Function. 2004;**22**(2):81-87. DOI: 10.1002/cbf.1059

[48] Spiller F, Carlos D, Souto FO, de Freitas A, Soares FS, Vieira SM, et al. alpha1-Acid glycoprotein decreases neutrophil migration and increases susceptibility to sepsis in diabetic mice. Diabetes. 2012;**61**(6):1584-1591. DOI: 10.2337/db11-0825

[49] Veenstra M, Ransohoff RM. Chemokine receptor CXCR2: Physiology regulator and neuroinflammation controller? Journal of Neuroimmunology. 2012;**246**(1-2):1-9. DOI: 10.1016/j.jneuroim.2012.02.016

[50] Haurogne K, Pavlovic M, Rogniaux H, Bach JM, Lieubeau B. Type 1 diabetes prone NOD mice have diminished Cxcr1 mRNA expression in polymorphonuclear neutrophils and CD4+ T lymphocytes. PLoS One. 2015;**10**(7):1-16. DOI: 10.1371/journal.pone.0134365

[51] Dubey M, Singh AK, Awasthi D, Nagarkoti S, Kumar S, Ali W, et al. L-Plastin S-glutathionylation promotes reduced binding to beta-actin and affects neutrophil functions. Free Radical Biology & Medicine. 2015;**86**:1-15. DOI: 10.1016/j.freeradbiomed.2015.04.008

[52] Arpin M, Friederich E, Algrain M, Vernel F, Louvard D. Functional differences between L- and T-plastin isoforms. The Journal of Cell Biology. 1994;**127**(6 Pt 2):1995-2008

[53] de Oliveira Martins J, Meyer-Pflug AR, Alba-Loureiro TC, Melbostad H, Costa da Cruz JW, Coimbra R, et al. Modulation of lipopolysaccharide-induced acute lung inflammation: Role of insulin. Shock. 2006;**25**(3):260-266. DOI: 10.1097/01.shk.0000194042.18699.b4

[54] Kuwabara WMT, Yokota CNF, Curi R, Alba-Loureiro TC. Obesity and type 2 diabetes mellitus induce lipopolysaccharide tolerance in rat neutrophils. Scientific Reports. 2018;**8**(1):1-13. DOI: 10.1038/s41598-018-35809-2

[55] Schuetz P, Castro P, Shapiro NI. Diabetes and sepsis: Preclinical findings and clinical relevance. Diabetes Care. 2011;**34**(3):771-778. DOI: 10.2337/dc10-1185

[56] Wierusz-Wysocka B, Wysocki H, Wykretowicz A, Klimas R. The influence of increasing glucose concentrations on selected functions of polymorphonuclear neutrophils. Acta Diabetologica Latina. 1988;**25**(4):283-288

[57] Walrand S, Guillet C, Boirie Y, Vasson MP. Insulin differentially regulates monocyte and polymorphonuclear neutrophil functions in healthy young and elderly humans. The Journal of Clinical Endocrinology and Metabolism. 2006;**91**(7):2738-2748. DOI: 10.1210/jc.2005-1619

[58] Cavalot F, Anfossi G, Russo I, Mularoni E, Massucco P, Burzacca S, et al. Insulin, at physiological concentrations, enhances the polymorphonuclear leukocyte chemotactic properties. Hormone and Metabolic Research. 1992;**24**(5):225-228. DOI: 10.1055/s-2007-1003298

[59] Oldenborg PA, Sehlin J. Insulin-stimulated chemokinesis in normal human neutrophils is dependent on D-glucose concentration and sensitive to inhibitors of tyrosine kinase and phosphatidylinositol 3-kinase. Journal of Leukocyte Biology. 1998;**63**(2):203-208

[60] Oldenborg PA, Sehlin J. Hyperglycemia in vitro attenuates insulin-stimulated chemokinesis in normal human neutrophils. Role of protein kinase C activation. Journal of Leukocyte Biology. 1999;**65**(5):635-640

[61] Okouchi M, Okayama N, Imai S, Omi H, Shimizu M, Fukutomi T, et al. High insulin enhances neutrophil transendothelial migration through increasing surface expression of platelet endothelial cell adhesion molecule-1 via activation of mitogen activated protein kinase. Diabetologia. 2002;**45**(10):1449-1456. DOI: 10.1007/s00125-002-0902-x

[62] Toure F, Zahm JM, Garnotel R, Lambert E, Bonnet N, Schmidt AM, et al. Receptor for advanced glycation end-products (RAGE) modulates neutrophil adhesion and migration on glycoxidated extracellular matrix. The Biochemical Journal. 2008;**416**(2):255-261. DOI: 10.1042/BJ20080054

[63] Singh VP, Bali A, Singh N, Jaggi AS. Advanced glycation end products and diabetic complications. The Korean Journal of Physiology & Pharmacology. 2014;**18**(1):1-14. DOI: 10.4196/kjpp.2014.18.1.1

[64] Collison KS, Parhar RS, Saleh SS, Meyer BF, Kwaasi AA, Hammami MM, et al. RAGE-mediated neutrophil dysfunction is evoked by advanced glycation end products (AGEs). Journal of Leukocyte Biology. 2002;**71**(3):433-444. DOI: 10.1189/jlb.71.3.433

[65] Sannomiya P, Oliveira MA, Fortes ZB. Aminoguanidine and the prevention of leukocyte dysfunction in diabetes mellitus: A direct vital microscopic study. British Journal of Pharmacology. 1997;**122**(5):894-898. DOI: 10.1038/sj.bjp.0701448

[66] Tian M, Qing C, Niu Y, Dong J, Cao X, Song F, et al. Effect of aminoguanidine intervention on neutrophils in diabetes inflammatory cells wound healing. Experimental and Clinical Endocrinology & Diabetes. 2013;**121**(10):635-642. DOI: 10.1055/s-0033-1351331

[67] Adela R, Nethi SK, Bagul PK, Barui AK, Mattapally S, Kuncha M, et al. Hyperglycaemia enhances nitric oxide production in diabetes: A study from south Indian patients. PLoS One. 2015;**10**(4):1-17. DOI: 10.1371/journal.pone.0125270

[68] Assmann TS, Brondani LA, Boucas AP, Rheinheimer J, de Souza BM, Canani LH, et al. Nitric oxide levels in patients with diabetes mellitus: A systematic review and meta-analysis. Nitric Oxide. 2016;**61**:1-9. DOI: 10.1016/j.niox.2016.09.009

[69] Nolan S, Dixon R, Norman K, Hellewell P, Ridger V. Nitric oxide regulates neutrophil migration through microparticle formation. The American Journal of Pathology. 2008;**172**(1):265-273. DOI: 10.2353/ajpath.2008.070069

[70] Benjamim CF, Ferreira SH, Cunha FQ. Role of nitric oxide in the failure of neutrophil migration in sepsis. The Journal of Infectious Diseases. 2000;**182**(1):214-223. DOI: 10.1086/315682

[71] Hochepied T, Berger FG, Baumann H, Libert C. Alpha(1)-acid glycoprotein: An acute phase protein with inflammatory and immunomodulating properties. Cytokine & Growth Factor Reviews. 2003;**14**(1):25-34. DOI: 10.1016/S1359-6101(02)00054-0

[72] Laine E, Couderc R, Roch-Arveiller M, Vasson MP, Giroud JP, Raichvarg D. Modulation of human polymorphonuclear neutrophil functions by alpha 1-acid glycoprotein. Inflammation. 1990;**14**(1):1-9

[73] Mestriner FL, Spiller F, Laure HJ, Souto FO, Tavares-Murta BM, Rosa JC, et al. Acute-phase protein alpha-1-acid glycoprotein mediates neutrophil migration failure in sepsis by a nitric oxide-dependent mechanism. Proceedings of the National Academy of Sciences of the United States of America. 2007;**104**(49):19595-19600. DOI: 10.1073/pnas.0709681104

[74] Carlos D, Spiller F, Souto FO, Trevelin SC, Borges VF, de Freitas A, et al. Histamine h2 receptor signaling in the pathogenesis of sepsis: Studies in a murine diabetes model. Journal of Immunology. 2013;**191**(3):1373-1382. DOI: 10.4049/jimmunol.1202907

[75] Bury TB, Corhay JL, Radermecker MF. Histamine-induced inhibition of neutrophil chemotaxis and T-lymphocyte proliferation in man. Allergy. 1992;**47**(6):624-629

[76] Patel L, Buckels AC, Kinghorn IJ, Murdock PR, Holbrook JD, Plumpton C, et al. Resistin is expressed in human macrophages and directly regulated by PPAR gamma activators. Biochemical and Biophysical Research Communications. 2003;**300**(2):472-476. DOI: 10.1016/S0006-291X(02)02841-3

[77] Kusminski CM, McTernan PG, Kumar S. Role of resistin in obesity, insulin resistance and type II diabetes.

Clinical Science. 2005;**109**(3):243-256. DOI: 10.1042/CS20050078

[78] Cohen G, Ilic D, Raupachova J, Horl WH. Resistin inhibits essential functions of polymorphonuclear leukocytes. Journal of Immunology. 2008;**181**(6):3761-3768. DOI: 10.4049/jimmunol.181.6.3761

[79] Hodges SK, Teague AM, Dasari PS, Short KR. Effect of obesity and type 2 diabetes, and glucose ingestion on circulating spexin concentration in adolescents. Pediatric Diabetes. 2018;**19**(2):212-216. DOI: 10.1111/pedi.12549

[80] Hatanaka E, Monteagudo PT, Marrocos MS, Campa A. Neutrophils and monocytes as potentially important sources of proinflammatory cytokines in diabetes. Clinical and Experimental Immunology. 2006;**146**(3):443-447. DOI: 10.1111/j.1365-2249.2006.03229.x

[81] Chao WC, Yen CL, Wu YH, Chen SY, Hsieh CY, Chang TC, et al. Increased resistin may suppress reactive oxygen species production and inflammasome activation in type 2 diabetic patients with pulmonary tuberculosis infection. Microbes and Infection. 2015;**17**(3):195-204. DOI: 10.1016/j.micinf.2014.11.009

[82] Wykretowicz A, Wierusz-Wysocka B, Wysocki J, Szczepanik A, Wysocki H. Impairment of the oxygen-dependent microbicidal mechanisms of polymorphonuclear neutrophils in patients with type 2 diabetes is not associated with increased susceptibility to infection. Diabetes Research and Clinical Practice. 1993;**19**(3):195-201. DOI: 10.1016/0168-8227(93)90114-K

[83] Gyurko R, Siqueira CC, Caldon N, Gao L, Kantarci A, Van Dyke TE. Chronic hyperglycemia predisposes to exaggerated inflammatory response and leukocyte dysfunction in Akita mice. Journal of Immunology.

2006;**177**(10):7250-7256. DOI: 10.4049/jimmunol.177.10.7250

[84] Zamakhchari MF, Sima C, Sama K, Fine N, Glogauer M, Van Dyke TE, et al. Lack of p47(phox) in akita diabetic mice is associated with interstitial pneumonia, fibrosis, and oral inflammation. The American Journal of Pathology. 2016;**186**(3):659-670. DOI: 10.1016/j.ajpath.2015.10.026

[85] Singer M, Deutschman CS, Seymour CW, Shankar-Hari M, Annane D, Bauer M, et al. The third international consensus definitions for sepsis and septic shock (sepsis-3). Journal of the American Medical Association. 2016;**315**(8):801-810. DOI: 10.1001/jama.2016.0287

[86] Crosara-Alberto DP, Darini AL, Inoue RY, Silva JS, Ferreira SH, Cunha FQ. Involvement of NO in the failure of neutrophil migration in sepsis induced by *Staphylococcus aureus*. British Journal of Pharmacology. 2002;**136**(5):645-658. DOI: 10.1038/sj.bjp.0704734

[87] Arraes SM, Freitas MS, da Silva SV, de Paula Neto HA, Alves-Filho JC, Auxiliadora Martins M, et al. Impaired neutrophil chemotaxis in sepsis associates with GRK expression and inhibition of actin assembly and tyrosine phosphorylation. Blood. 2006;**108**(9):2906-2913. DOI: 10.1182/blood-2006-05-024638

[88] Shah BR, Hux JE. Quantifying the risk of infectious diseases for people with diabetes. Diabetes Care. 2003;**26**(2):510-513. DOI: 10.2337/diacare.26.2.510

[89] Filgueiras LR Jr, Martins JO, Serezani CH, Capelozzi VL, Montes MB, Jancar S. Sepsis-induced acute lung injury (ALI) is milder in diabetic rats and correlates with impaired NFkB activation. PLoS One. 2012;7(9):1-9. DOI: 10.1371/journal.pone.0044987

[90] Frydrych LM, Bian G, Fattahi F, Morris SB, O'Rourke RW, Lumeng CN, et al. GM-CSF Administration improves defects in innate immunity and sepsis survival in obese diabetic mice. Journal of Immunology. 2019;**202**(3):931-942. DOI: 10.4049/jimmunol.1800713

[91] Hanses F, Park S, Rich J, Lee JC. Reduced neutrophil apoptosis in diabetic mice during staphylococcal infection leads to prolonged Tnfalpha production and reduced neutrophil clearance. PLoS One. 2011;**6**(8):1-10. DOI: 10.1371/journal.pone.0023633

[92] Jeon CY, Murray MB. Diabetes mellitus increases the risk of active tuberculosis: A systematic review of 13 observational studies. PLoS Medicine. 2008;**5**(7):1091-1101. DOI: 10.1371/journal.pmed.0050152

[93] Andrade BB, Kumar NP, Sridhar R, Banurekha VV, Jawahar MS, Nutman TB, et al. Heightened plasma levels of heme oxygenase-1 and tissue inhibitor of metalloproteinase-4 as well as elevated peripheral neutrophil counts are associated with TB-diabetes comorbidity. Chest. 2014;**145**(6):1244-1254. DOI: 10.1378/chest.13-1799

[94] Prada-Medina CA, Fukutani KF, Pavan Kumar N, Gil-Santana L, Babu S, Lichtenstein F, et al. Systems immunology of diabetes-tuberculosis comorbidity reveals signatures of disease complications. Scientific Reports. 2017;**7**(1):1-16. DOI: 10.1038/s41598-017-01767-4

[95] Raposo-Garcia S, Guerra-Laso JM, Garcia-Garcia S, Juan-Garcia J, Lopez-Fidalgo E, Diez-Tascon C, et al. Immunological response to mycobacterium tuberculosis infection in blood from type 2 diabetes patients. Immunology Letters. 2017;**186**:41-45. DOI: 10.1016/j.imlet.2017.03.017

[96] Podell BK, Ackart DF, Obregon-Henao A, Eck SP, Henao-Tamayo M,

Richardson M, et al. Increased severity of tuberculosis in Guinea pigs with type 2 diabetes: A model of diabetes-tuberculosis comorbidity. The American Journal of Pathology. 2014;**184**(4):1104-1118. DOI: 10.1016/j.ajpath.2013.12.015

[97] Cheekatla SS, Tripathi D, Venkatasubramanian S, Nathella PK, Paidipally P, Ishibashi M, et al. NK-CD11c+ cell crosstalk in diabetes enhances IL-6-mediated inflammation during mycobacterium tuberculosis infection. PLoS Pathogens. 2016;**12**(10):1-24. DOI: 10.1371/journal.ppat.1005972

[98] Joshi N, Caputo GM, Weitekamp MR, Karchmer AW. Infections in patients with diabetes mellitus. The New England Journal of Medicine. 1999;**341**(25):1906-1912. DOI: 10.1056/NEJM199912163412507

[99] Torres A, Blasi F, Dartois N, Akova M. Which individuals are at increased risk of pneumococcal disease and why? Impact of COPD, asthma, smoking, diabetes, and/or chronic heart disease on community-acquired pneumonia and invasive pneumococcal disease. Thorax. 2015;**70**(10):984-989. DOI: 10.1136/thoraxjnl-2015-206780

[100] Koh GC, Peacock SJ, van der Poll T, Wiersinga WJ. The impact of diabetes on the pathogenesis of sepsis. European Journal of Clinical Microbiology & Infectious Diseases. 2012;**31**(4):379-388. DOI: 10.1007/s10096-011-1337-4

[101] Martinez N, Ketheesan N, Martens GW, West K, Lien E, Kornfeld H. Defects in early cell recruitment contribute to the increased susceptibility to respiratory Klebsiella pneumoniae infection in diabetic mice. Microbes and Infection. 2016;**18**(10):649-655. DOI: 10.1016/j.micinf.2016.05.007

[102] Siu LK, Yeh KM, Lin JC, Fung CP, Chang FY. Klebsiella pneumoniae liver abscess: A new invasive syndrome. The Lancet Infectious Diseases. 2012;**12**(11):881-887. DOI: 10.1016/S1473-3099(12)70205-0

[103] Dovi JV, He LK, DiPietro LA. Accelerated wound closure in neutrophil-depleted mice. Journal of Leukocyte Biology. 2003;**73**(4):448-455. DOI: 10.1189/jlb.0802406

[104] Fadini GP, Menegazzo L, Rigato M, Scattolini V, Poncina N, Bruttocao A, et al. NETosis delays diabetic wound healing in mice and humans. Diabetes. 2016;**65**(4):1061-1071. DOI: 10.2337/db15-0863

[105] Wong SL, Demers M, Martinod K, Gallant M, Wang Y, Goldfine AB, et al. Diabetes primes neutrophils to undergo NETosis, which impairs wound healing. Nature Medicine. 2015;**21**(7):815-819. DOI: 10.1038/nm.3887

[106] Yates C, May K, Hale T, Allard B, Rowlings N, Freeman A, et al. Wound chronicity, inpatient care, and chronic kidney disease predispose to MRSA infection in diabetic foot ulcers. Diabetes Care. 2009;**32**(10):1907-1909. DOI: 10.2337/dc09-0295

[107] Joshi MB, Lad A, Bharath Prasad AS, Balakrishnan A, Ramachandra L, Satyamoorthy K. High glucose modulates IL-6 mediated immune homeostasis through impeding neutrophil extracellular trap formation. FEBS Letters. 2013;**587**(14):2241-2246. DOI: 10.1016/j.febslet.2013.05.053

[108] Riyapa D, Buddhisa S, Korbsrisate S, Cuccui J, Wren BW, Stevens MP, et al. Neutrophil extracellular traps exhibit antibacterial activity against burkholderia pseudomallei and are influenced by bacterial and host factors. Infection and Immunity. 2012;**80**(11):3921-3929. DOI: 10.1128/IAI.00806-12

[109] You Q , He DM, Shu GF, Cao B, Xia YQ , Xing Y, et al. Increased formation of neutrophil extracellular traps is associated with gut leakage in patients with type 1 but not type 2 diabetes. Journal of Diabetes. 2018:1-9. DOI: 10.1111/1753-0407.12892

[110] Yano H, Kinoshita M, Fujino K, Nakashima M, Yamamoto Y, Miyazaki H, et al. Insulin treatment directly restores neutrophil phagocytosis and bactericidal activity in diabetic mice and thereby improves surgical site *Staphylococcus aureus* infection. Infection and Immunity. 2012;**80**(12):4409-4416. DOI: 10.1128/IAI.00787-12

# 7

# Resident Memory T Cells

*Hasan Akbaba*

## Abstract

Until recently, T cells were thought to remain in circulation until recruitment of the inflammation and only a small number of T cells remained in the peripheral tissues without inflammation. However, studies have found that a group of T cells settled in the tissues and remained there for a long time. Those cells are named as tissue-resident memory T cells (TRM). TRM cells are transcriptionally, phenotypically, and functionally distinct from other T cells, which recirculate between blood, secondary lymphoid organs, and non-lymphoid tissues. They undergo a distinct proliferation that discriminates them from circulating T cells and their main cell surface markers are CD69, CD103, and CD49a. Upon exposure to the same or similar diseases, TRM cells provide a first line of adaptive cellular defense against infection in peripheral non-lymphoid tissues, such as skin, lungs, digestive, and urogenital tracts. This approach forms the basis of a novel vaccination strategy called "prime and pull", which ensures long-term local immunity. On the other hand, abnormal activated and malignant TRM may contribute to numerous human inflammatory diseases such as psoriasis and vitiligo. Here in this chapter, we aimed to emphasize TRM cell location, migration, phenotypic structure, maintenance, and diseases associated with TRM cells.

**Keywords:** resident memory T cell, CD8+ TRM, CD69, CD103, CD49a, prime and pull, autoreactive human disease

## 1. Introduction

Tissue-resident memory T cells were discovered about a decade ago. Before the discovery of TRM cells and acceptance as a new subset of T cell, memory T cells have been subdivided into two populations: effector memory and central memory T cell [1, 2]. Traditionally, it was thought that T cells taken into the tissues during infection and leave the tissue after the pathogen clearance or undergo apoptosis [3]. However, at the beginning of this millennium, it was observed that some CD8+ T cells remain long-term in the tissues after infection.

The discovery of antigen-specific CD8+ T cells located in the lung after influenza virus infection was the first example of phenomenon [4]. Later, this finding was also observed in other non-lymphoid tissues after infections with Listeria and vesicular stomatitis virus [5, 6]. Eventually, TRM cells have been described in almost all organs and can be either CD4+ or CD8+ but tissue residency has been predominantly described for memory CD8+ T cells [7]. The term "TRM cells" were used to refer to CD8+ cells, unless otherwise specified in this chapter.

The retention of TRM cells is based on two mechanisms. First, TRM cells do not express lymph node homing molecules, which are required for tissue exit such as CD62L, CCR7, and S1PR1. Second TRM cells express adhesion molecules to their host tissue such as CD103 and CD49a [8–12]. Not all of these markers are essential for TRM identification and function of many of them are still not fully understood.

The major function of TRM cells is to establish frontline defense against previously encountered pathogens in barrier tissues where they first encounter [13, 14]. Due to their robust systemic responses, TRM cells provide superior protection compared with circulating memory T cells in peripheral tissues [15–17]. However, dysregulation of TRM can contribute to human autoimmune and inflammatory diseases such as psoriasis, vitiligo, and multiple sclerosis [18–20].

In this chapter, we aimed to emphasize TRM cell location, migration, phenotypic structure, maintenance, and diseases associated with TRM cells. We discuss the TRM cells in a basic and perceptible form as a whole, where there is no unity due to a large number of tissue variations use. We have reviewed the subject not only on the molecular level, but also on the perspective of disease formation and therapeutic usage.

## 2. Location

T cells can be distinguished based to their microenvironment or their location in the host tissues and thereby it is possible to classify them as TRM cells or other T cell subsets [21–23]. TRM cells are easily identified in the tissues that have direct exposure to the pathogens such as the gut, skin, lungs, and reproductive system, where they receive signals that are required for their unique development program from these microenvironments [20, 24–27].

TRM cells have different phenotypes that show heterogeneity depending on the host tissue microenvironment. Requirement for TRM generation, proliferation, migration, and maintenance vary in different kind of tissues [9, 25, 26]. In particular, the majority of TRM cells are CD8+ memory T cells, and the TRM cell population in the skin is known as CD103+ and Cd69+. However, CD4+ TRM cell populations have been identified in the skin, lungs, reproductive tract, and salivary glands. Similar to CD8 TRM cells, they express the surface molecules CD69 but expression of CD103 is low or negative [28–31]. These requirements will be detailed below according to tissue types.

The locations of the TRM cell can be classified according to host tissues as shown in **Figure 1**.

The skin is one of the primary barrier tissues against infectious agents. Epidermis, dermis, and subcutaneous fatty region form a 3-layer structure of the skin and

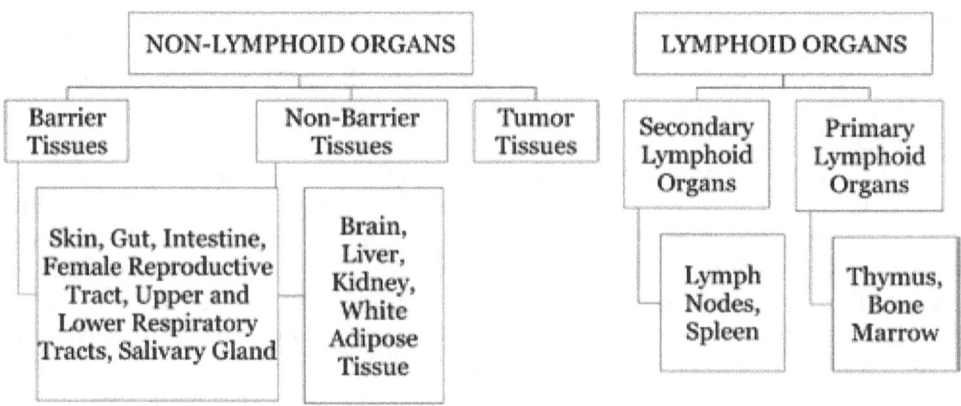

**Figure 1.**
*Classification of TRM cell locations according to their host tissue.*

TRM formation has been shown in all layers [32–34]. The skin has very complex cell populations and hosts both natural and adaptive immune system cells. These immune system cells provide a biological barrier to invasive pathogens. CD8+ TRM constitutes the majority of the memory T cell population in the epidermis. CD8+ TRM cells are commonly resident in the skin and their numbers increase rapidly when they are exposed with the infectious agents. Skin TRM cells may easily characterized due to their surface markers such as marker CD69, CD103, and CD49a [9, 27, 35]. These markers and others will be described in detail in terms of their function.

The intestinal mucosa consists of a layer of single epithelial cells and provides a barrier tissue against infectious agents. This layer is also considered as an immunological site for the maintenance of TRM cells. Following intestinal infections, a significant number of pathogen-specific TRM cells have been shown to form in the intraepithelial compartment [36, 37].

The female reproductive tract (FRT) is another organ that is directly exposed to external pathogens. FGT can be divided into two parts. Upper female reproductive tract consists of endometrium and endocervix and lower FRT consists of vagina and ectocervix. FRT is a variable tissue that undergoes significant cyclic changes in women. Under the control of estrogen and progesterone hormones, growth, differentiation, and degeneration occurs periodically [38, 39]. Although this suggests that anatomical sites are limited for the localization of TRM cells, it has been showed that numerous immune system cells, including memory T cells are present throughout FRT. Generation of FRT TRM cells is a promising vaccination strategy against HSV-2, and potentially against other sexually transmitted infections such as HIV and HPV [16, 39, 40].

Respiratory tract (RT) is also a structure which is directly exposed to external pathogens. RT can also be divided into two parts as upper (URT) and lower (LRT). Most common airborne pathogens in humans primarily infect URT [41, 42]. URT contains lymph nodes known as tonsils, which contain B cell follicles and T cell subsets. URT is considered a mucosal inductive region for humoral and cellular immune responses. Although the effector CD4+ T cells predominate the tonsils, the presence and the localization of TRM cells is also shown in the lungs [15, 43].

Salivary glands are exocrine epithelial tissues, which are the targets of viral infections. The presence of TRM cells in these tissues has also been shown in various studies [28, 44].

The liver is an organ, which is the member of the immune system. Through the portal vein, antigen-rich blood enters the liver and encounters the immune system cells that are resident in the tissue [22, 45, 46]. Studies have shown that CD8+ TRM cells are established in the liver especially after systemic infection or vaccination [47, 48].

Due to the presence of a blood-brain barrier, immune cells are not thought to be resident in the central nervous system [49]. However, after clearing a viral infection in the central nervous system, some of the antigen-specific CD8+ T cells maintained in the brain as TRM cells [50].

The kidney has a very high amount of blood vessels and has a very high circulating volume. This helps to eliminate toxins from the body. Therefore, healthy kidneys are not suitable tissues for the localization of immune system cells. Even so, it has been shown that a small number of resident TRM cells may be present in the kidney. White adipose tissue is another tissue in which TRM cells have been shown to be resident and they act as a reservoir of TRM cells [51–53].

CD8+ TRM cells have been reported in solid tumors [54]. Studies have shown that infiltrating T lymphocytes (TIL) are phenotypically similar to TRM cells that TRM cells from neighboring peripheral tissues could infiltrate into solid tumors [55, 56]. It was found that presence of CD8+ TRM cells is associated with good prognosis in various cancers [57].

Secondary lymphoid organs and lymph nodes are the tissues where TCM and TEM cells are more common and pass through. However, recent studies have shown that a small number of non-circulating memory T cells are present in these tissues. TRM cells in SLO show phenotypic characterization similar to those in non-lymphoid tissues [1, 58].

Primary lymphoid organs (PLO) are bone marrow and thymus. Antigen-specific TRM cells have also been found in these tissues and have been shown to facilitate long-term maintenance in the PLO. TRM cells in the PLO express CD69 and CD103 as a characteristic of TRM phenotype [59–61].

## 3. Migration

Circulation of T cell in the blood, secondary lymphoid organs, and non-lymphoid tissues is a complex system. Numerous receptors, ligands, chemokines, cytokines, and transcription factors has a role on this [31, 32]. T cells can be classified according to the organs or tissues in which they recirculate. Schematic illustration for migration of T cell subsets is shown in **Figure 2**.

- Naive T cells: recirculate in the blood, secondary lymphoid organs, and non-lymphoid tissues [62, 63].

- Effector memory T cells: recirculate in the blood, secondary lymphoid organs, and non-lymphoid tissues, same as naive T cells.

- Central memory T cells: recirculate between nonlymphoid tissues, lymph, and lymph nodes [64, 65].

- Tissue-resident memory T cells: do not recirculate between blood, secondary lymphoid organs, nonlymphoid tissues, but may migrate within the tissue it settled [8, 11, 66, 67].

CC-chemokine receptor 7 (CCR7), CD69, CD49, S1PR1, KLF2, and integrins are the main factors responsible for the migration of T cell subsets. The role of these factors may differ depending on the location of the host tissue [68, 69]. These will be further explained in more detail in phenotype and localization parts.

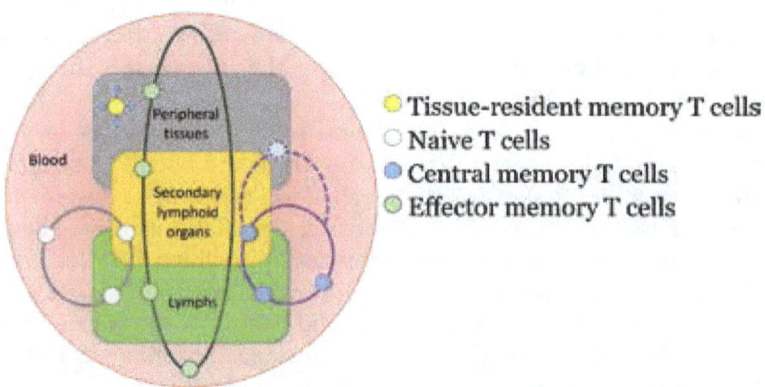

**Figure 2.**
*Schematic illustration of circulation and migration of T cell subsets.*

## 4. TRM markers

In order to distinguish TRM cells from other T cell subsets, in most of the studies in both mice and humans, identification markers such as CD103, CD69, Cd49a, and CD44 have been widely investigated.

### 4.1 CD103

αEβ7 integrin (CD103) was first discovered in the late 1980s. After that several new monoclonal antibodies were produced as a specific marker for intestinal intraepithelial T cells in humans, mice, and rats, presumably contributing to their tissue-specific localization [70]. Integrins are transmembrane αβ heterodimers that bind to extracellular matrix components and to cellular counter receptors. They have important roles on cell localization, migration, and signaling and are important for T lymphocyte adhesion and stimulation [71].

Following the discovery of the ligand called E-cadherin, interest in CD103 has been increased considerably. E-cadherin is a transmembrane protein with an extracellular region containing extracellular cadherin domain repeats, which mediates cell-cell adhesion by homodimerizing in trans with E-cadherin domains of neighboring cells [72].

CD103 is important in adhesion as well as T cell activation and TGF-B induced defense in tumor microenvironment. In TGF-B environment, CD103 TRM cells have been shown to release more efficient granzyme. Although CD103 is an important marker, CD103 alone is not sufficient to detect TRM cells. CD103 negative TRM cells were found in several tissues. Furthermore, there are different types of CD103 T cells such as CD4 CD103 T cells and CD8 CD103 Treg cells.

### 4.2 CD69

CD8+ TRM cells can be characterized by their expression of the surface molecules CD69 and CD103. These markers are usually not expressed on circulation T cells [73]. CD69 is a type II C-lectin membrane receptor with a scarce expression in resting lymphocytes that is rapidly induced upon cell activation [74]. Because of these features, CD69 was considered as early activation antigen of immune cells. However, recent studies have shown that this molecule is an important indicator of TRM differentiation as well as activation of the immune response.

CD69 has been found to suppress the activity of sphingosine-1 phosphate receptor 1 (S1P1), helping the TRM cells that remain in peripheral tissues [75]. The S1P1 receptor/gene, originally known as endothelial differentiation gene 1, acts by binding with a bioactive signaling molecule S1P1 [76]. It was suggested that CD69 expression might help retaining TRM cells in peripheral tissues by suppressing the activity of S1P1. Decreased expression of transcription factor of KLF2 is another factor affecting S1P1 expression to remain down-regulated in TRM cells [77, 78].

Moreover, CD69 expression is not limited to TRM cells and is not essential for TRM formation. CD69 has also been shown to be expressed in cells such as natural killer cells, dendritic cells, and in the absence of CD69, TRM formation decreased but is not completely eliminated [32, 79]. Therefore, CD69 is a good TRM marker, but it is not sufficient to be the sole determinant.

### 4.3 CD49a

CD49a or integrin α1 paired with CD29 (integrin-β1) to form very late antigen (VLA-1). VLA-1 is a collagen-binding integrin and receptor for collagen and laminin such as ColIV and ColI [9, 80, 81].

Collagen IV enriched in the basement membrane separating epidermis and dermis. CD49a is therefore a good marker for skin TRM cells. In human skin epithelia, CD8+ CD49a+ TRM cells produced interferon-γ, whereas CD8+ CD49a TRM cells produced interleukin-17 (IL-17). It has been reported that CD8+ T cells with a TRM phenotypes (CD103+ and CD49a+) are present in solid tumors as well as lung interstitium [9, 35, 82].

VLA1 is a receptor not only involved in adhesion but also to migration and survival. In the formation and proliferation of TRM cells, CD49a together with CD103 and CD69 are the most determinative markers of TRM presence.

## 4.4 CD44

The CD44 antigen is a cell-surface glycoprotein involved in cell-cell interactions, cell adhesion, and migration [83]. The most well-studied function of CD44 is as a receptor for hyaluronic acid, a component of the extracellular matrix. In regard to accessing peripheral tissues during an immune challenge, CD44 can bind hyaluronic acid expressed on vascular endothelial cells and facilitate transmigration. CD44 is a classical marker of previous activation, expressed on newly generated effector cells as well as resting memory cells [23, 84, 85].

It is important to specify that TRM cells express different markers depending on the host tissues. It should not be ignored that there may be some differences between TRM subsets in various tissue types. The results obtained by using in vivo techniques such as parabiosis, organ transplantation, using transgenic mice, and bone marrow chimera techniques were more effective in the identification TRM cell proliferation. The main factors that enable scientists to identify TRM cells as a subset of T cells have been obtained by these methods.

### 4.4.1 Parabiosis

Parabiosis is a surgical process that allows the sharing of blood circulation in two organisms. Bringing the skin of the two animals, in particular mice, together stimulate the capillary blood vessel formation in this region. Blood and immune cells circulate between parabiotic partners [86]. Therefore, migration or residence can be examined by investigating whether the immune system cell in one organism is in equilibrium with the other.

### 4.4.2 Bone marrow chimera (BMC)

BMC is another widely used technique to study donor organism, which has congenitally distinctive or labeled bone marrow, and a recipient organism, which have been irradiated, thus losing its all bone marrow-derived cells (lymphocytes) are two component of this method. Then, bone marrow cells of donor organism are transferred to the recipient organism [87, 88].

### 4.4.3 Organ transplantation

Transplantation is a similar approach to BMC in TRM cell studies. In this method, organ or skin graft of the donor organism is transplanted into the recipient. The equilibrium between the established T cell populations of donor and recipient organisms are examined to investigate the TRM cells. Moreover, TRM cells have important roles in organ transplantation and tissue rejection [89, 90].

### 4.4.4 Transgenic organism

Transgenic organisms are widely used in TRM studies. Numerous studies have been performed using knockout mice where proteins involved in tissue localization or tissue exit cannot be expressed [32, 57, 91, 92].

## 5. Phenotype

There is not a single phenotypic character to be used to identify TRM cells. Many researchers have examined the TRM cell phenotype in different tissues including lungs, liver, lymphoid sites, skin, and intestines both in mice and humans.

Characteristically, TRM cells express CD103 and CD69. CD49a, which binds to the extracellular collagen and laminin, can be added to these two for the skin tissue [21, 23, 93]. TRM cells do not express or express very low levels of lymph node homing molecules which are required for tissue exit such as CD62L, CCR7, and S1PR1 and it is critical for TRM cell tissue residency [1, 15, 53, 67, 69]. S1P1 is mediated by the downregulation of the transcription factor KLF2 [93].

TRM cells also express cluster of chemokines and chemokine receptors including CXCR3 and CCR6, and was able to produce chemokine ligands such as CCL19 andCCL21 [2, 93, 94].

Tissue microenvironment also promotes TRM differentiation. TRM precursors that are KLRG1 negative, are more likely to differentiate into TRM cells [53, 55].

Broad range of transcription factors is associated with TRM formation. Most common transcription factors are AHR (aryl hydrocarbon receptor), Notch, Blimb1, Hobit, Eomes, and T-bet [30, 95]. These phenotypic structures are illustrated in **Figure 3** and each is described in detail in **Table 1**.

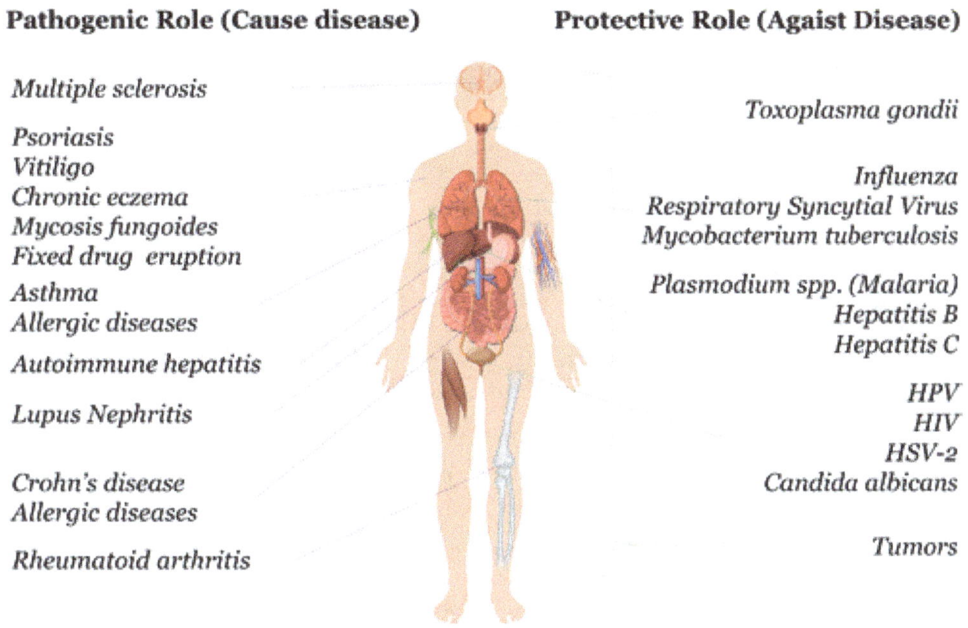

| Pathogenic Role (Cause disease) | Protective Role (Agaist Disease) |
|---|---|
| Multiple sclerosis | Toxoplasma gondii |
| Psoriasis | |
| Vitiligo | Influenza |
| Chronic eczema | Respiratory Syncytial Virus |
| Mycosis fungoides | Mycobacterium tuberculosis |
| Fixed drug eruption | |
| Asthma | Plasmodium spp. (Malaria) |
| Allergic diseases | Hepatitis B |
| | Hepatitis C |
| Autoimmune hepatitis | |
| | HPV |
| Lupus Nephritis | HIV |
| | HSV-2 |
| Crohn's disease | Candida albicans |
| Allergic diseases | |
| Rheumatoid arthritis | Tumors |

**Figure 3.**
*Schematic illustration of some of the most common, receptors, transcription factors, ligands, and molecules involved in differentiation and maintenance of TRM cells and their regulation for TRM formation.*

| Marker | Function | Regulation |
|---|---|---|
| CD103 (integrin αEβ7) | CD103 is as a receptor for E-cadherin, an adherent junctional protein interlocking epithelial cells [96] | ↑ |
| CD49a (integrin α1β1) | CD49a pairs with CD29 (integrin β1) to form the heterodimer called VLA-1 which is a collagen-binding integrin [35] | ↑ |
| CD69 | Human transmembrane C-Type lectin protein. CD69 is a lymphoid activation antigen whose rapid expression makes it amenable for the early detection of T-cell activation and for subset activation analyses [97] | ↑ |
| Krüppel-like Factor 2 (KLF2) | Klf2 also plays a role in T-cell differentiation and regulate the migration of mature thymocytes from the thymus and to control the circulation of peripheral T cells. In the absence of Klf2, mature T cells exist in an activated state and are more prone to apoptosis [98] | ↓ |
| Ki67 | Function of the Ki67 protein is still unclear. Ki67 protein has been widely used as a proliferation marker that is expressed by cells mitotic phases [99–101] | ↓ |
| Killer cell lectin-like receptor subfamily G member 1 (KLRG1) | KLRG1 is expressed by NK and T-cell subsets and recognizes members of the classical cadherin family. KLRG1 is widely used as a lymphocyte differentiation marker in both humans and mice [102] | ↑ |
| C-C chemokine receptor type 7 (CCR7) | CCR7 is a chemokine receptor which regulates T cell trafficking and compartmentalization within secondary lymphoid organs [103] | ↓ |
| Sphingosine-1-phosphate receptor 1 (S1PR1) | S1PR1 was implicated in lymphocyte trafficking and it has an important role in regulating endothelial cell cytoskeletal structure, migration, and T cell maturation [104] | ↓ |
| Chemokine receptor 3 (CXCR3) | CXCR3 plays a role to regulate leukocyte trafficking. Ligand that binds to CXCR3 induces cellular responses, such as integrin activation, cytoskeletal changes and chemotactic migration [94] | ↑ |
| CD62L (L-selectin) | L-selectin is an adhesion molecule that regulates both the migration of leukocytes at sites of inflammation and the recirculation of lymphocytes between blood and lymphoid tissues [105] | ↓ |
| Chemokine ligand 21 (CCL21) | CCL21 is a high affinity functional ligand for chemokine receptor 7 [106] | ↓ |
| Eomesodermin (Eomes) and T-bet | Downregulation of T-bet and Eomes enables increased TGF-β responsiveness, thereby creating a feedback loop that promotes TRM differentiation [30] | ↓ |
| Blimp-1 and Hobit | Loss incompatible with development of tissue-resident cell types; in combination enforces tissue retention by depression of KLF2, S1PR1, and CCR7 [69] | ↑ |
| Aryl hydrocarbon receptor (Ahr) | is required for long-term persistence of $T_{RM}$ as a survival pathway for T cells residing in the epidermis [33] | ↑ |
| Notch | Required for maintenance of CD8 $T_{RM}$; proposed to control metabolic functions in $T_{RM}$ and CD103 expression [23] | ↑ |

**Table 1.**
*Detailed explanations of receptors, transcription factors, ligands, and molecules involved in formation and migration of TRM.*

## 6. TRM and diseases

TRM cells may assume pathogenic roles if they become over-sensitized or autore-activated. However, TRM cells are the first line protector of the immune system against the pathogen at the same time. Therefore, they play or stimulate to play an important role in effective treatment or vaccination. **Figure 4** summarizes the diseases associated with TRM cells both in the perspectives of pathogenic and protective roles.

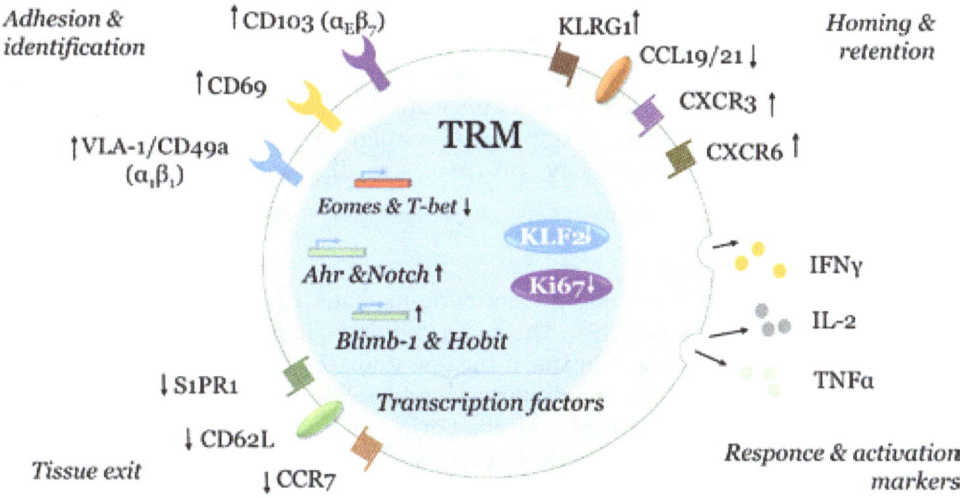

**Figure 4.**
*Illustration of some of the TRM-associated diseases that has been reported.*

## 6.1 Pathogenic roles

### 6.1.1 Psoriasis

Psoriasis is a common chronic inflammatory skin disease with a spectrum of clinical phenotypes and results from the interplay of genetic, environmental, and immunological factors [107]. Psoriasis can be divided into five types. The most common is plaque psoriasis, which causes itching and pain due to plaque formation. This type also maintains large areas of erythema or scaling of the skin, causing deformation of the skin [108]. Many studies showed that the chronic inflammation observed in psoriasis arises from an uncontrolled proliferation of T cells [66, 109]. Resident T cells play a role in the formation and recurrence of psoriatic lesions. Psoriasis lesion can be triggered and sustained by the local network of skin-resident immune cells in mouse models [110].

In recent studies, TRM cells were identified in healthy skin but were increased in psoriatic lesions. And these TRM cells have been found to produce perforin and IFN-gamma and to secrete IL-17 which is responsible for unwanted symptoms [111]. Demarcated, inflamed, and hyperproliferative plaques are maintained by interleukin-23 (IL-23) and IL-17 in psoriasis [41, 112].

For the treatment of psoriasis, an autoimmune disease, various immunosuppressive drugs, neutralizing antibodies, and cytokines have been tried for the treatment [42, 113–116]. These therapies have not been fully successful nowadays due to the systemic side-effects and the presence of autoreactive resident T cells in tissues without lesions.

### 6.1.2 Vitiligo

Another disease with several patchy appearance lesions in the skin like psoriasis is Vitiligo. These two diseases are often confused with each other. Vitiligo is an auto-reactive T cell-mediated disease in which immune cells target and kill melanocytes, leading to depigmentation of the skin [73].

Vitiligo lesions recur in the same areas of the skin and this is a sign of the presence of resident autoimmune memory [117]. Recent studies have shown the presence of melanocyte-specific TRM cells in skin tissues with vitiligo. These  TRM cells are CD8+ cells secreting IFNg and TNFα and expressing common TRM markers such as CD69, CD103, and CXCR3 [19, 118]. In a mouse vitiligo model, it was showed that neutralization of the IL-15 receptor by anti-CD122 antibody decreases the IFNg production from TRM cells and leads to repigmentation of the lesion [91]. Currently, there is no FDA-approved vitiligo treatment and such studies targeting TRM cells are likely to have prosperous results in the future.

### 6.1.3 Multiple sclerosis

Multiple sclerosis (MS) is a chronic, immune-mediated, demyelinating disorder of the central nervous system [119]. The brain is not a frequently visited tissue for immune cells due to its barriers. In one of the few studies in this field, CD8+ TRM cells that persist within the brain after an acute systemic vesicular stomatitis virus infection were characterized [120]. These cells were not in equilibrium with circulating T cells as evidence for TRM establishment in the brain tissue [50]. However, the mechanism for the generation and maintenance of TRM cells in the brain remains unclear.

### 6.1.4 Asthma

Asthma, other allergic airway diseases are inflammatory lung diseases that are related to the TRM cells. Asthma is a heterogeneous disease and is characterized by chronic airway inflammation, increased susceptibility to respiratory viral infection, and altered airway microbiology [121, 122]. The lungs have been widely investigated for TRM cell formation due to their exposure to the external environment and recurrent infections. In one of those studies, house dust mite HDM-specific memory cells have been identified as central memory cells in the lymphoid organs and TRM cells in the lung [123].

The majority of T cells in the human lung are TRM cells. TRM cells provide important roles in the protection against asthma, multiple respiratory pathogens, and other allergic diseases and might be contributed for developing new therapies and vaccines [25, 26].

### 6.1.5 Rheumatoid arthritis

Rheumatoid arthritis is a chronic autoimmune disease which can cause cartilage and bone damage, progressive articular damage, as well as functional loss disability [124–126]. Rheumatoid arthritis, is known largely a disease of the joints, however many organs and systems are effected, including the pulmonary, cardiovascular, ocular, and cutaneous systems [127].

Recurrence of arthritis in the joints is the key for the treatment of human rheumatoid arthritis. The disease is propagated through resident cells in the synovium of the joint, resident synovial cells that interact with the infiltrating immune cells and transition from acute synovitis to chronic RA [128]. The link between recurrence and residency suggests the presence of TRM cells. Studies have shown that TRM formation was induced in the enthesis. The enthesis is the region at the junction between tendon and bone. This zone was shown to contain a unique population of resident T cells, when activated by the cytokine interleukin-23 and can cause pathogenesis [129, 130].

### 6.1.6 Crohn's disease

Crohn disease (CD) is an inflammatory condition of the gastrointestinal (GI) tract, characterized by unpredictable periods of symptomatic relapses and remissions [131]. It has been suggested that CD has clinical similarities with TRM-mediated skin diseases. The skin lesion is similar "skip lesions" in the gut seen in CD [3, 67]. The use of immunosuppressive drugs for the treatment of CD can be considered as another similarity. However, the presence of a direct link between CD and TRM formation should be investigated.

Some of the other diseases that are related to the TRM formation are mycosis fungoides, contact dermatitis, chronic eczema, and fixed drug eruption and all needs to be further investigated.

## 6.2 Protective roles

Autoreactive TRM cells may contribute to the pathogenesis of autoimmune, atopic, and allergic diseases as described above. In contrast, they can provide rapid and efficient protection against wide range of pathogens and various types of tumors. Malaria, HSV, and cancer must be emphasized due to the role of TRM cell mediated treatment and vaccination strategies.

Malaria is a vector-borne parasitic tropical disease found in 91 countries worldwide [132]. *Plasmodium falciparum* (PF) is the dominant specie that produces high levels of parasites in critical organs and cause severe anemia, especially in African children, in whom. Malaria affected an estimated 216 million people causing 445,000 deaths in 2016 [133] around the World and the vast majority of malaria deaths occur in developing countries. Over the years, extensive research has been conducted on the prevention and treatment of malaria. However, increasing drug and insecticide resistance and threatens the successes. Moreover, the results obtained from current vaccine studies have not been sufficient to prevent malaria.

Development of a broadly protective vaccine is required for the eradication of Malaria. For this purpose, TRM cell-mediated vaccination strategies can be very promising. Researchers identified that memory CD8+ T cells that expressed the gene signature of TRM cells and remained permanently within the liver [45, 48].

A recent study explored the mechanism of action of a newly developed malaria vaccine, *Plasmodium falciparum* sporozoites (PfSPZ), which has exhibited very promising efficacy in human clinical trials. The efficacy of this vaccine has been shown to be due to TRM formation within the liver was 100-fold higher [47]. Researcher also showed that this TRM cells within the liver can also be generated by a "prime and trap" or "prime and pull" vaccination strategy [16, 22].

This strategy has two stages. First is the conventional vaccination to obtain systemic T cell responses (prime), second is recruitment of activated T cells via topical chemokine application to the desired tissue (pull), where such TRM cells were established and mediate long-term protective immunity [16, 102, 134]. The robust protective immunity provided by memory T cells localized in peripheral tissues, together with localized memory T cells, provides hope that site-specific vaccination strategies can be developed [135].

Development of a T cells mediated vaccines are required for efficacious protection. Due to their robust systemic responses, TRM cells provide superior protection compared with circulating memory T cells in peripheral tissues [136]. Recent studies focused on TRM establishment of training to protect against infection agent where they first contact [40].

The female genital tract, which is a portal of entry for sexually transmitted infections such as HIV and HSV. In a recent study "prime and pull" strategy was used against HSV-2 infection in female genital tract. In this study, mice were infected by attenuated strain of HSV-2 subcutaneously and topical application of chemokines CXCL9 and CXCL10 have been used to recruit TRM cells in the vagina to prevent the development of clinical disease for further infections [16].

TRM-mediated vaccine development researches against infectious agents are not limited to PF HSV and HIV. Moreover, vaccine studies are being carried out in order to provide first step protection against many infectious agents such as influenza, varicella, Human papillomavirus (HPV), toxoplasma, etc. [8, 38, 43, 137, 138].

In the context of TRM cells, cancer should also be emphasized. Currently, developed cancer vaccines are generally aimed for the treatment and the number of prophylactic vaccines is relatively low. Therefore, vaccination studies for the formation of TRM against cancer are very promising.

Recent studies suggest that TRM cells also play a vital part in cancer surveillance [57, 139]. It was demonstrated in many studies that TRM cells generated by vaccines can protect against tumor challenge [10, 55, 140, 141]. Formation of CD8 + T cells is one of the main objectives in cancer vaccine development against solid tumors. The type of CD8+ T cells that can migrate and localize in tumor microenvironments are TRM cells. [55]. It was found that presence of CD8+ TRM cells is associated with good prognosis in various cancers [57]. TRM cells can act in three major ways against solid tumors [73].

- TRM cells can express cytokines: TRM cells can produce cytokines such as perforin and granzyme B, and other effector molecules such as IFNγ and TNFα and eliminate tumor cells [10, 73].

- TRM cells may promote tumor-immune equilibrium: CD8+ TRM cells can contribute tumor immunosurveillance and they prevent tumor outgrowth without completely eliminating cancerous cells [73, 142, 143].

- TRM cells express inhibitory checkpoint molecules: TRM cells also predominantly express checkpoint receptors such as programmed cell death protein-1 (PD-1), cytotoxic T-lymphocyte-associated protein-4 (CTLA-4), and T-cell immunoglobulin and mucin-domain containing-3 (Tim-3) [55, 80].

It is becoming increasingly clear that TRM cells play an integral role in tumor surveillance in both animal models and human cancers. However, the role of TRM cells in solid human cancers should be further investigated.

## 7. Conclusion

The knowledge about TRM cells is at an early stage. Moreover, it has been revealed only in recent decades that TRM cells are unique subsets. It was found that TRM cells become resident by their phenotypic characteristics by adopting the microenvironment of the host tissue. TRM cells are transcriptionally, phenotypically, and functionally distinct from other circulating T cell subsets.

TRM cells have different phenotypes show heterogeneity depending on the host tissue microenvironment. Requirement for TRM generation, proliferation, migration, and maintenance vary in different kind of tissues. In order to distinguish TRM cells from other T cell subsets, in most of the studies in both mice and humans, identification markers such as CD103, CD69, and Cd49a were the most common ones.

TRM cells may assume pathogenic roles if they become over-sensitized or auto-reactivated. However, TRM cells are the first line protector of the immune system against the pathogen at the same time. Therefore, they play or stimulate to play an important role in effective treatment or vaccination. It was found that presence of CD8+ TRM cells is associated with good prognosis in various cancers.

Unlike other T cell subsets, TRM cells are not present in the blood. This is one of the major logistical barriers to the study of TRM cells. Therefore, TRM studies in humans have been limited due to the need for biopsy. In human NLT tissues, TRM isolation should be performed in a small biopsy volume, they should be phenotypically redefined and distinctive surface markers should be identified for humans. However, TRM cell-mediated vaccination and effective T cell treatments against solid tumors can be achieved by overcoming these problems in the following years.

## Author details

Hasan Akbaba
Faculty of Pharmacy, Ege University, Izmir, Turkey

*Address all correspondence to: hasan.akbaba@ege.edu.tr

# References

[1] Rosato PC, Beura LK, Masopust D. Tissue resident memory T cells and viral immunity. Current Opinion in Virology. 2017;**22**:44-50. DOI: 10.1016/j. coviro.2016.11.011

[2] Schenkel JM, Masopust D. Tissue-resident memory T cells. Immunity. 2014;**41**:886-897. DOI: 10.1016/j. immuni.2014.12.007

[3] Hill C. Resident cells in human disease. Science Translational Medicine. 2015;**73**:389-400. DOI: 10.1530/ERC-14- 0411.Persistent

[4] Hogan RJ, Usherwood EJ, Zhong W, Roberts AD, Dutton RW, Harmsen AG, et al. Activated antigen-specific CD8+ T cells persist in the lungs following recovery from respiratory virus infections. Journal of Immunology. 2001;**166**:1813-1822. DOI: 10.4049/jimmunol.166.3.1813

[5] Masopust D. Preferential localization of effector memory cells in nonlymphoid tissue. Science. 2001;**291**:2413-2417. DOI: 10.1126/science.1058867

[6] Wei C-H, Trenney R, Sanchez-Alavez M, Marquardt K, Woodland DL, Henriksen SJ, et al. Tissue-resident memory CD8+ T cells can be deleted by soluble, but not cross-presented antigen. Journal of Immunology. 2005;**175**:6615- 6623. DOI: 10.4049/jimmunol.175.10.6615

[7] Moon JJ, Chu HH, Hataye J, Pagán AJ, Pepper M, McLachlan JB, et al. Tracking epitope-specific T cells. Nature Protocols. 2009;**4**:565-581. DOI: 10.1038/nprot.2009.9

[8] Gebhardt T, Mueller SN, Heath WR, Carbone FR. Peripheral tissue surveillance and residency by memory T cells. Trends in Immunology. 2013;**34**:27-32. DOI: 10.1016/j.it.2012.08.008

[9] Cheuk S, Schlums H, Gallais Sérézal I, Martini E, Chiang SC, Marquardt N, et al. CD49a expression defines tissue-resident CD8+ T cells poised for cytotoxic function in human skin. Immunity. 2017;**46**:287-300. DOI: 10.1016/j.immuni.2017.01.009

[10] Dumauthioz N, Labiano S, Romero P. Tumor resident memory T cells: New players in immune surveillance and therapy. Frontiers in Immunology. 2018;**9**:1-6. DOI: 10.3389/fimmu.2018.02076

[11] Carbone FR, Mackay LK, Heath WR, Gebhardt T. Distinct resident and recirculating memory T cell subsets in non-lymphoid tissues. Current Opinion in Immunology. 2013;**25**:329-333. DOI: 10.1016/j.coi.2013.05.007

[12] Sallusto F, Geginat J, Lanzavecchia A. Central memory and effector memory T cell subsets: Function, generation, and maintenance. Annual Review of Immunology. 2004;**22**:745-763. DOI: 10.1146/annurev. immunol.22.012703.104702

[13] Slütter B, Pewe LL, Kaech SM, Harty JT. Lung airway-surveilling CXCR3hi memory CD8+ T cells are critical for protection against influenza A virus. Immunity. 2013;**39**:939-948. DOI: 10.1016/j.immuni.2013.09.013

[14] Wu T, Hu Y, Lee Y-T, Bouchard KR, Benechet A, Khanna K, et al. Lung-resident memory CD8 T cells (TRM) are indispensable for optimal cross-protection against pulmonary virus infection. Journal of Leukocyte Biology. 2014;**95**:215-224. DOI: 10.1189/jlb.0313180

[15] Gilchuk P, Hill TM, Guy C, McMaster SR, Boyd KL, Rabacal WA, et al. A distinct lung-interstitium-resident memory CD8+ T cell subset confers enhanced protection to lower

respiratory tract infection. Cell Reports. 2016;**16**:1800-1809. DOI: 10.1016/j. celrep.2016.07.037

[16] Shin H, Iwasaki A. A vaccine strategy that protects against genital herpes by establishing local memory T cells. Nature. 2012;**491**:463-467. DOI: 10.1038/nature11522

[17] Steinert EM, Schenkel JM, Fraser KA, Beura LK, Manlove LS, Igyártó BZ, et al. Quantifying memory CD8 T cells reveals regionalization of immunosurveillance. Cell. 2015;**161**:737-749. DOI: 10.1016/j.cell.2015.03.031

[18] Jiang X, Clark RA, Liu L, Wagers AJ, Fuhlbrigge RC, Kupper TS. Skin infection generates non-migratory memory CD8+ TRM cells providing global skin immunity. Nature. 2012;**483**:227-231. DOI: 10.1038/nature10851

[19] Boniface K, Jacquemin C, Darrigade AS, Dessarthe B, Martins C, Boukhedouni N, et al. Vitiligo skin is imprinted with resident memory CD8 T cells expressing CXCR3. The Journal of Investigative Dermatology. 2018;**138**:355-364. DOI: 10.1016/j. jid.2017.08.038

[20] Omenetti S, Bussi C, Metidji A, Iseppon A, Lee S, Tolaini M, et al. The intestine harbors functionally distinct homeostatic tissue-resident and inflammatory Th17 cells. Immunity. 2019;**51**:77-89.e6. DOI: 10.1016/j. immuni.2019.05.004

[21] Takamura S. Niches for the long-term maintenance of tissue-resident memory T cells. Frontiers in Immunology. 2018;**9**. DOI: 10.3389/ fimmu.2018.01214

[22] Fernandez-Ruiz D, Ng WY, Holz LE, Ma JZ, Zaid A, Wong YC, et al. Liver-resident memory CD8+T cells form a front-line defense against malaria liver-stage infection. Immunity.

2016;**45**:889-902. DOI: 10.1016/j. immuni.2016.08.011

[23] Topham DJ, Reilly EC. Tissue-resident memory CD8+T cells: From phenotype to function. Frontiers in Immunology. 2018;**9**:515-525. DOI: 10.3389/fimmu.2018.00515

[24] Skulska K, Wegrzyn AS, Chelmonska-Soyta A, Chodaczek G. Impact of tissue enzymatic digestion on analysis of immune cells in mouse reproductive mucosa with a focus on γδ T cells. Journal of Immunological Methods. 2019;**474**:112665. DOI: 10.1016/j.jim.2019.112665

[25] Bull NC, Kaveh DA, Garcia- Pelayo MC, Stylianou E, McShane H, Hogarth PJ. Induction and maintenance of a phenotypically heterogeneous lung tissue-resident CD4+ T cell population following BCG immunisation. Vaccine. 2018;**36**:5625-5635. DOI: 10.1016/j. vaccine.2018.07.035

[26] Snyder ME, Farber DL. Human lung tissue resident memory T cells in health and disease. Current Opinion in Immunology. 2019;**59**:101-108. DOI: 10.1016/j.coi.2019.05.011

[27] Zaric M, Becker PD, Hervouet C, Kalcheva P, Ibarzo Yus B, Cocita C, et al. Long-lived tissue resident HIV-1 specific memory CD8+ T cells are generated by skin immunization with live virus vectored microneedle arrays. Journal of Controlled Release. 2017;**268**:166-175. DOI: 10.1016/j. jconrel.2017.10.026

[28] Thom JT, Weber TC, Walton SM, Torti N, Oxenius A. The salivary gland acts as a sink for tissue-resident memory CD8+ T cells, facilitating protection from local cytomegalovirus infection. Cell Reports. 2015;**13**:1125-1136. DOI: 10.1016/j.celrep.2015.09.082

[29] Shelke AR, Roscoe JA, Morrow GR, Colman LK, Banerjee TK, Kirshner JJ.

基因的改变NIH public access. Bone. 2008;**23**:1-7. DOI: 10.1038/jid.2014.371

[30] Mackay LK, Kallies A. Transcriptional regulation of tissue-resident lymphocytes. Trends in Immunology. 2017;**38**:94-103. DOI: 10.1016/j.it.2016.11.004

[31] Gebhardt T, Wakim LM, Eidsmo L, Reading PC, Heath WR, Carbone FR. Memory T cells in nonlymphoid tissue that provide enhanced local immunity during infection with herpes simplex virus. Nature Immunology. 2009;**10**: 524-530. DOI: 10.1038/ni.1718

[32] MacKay LK, Rahimpour A, Ma JZ, Collins N, Stock AT, Hafon ML, et al. The developmental pathway for CD103 + CD8+ tissue-resident memory T cells of skin. Nature Immunology. 2013;**14**: 1294-1301. DOI: 10.1038/ni.2744

[33] Zaid A, Mackay LK, Rahimpour A, Braun A, Veldhoen M, Carbone FR, et al. Persistence of skin-resident memory T cells within an epidermal niche. Proceedings of the National Academy of Sciences. 2014;**111**:5307-5312. DOI: 10.1073/pnas.1322292111

[34] Ø Gadsbøll A-S, Jee MH, Funch AB, Alhede M, Mraz V, Weber JF, et al. Pathogenic CD8+ epidermis-resident memory T cells displace dendritic epidermal T cells in allergic dermatitis. The Journal of Investigative Dermatology. 2019;**xx**:xx-xx. DOI: 10.1016/j.jid.2019.07.722

[35] Roberts A, Brolin RE, Ebert EC. Integrin α1β1 (VLA-1) mediates adhesion of activated intraepithelial lymphocytes to collagen. Immunology. 1999;**97**:679-685. DOI: 10.1046/j.1365-2567.1999.00812

[36] Hegazy AN, West NR, Stubbington MJT, Wendt E, Suijker KIM, Datsi A, et al. Circulating and tissue-resident CD4+ T cells with reactivity to intestinal microbiota are abundant in healthy individuals and function is altered during inflammation. Gastroenterology. 2017;**153**:1320-1337. e16. DOI: 10.1053/j.gastro.2017.07.047

[37] Fu YY, Egorova A, Sobieski C, Kuttiyara J, Calafiore M, Takashima S, et al. T cell recruitment to the intestinal stem cell compartment drives immune-mediated intestinal damage after allogeneic transplantation. Immunity. 2019;**51**:90-103.e3. DOI: 10.1016/j. immuni.2019.06.003

[38] Doorbar J. Host control of human papillomavirus infection and disease. Best Practice & Research. Clinical Obstetrics & Gynaecology. 2018;**47**:27-41. DOI: 10.1016/j.bpobgyn.2017.08.001

[39] Çuburu N, Graham BS, Buck CB, Kines RC, Pang YYS, Day PM, et al. Intravaginal immunization with HPV vectors induces tissue-resident CD8+ T cell responses. The Journal of Clinical Investigation. 2012;**122**:4606-4620. DOI: 10.1172/JCI63287

[40] Farber DL. Training T cells for tissue residence. Science. 2019;**366**:188-189. DOI: 10.1126/science.aaz3289

[41] Hueber W, Patel DD, Dryja T, Wright AM, Koroleva I, Bruin G, et al. Effects of AIN457, a fully human antibody to interleukin-17A, on psoriasis, rheumatoid arthritis, and uveitis. Science Translational Medicine. 2010;**2**:1-11. DOI: 10.1126/scitranslmed.3001107

[42] Papp KA, Merola JF, Gottlieb AB, Griffiths CEM, Cross N, Peterson L, et al. Dual neutralization of both interleukin 17A and interleukin 17F with bimekizumab in patients with psoriasis: Results from BE ABLE 1, a 12-week randomized, double-blinded, placebo-controlled phase 2b trial. Journal of the American Academy of Dermatology. 2018;**79**:277-286.e10. DOI: 10.1016/j. jaad.2018.03.037

[43] Van Braeckel-Budimir N, Varga SM, Badovinac VP, Harty JT. Repeated

antigen exposure extends the durability of influenza-specific lung-resident memory CD8+ T cells and heterosubtypic immunity. Cell Reports. 2018;**24**:3374- 3382.e3. DOI: 10.1016/j.celrep.2018.08.073

[44] Hofmann M, Pircher H. E-cadherin promotes accumulation of a unique memory CD8 T-cell population in murine salivary glands. Proceedings of the National Academy of Sciences of the United States of America. 2011;**108**:16741-16746. DOI: 10.1073/pnas.1107200108

[45] Walk J, Stok JE, Sauerwein RW. Can patrolling liver-resident T cells control human malaria parasite development? Trends in Immunology. 2019;**40**:186-196. DOI: 10.1016/j.it.2019.01.002

[46] McNamara HA, Cai Y, Wagle MV, Sontani Y, Roots CM, Miosge LA, et al. Up-regulation of LFA-1 allows liver-resident memory T cells to patrol and remain in the hepatic sinusoids. Science Immunology. 2017;**2**:eaaj1996. DOI: 10.1126/sciimmunol.aaj1996

[47] Ishizuka AS, Lyke KE, DeZure A, Berry AA, Richie TL, Mendoza FH, et al. Protection against malaria at 1 year and immune correlates following PfSPZ vaccination. Nature Medicine. 2016;**22**:614-623. DOI: 10.1038/nm.4110

[48] Nlinwe ON, Kusi KA, Adu B, Sedegah M. T-cell responses against malaria: Effect of parasite antigen diversity and relevance for vaccine development. Vaccine. 2018;**36**:2237-2242. DOI: 10.1016/j.vaccine.2018.03.023

[49] Erel-Akbaba G, Carvalho LA, Tian T, Zinter M, Akbaba H, Obeid PJ, et al. Radiation-induced targeted nanoparticle-based gene delivery for brain tumor therapy. ACS Nano. 2019;**13**(4):4028-4040 doi:10.1021/acsnano.8b08177

[50] Wakim LM, Woodward-Davis A, Bevan MJ. Memory T cells persisting within the brain after local infection show functional adaptations to their tissue of residence. Proceedings of the National Academy of Sciences of the United States of America. 2010;**107**:17872-17879. DOI: 10.1073/pnas.1010201107

[51] Friedersdorff F, Dornieden T, Sattler A, Bergmann Y, Ruhm A, Schlomm T, et al. Tissue-resident memory CD8+ T cells in the kidney—Implications for renal transplantation. European Urology Supplements. 2019;**18**:e1654. DOI: 10.1016/s1569-9056(19)31200-x

[52] Watanabe R. Protective and pathogenic roles of resident memory T cells in human skin disorders. Journal of Dermatological Science. 2019;**95**:2-7. DOI: 10.1016/j.jdermsci.2019.06.001

[53] Pan Y, Tian T, Park CO, Lofftus SY, Mei S, Liu X, et al. Survival of tissue-resident memory T cells requires exogenous lipid uptake and metabolism. Nature. 2017;**543**:252-256. DOI: 10.1038/nature21379

[54] Amsen D, Van Gisbergen KPJM, Hombrink P, Van Lier RAW. Tissue-resident memory T cells at the center of immunity to solid tumors. Nature Immunology. 2018;**19**:538-546. DOI: 10.1038/s41590-018-0114-2

[55] Djenidi F, Adam J, Goubar A, Durgeau A, Meurice G, de Montpréville V, et al. CD8+ CD103+ tumor–infiltrating lymphocytes are tumor-specific tissue-resident memory T cells and a prognostic factor for survival in lung cancer patients. Journal of Immunology. 2015;**194**:3475-3486. DOI: 10.4049/jimmunol.1402711

[56] Ganesan AP, Clarke J, Wood O, Garrido-Martin EM, Chee SJ, Mellows T, et al. Tissue-resident memory features are linked to the magnitude of cytotoxic T cell responses in human lung cancer. Nature Immunology. 2017;**18**:940-950. DOI: 10.1038/ni.3775

[57] Vesely MD, Kershaw MH, Schreiber RD, Smyth MJ. Natural innate and adaptive immunity to cancer. Annual Review of Immunology. 2011;**29**:235-271. DOI: 10.1146/annurev-immunol-031210-101324

[58] Schenkel JM, Fraser KA, Masopust D. Cutting edge: Resident memory CD8 T cells occupy frontline niches in secondary lymphoid organs. Journal of Immunology. 2014;**192**:2961- 2964. DOI: 10.4049/jimmunol.1400003

[59] Cowan JE, McCarthy NI, Anderson G. CCR7 controls thymus recirculation, but not production and emigration, of Foxp3+ T cells. Cell Reports. 2016;**14**:1041-1048. DOI: 10.1016/j.celrep.2016.01.003

[60] Di Rosa F. Two niches in the bone marrow: A hypothesis on life-long T cell memory. Trends in Immunology. 2016;**37**:503-512. DOI: 10.1016/j.it.2016.05.004

[61] Casorati G, Locatelli F, Pagani S, Garavaglia C, Montini E, Lisini D, et al. Bone marrow-resident memory T cells survive pretransplant chemotherapy and contribute to early immune reconstitution of patients with acute myeloid leukemia given mafosfamide-purged autologous bone marrow transplantation. Experimental Hematology. 2005;**33**:212-218. DOI: 10.1016/j.exphem.2004.10.008

[62] Von Andrian UH, Mempel TR. Homing and cellular traffic in lymph nodes. Nature Reviews. Immunology. 2003;**3**:867-878. DOI: 10.1038/nri1222

[63] Von Andrian UH, Mackay CR. T-cell function and migration. Two sides of the same coin. The New England Journal of Medicine. 2000;**343**:1020-1034. DOI: 10.1056/NEJM200010053431407

[64] Mueller SN, Gebhardt T, Carbone FR, Heath WR. Memory T cell subsets, migration patterns, and tissue residence. Annual Review of Immunology. 2013;**31**:137-161. DOI: 10.1146/annurev immunol-032712-095954

[65] Zhang Q, Lakkis FG. Memory T cell migration. Frontiers in Immunology. 2015;**6**:504-510. DOI: 10.3389/fimmu.2015.00504

[66] Gudjonsson JE, Johnston A, Sigmundsdottir H, Valdimarsson H. Immunopathogenic mechanisms in psoriasis. Clinical and Experimental Immunology. 2004;**135**:1-8. DOI: 10.1111/j.1365-2249.2004.02310.x

[67] Islam SA, Luster AD. T cell homing to epithelial barriers in allergic disease. Nature Medicine. 2012;**18**:705-715. DOI: 10.1038/nm.2760

[68] Masopust D, Choo D, Vezys V, Wherry EJ, Duraiswamy J, Akondy R, et al. Dynamic T cell migration program provides resident memory within intestinal epithelium. The Journal of Experimental Medicine. 2010;**207**:553-564. DOI: 10.1084/jem.20090858

[69] Mueller SN, Mackay LK. Tissue-resident memory T cells: Local specialists in immune defence. Nature Reviews. Immunology. 2016;**16**:79-89. DOI: 10.1038/nri.2015.3

[70] Hardenberg JHB, Braun A, Schön MP. A Yin and Yang in epithelial immunology: The roles of the α E (CD103)β 7 integrin in T cells. The Journal of Investigative Dermatology. 2018;**138**:23-31. DOI: 10.1016/j.jid.2017.05.026

[71] Agace WW, Higgins JMG, Sadasivan B, Brenner MB, Parker CM. T-lymphocyte—Epithelial-cell interactions: Integrin α E (CD103) β7, LEEP-CAM and chemokines. Current Opinion in Cell Biology. 2000;**12**:563-568. DOI: 10.1016/s0955-0674(00)00132-0

[72] Venhuizen J-H, Jacobs FJC, Span PN, Zegers MM. P120 and E-cadherin: Double-edged swords in tumor metastasis. Seminars in Cancer Biology. 2019;**xx**:1-14. DOI: 10.1016/j.semcancer.2019.07.020

[73] Park SL, Gebhardt T, Mackay LK. Tissue-resident memory T cells in cancer immunosurveillance. Trends in Immunology. 2019;**40**:735-747. DOI: 10.1016/j.it.2019.06.002

[74] González-Amaro R, Cortés JR, Sánchez-Madrid F, Martín P. Is CD69 an effective brake to control inflammatory diseases? Trends in Molecular Medicine. 2013;**19**:625-632. DOI: 10.1016/j.molmed.2013.07.006

[75] Bankovich AJ, Shiow LR, Cyster JG. CD69 suppresses sphingosine 1-phosophate receptor-1 (S1P1) function through interaction with membrane helix 4. The Journal of Biological Chemistry. 2010;**285**:22328-22337. DOI: 10.1074/jbc.M110.123299

[76] Luo Z, Gu J, Dennett RC, Gaehle GG, Perlmutter JS, Chen DL, et al. Automated production of a sphingosine-1 phosphate receptor 1 (S1P1) PET radiopharmaceutical [11C]CS1P1 for human use. Applied Radiation and Isotopes. 2019;**152**:30-36. DOI: 10.1016/j.apradiso.2019.06.029

[77] Shiow LR, Rosen DB, Brdičková N, Xu Y, An J, Lanier LL, et al. CD69 acts downstream of interferon-α/β to inhibit S1P 1 and lymphocyte egress from lymphoid organs. Nature. 2006;**440**:540-544. DOI: 10.1038/nature04606

[78] Skon CN, Lee J-Y, Anderson KG, Masopust D, Hogquist KA, Jameson SC. Transcriptional downregulation of S1pr1 is required for the establishment of resident memory CD8+ T cells. Nature Immunology. 2013;**14**:1285-1293. DOI: 10.1038/ni.2745

[79] Bieber T, Rieger A, Stingl G, Sander E, Wanek P, Strobel I. CD69, an early activation antigen on lymphocytes, is constitutively expressed by human epidermal langerhans cells. The Journal of Investigative Dermatology. 1992;**98**:771-776. DOI: 10.1111/1523-1747.ep12499948

[80] Mami-Chouaib F, Blanc C, Corgnac S, Hans S, Malenica I, Granier C, et al. Resident memory T cells, critical components in tumor immunology. Journal for Immunotherapy of Cancer. 2018;**6**:1-10. DOI: 10.1186/s40425-018-0399-6

[81] Haddadi S, Thanthrige-Don N, Afkhami S, Khera A, Jeyanathan M, Xing Z. Expression and role of VLA-1 in resident memory CD8 T cell responses to respiratory mucosal viral-vectored immunization against tuberculosis. Scientific Reports. 2017;**7**:1-14. DOI: 10.1038/s41598-017-09909-4

[82] Ray SJ, Franki SN, Pierce RH, Dimitrova S, Koteliansky V, Sprague AG, et al. The collagen binding α1β1 integrin VLA-1 regulates CD8 T cell-mediated immune protection against heterologous influenza infection. Immunity. 2004;**20**:167-179. DOI: 10.1016/S1074-7613(04)00021-4

[83] Liu Y, Ma C, Zhang N. Tissue-specific control of tissue-resident memory T cells. Critical Reviews in Immunology. 2018;**38**:79-103. DOI: 10.1615/CritRevImmunol.2018025653

[84] Topham DJ, Reilly EC, Emo KL, Sportiello M. Formation and maintenance of tissue resident memory CD8+ T cells after viral infection 2019;**8**:1-9. DOI: 10.3390/pathogens 8040196

[85] Baaten BJG, Li CR, Bradley LM. Multifaceted regulation of T cells by CD44. Communicative & Integrative Biology. 2010;**3**:508-512. DOI: 10.4161/cib.3.6.13495

[86] Kamran P, Sereti KI, Zhao P, Ali SR, Weissman IL, Ardehali R. Parabiosis in mice: A detailed protocol. Journal of Visualized Experiments. 2013;**80**:1-5. DOI: 10.3791/50556

[87] Hartney JM, Robichaud A. Mouse models of allergic disease: Methods and protocols. Methods in Molecular Biology. 2013;**1032**:205-217. DOI: 10.1007/978-1-62703-496-8

[88] Brown CR, Reiner SL. Bone-marrow chimeras reveal hemopoietic and nonhemopoietic control of resistance to experimental lyme arthritis. Journal of Immunology. 2000;**165**:1446-1452. DOI: 10.4049/jimmunol.165.3.1446

[89] Benichou G, Gonzalez B, Marino J, Ayasoufi K, Valujskikh A. Role of memory T cells in allograft rejection and tolerance. Frontiers in Immunology. 2017;**8**:170-179. DOI: 10.3389/fimmu.2017.00170

[90] Beura LK, Rosato PC, Masopust D. Implications of resident memory T cells for transplantation. American Journal of Transplantation. 2017;**17**:1167-1175. DOI: 10.1111/ajt.14101

[91] Richmond JM, Strassner JP, Zapata LZ, Garg M, Riding RL, Refat MA, et al. Antibody blockade of IL-15 signaling has the potential to durably reverse vitiligo. Science Translational Medicine. 2018;**10**:3. DOI: 10.1126/scitranslmed.aam7710

[92] Lee Y-T, Suarez-Ramirez JE, Wu T, Redman JM, Bouchard K, Hadley GA, et al. Environmental and antigen receptor-derived signals support sustained surveillance of the lungs by pathogen-specific cytotoxic T lymphocytes. Journal of Virology. 2011;**85**:4085-4094. DOI: 10.1128/jvi.02493-10

[93] Wu H, Liao W, Li Q, Long H, Yin H, Zhao M, et al. Pathogenic role of tissue-resident memory T cells in autoimmune diseases. Autoimmunity Reviews. 2018;**17**:906-911. DOI: 10.1016/j.autrev.2018.03.014

[94] Van Raemdonck K, Van den Steen PE, Liekens S, Van Damme J, Struyf S. CXCR3 ligands in disease and therapy. Cytokine & Growth Factor Reviews. 2015;**26**:311-327. DOI: 10.1016/j.cytogfr.2014.11.009

[95] Mackay LK, Wynne-Jones E, Freestone D, Pellicci DG, Mielke LA, Newman DM, et al. T-box transcription factors combine with the cytokines TGF-β and IL-15 to control tissue-resident memory T cell fate. Immunity. 2015;**43**:1101-1111. DOI: 10.1016/j.immuni.2015.11.008

[96] Hadley GA, Bartlett ST, Via CS, Rostapshova EA, Moainie S. The epithelial cell-specific integrin, CD103 (alpha E integrin), defines a novel subset of alloreactive CD8+ CTL. Journal of Immunology. 1997;**159**:3748-3756

[97] Simms PE, Ellis TM. Utility of flow cytometric detection of CD69 expression as a rapid method for determining poly- and oligoclonal lymphocyte activation. Clinical and Diagnostic Laboratory Immunology. 1996;**3**:301-304

[98] Pearson R, Fleetwood J, Eaton S, Crossley M, Bao S. Krüppel-like transcription factors: A functional family. The International Journal of Biochemistry & Cell Biology. 2008;**40**:1996-2001. DOI: 10.1016/j.biocel.2007.07.018

[99] Sun X, Kaufman PD. Ki-67: More than a proliferation marker. Chromosoma. 2018;**127**:175-186. DOI: 10.1007/s00412-018-0659-8

[100] Sobecki M, Mrouj K, Camasses A, Parisis N, Nicolas E, Llères D, et al. The cell proliferation antigen Ki-67 organises heterochromatin. eLife. 2016;**5**:1-33. DOI: 10.7554/eLife.13722

[101] Miller I, Min M, Yang C, Tian C, Gookin S, Carter D, et al. Ki67 is a graded rather than a binary marker of proliferation versus quiescence. Cell Reports. 2018;**24**:1105-1112.e5. DOI: 10.1016/j.celrep.2018.06.110

[102] Gründemann C, Schwartzkopff S, Koschella M, Schweier O, Peters C, Voehringer D, et al. The NK receptor KLRG1 is dispensable for virus-induced NK and CD8+ T-cell differentiation and function in vivo. European Journal of Immunology. 2010;**40**:1303-1314. DOI: 10.1002/eji.200939771

[103] Sharma N, Benechet AP, Lefrancois L, Khanna KM. CD8 T cells enter the splenic T cell zones independently of CCR7, but the subsequent expansion and trafficking patterns of effector T cells after infection are dysregulated in the absence of CCR7 migratory cues. Journal of Immunology. 2015;**195**:5227- 5236. DOI: 10.4049/jimmunol.1500993

[104] Liu CH, Thangada S, Lee M, Van JR, Spiegel S, Hla T. Ligand-induced trafficking of the sphingosine-1-phosphate receptor EDG-1. Molecular Biology of the Cell. 1999;**10**:1179-1190. DOI: 10.1091/mbc.10.4.1179

[105] Grailer JJ, Kodera M, Steeber DA. L-selectin: Role in regulating homeostasis and cutaneous inflammation. Journal of Dermatological Science. 2009;**56**:141-147. DOI: 10.1016/j.jdermsci.2009.10.001

[106] Yoshida R, Nagira M, Kitaura M, Imagawa N, Imai T, Yoshie O. Secondary lymphoid-tissue chemokine is a functional ligand for the CC chemokine receptor CCR7. The Journal of Biological Chemistry. 1998;**273**:7118-7122. DOI: 10.1074/jbc.273.12.7118

[107] Di Meglio P, Villanova F, Nestle FO. Psoriasis. Cold Spring Harbor Perspectives in Medicine. 2014;**4**(8):1-30

[108] Meng S, Sun L, Wang L, Lin Z, Liu Z, Xi L, et al. Loading of water-insoluble celastrol into niosome hydrogels for improved topical permeation and anti-psoriasis activity. Colloids and Surfaces. B, Biointerfaces. 2019;**182**:110352. DOI: 10.1016/j.colsurfb.2019.110352

[109] Nickoloff BJ, Nestle FO. Recent insights into the immunopathogenesis of psoriasis provide new therapeutic opportunities. The Journal of Clinical Investigation. 2004;**113**:1664-1675. DOI: 10.1172/JCI200422147

[110] Boyman O, Conrad C, Tonel G, Gilliet M, Nestle FO. The pathogenic role of tissue-resident immune cells in psoriasis. Trends in Immunology. 2007;**28**:51-57. DOI: 10.1016/j.it.2006.12.005

[111] Boehncke WH, Schön MP. Psoriasis: Electrochemical behaviour of tin (II) chloride As a solid state ionic conductor. Lancet. 2015;**4**:169-177. DOI: 10.1016/S0140-6736(14)61909-7

[112] Papp KA, Langley RG, Lebwohl M, Krueger GG, Szapary P, Yeilding N, et al. Efficacy and safety of ustekinumab, a human interleukin-12/23 monoclonal antibody, in patients with psoriasis: 52-week results from a randomised, double-blind, placebo-controlled trial (PHOENIX 2). Lancet. 2008;**371**:1675-1684. DOI: 10.1016/S0140-6736(08)60726-6

[113] Rappersberger K, Meingassner JG, Fialla R, Födinger D, Sterniczky B, Rauch S, et al. Clearing of psoriasis by a novel immunosuppressive macrolide. The Journal of Investigative Dermatology. 1996;**106**:701-710. DOI: 10.1111/1523-1747.ep12345542

[114] Shan Y, Shi K, Qian X, Chang Z, Yang J, Gao Y, et al. Preclinical development of GR1501, a human monoclonal antibody that neutralizes interleukin-17A. Biochemical and Biophysical Research Communications. 2019;**517**:303-309. DOI: 10.1016/j.bbrc.2019.07.078

[115] Aleem D, Tohid H. Pro-inflammatory cytokines, biomarkers, genetics and the immune system: A mechanistic approach of depression and psoriasis. The Revista Colombiana de Psiquiatría. 2018;**47**:177-186. DOI: 10.1016/j.rcp.2017.03.002

[116] Dai H, Zhou Y, Tong C, Guo Y, Shi F, Wang YAO, et al. Restoration of CD3+CD56+ cell level improves skin lesions in severe psoriasis: A pilot clinical study of adoptive immunotherapy for patients with psoriasis using autologous cytokine-induced killer cells. Cytotherapy. 2018;**20**:1155-1163. DOI: 10.1016/j.jcyt.2018.07.003

[117] Liu LY, Strassner JP, Refat MA, Harris JE, King BA. Repigmentation in vitiligo using the Janus kinase inhibitor tofacitinib may require concomitant light exposure. Journal of the American Academy of Dermatology. 2017;**77**:675-682.e1. DOI: 10.1016/j.jaad.2017.05.043

[118] Cooke DM. Community college gerontology education: A natural role for occupational therapy. Occupational Therapy in Health Care. 1984;**1**:23-30. DOI: 10.1080/J003v01n01_05

[119] Brownlee WJ, Hardy TA, Fazekas F, Miller DH. Diagnosis of multiple sclerosis: Progress and challenges. Lancet. 2017;**389**:1336-1346. DOI: 10.1016/S0140-6736(16)30959-X

[120] Hussain RZ, Hayardeny L, Cravens PC, Yarovinsky F, Eagar TN, Arellano B, et al. Immune surveillance of the central nervous system in multiple sclerosis—Relevance for therapy and experimental models. Journal of Neuroimmunology. 2014;**276**:9-17. DOI: 10.1016/j.jneuroim.2014.08.622

[121] Gans MD, Gavrilova T. Understanding the immunology of asthma: Pathophysiology, biomarkers, and treatments for asthma endotypes. Paediatric Respiratory Reviews. 2019;**xx**;xx-xx. DOI: 10.1016/j.prrv.2019.08.002

[122] Gibson PG, Yang IA, Upham JW, Reynolds PN, Hodge S, James AL, et al. Effect of azithromycin on asthma exacerbations and quality of life in adults with persistent uncontrolled asthma (AMAZES): A randomised, double-blind, placebo-controlled trial. Lancet. 2017;**390**:659-668. DOI: 10.1016/S0140-6736(17)31281-3

[123] Hondowicz BD, An D, Schenkel JM, Kim KS, Steach HR, Krishnamurty AT, et al. Interleukin- 2-dependent allergen-specific tissue-resident memory cells drive asthma. Immunity. 2016;**44**:155-166. DOI: 10.1016/j.immuni.2015.11.004

[124] McInnes IB, Schett G. Pathogenetic insights from the treatment of rheumatoid arthritis. Lancet. 2017;**389**:2328-2337. DOI: 10.1016/S0140-6736(17)31472-1

[125] Smolen JS, Aletaha D, McInnes IB. Therapies for bone R. Lancet (London, England). 2016;**388**:2023-2038. DOI: 10.1016/S0140-6736(16)30173-8

[126] Klareskog L, Irinel A, Catrina SP. Rheumatoid arthritis chronotherapy. European Musculoskeletal Review. 2012;**7**:29-32. DOI: 10.1016/S0140-6736(09)60008-8

[127] Deane KD, Holers VM. The natural history of rheumatoid arthritis. Clinical Therapeutics. 2019;**41**:1256-1269. DOI: 10.1016/j.clinthera.2019.04.028

[128] Venuturupalli S. Immune mechanisms and novel targets in rheumatoid arthritis. Immunology and Allergy Clinics of North America. 2017;**37**:301-313. DOI: 10.1016/j.iac.2017.01.002

[129] Lories RJ, McInnes IB. Primed for inflammation: Enthesis-resident T cells.

Nature Medicine. 2012;**18**:1018-1019. DOI: 10.1038/nm.2854

[130] Sherlock JP, Joyce-Shaikh B, Turner SP, Chao CC, Sathe M, Grein J, et al. IL-23 induces spondyloarthropathy by acting on ROR-γt+ CD3+ CD4– CD8– entheseal resident T cells. Nature Medicine. 2012;**18**:1069-1076. DOI: 10.1038/nm.2817

[131] Hagen JW, Swoger JM, Grandinetti LM. Cutaneous manifestations of Crohn disease. Dermatologic Clinics. 2015;**33**:417-431. DOI: 10.1016/j.det.2015.03.007

[132] Ashley EA, Pyae Phyo A, Woodrow CJ. Malaria. Lancet. 2018;**391**: 1608-1621. DOI: 10.1016/S0140- 6736(18)30324-6

[133] Plewes K, Leopold SJ, Kingston HWF, Dondorp AM. Malaria: What's new in the management of malaria? Infectious Disease Clinics of North America. 2019;**33**:39-60. DOI: 10.1016/j.idc.2018.10.002

[134] Khan AA, Srivastava R, Chentoufi AA, Kritzer E, Chilukuri S, Garg S, et al. Bolstering the number and function of HSV-1–specific CD8+ effector memory T cells and tissue-resident memory T cells in latently infected trigeminal ganglia reduces recurrent ocular herpes infection and disease. Journal of Immunology. 2017;**199**:186- 203. DOI: 10.4049/jimmunol.1700145

[135] Woodland DL, Kohlmeier JE. Migration, maintenance and recall of memory T cells in peripheral tissues. Nature Reviews. Immunology. 2009;**9**:153-161. DOI: 10.1038/nri2496

[136] Schenkel JM, Fraser KA, Vezys V, Masopust D. Sensing and alarm function of resident memory CD8+ T cells. Nature Immunology. 2013;**14**: 9-14. DOI: 10.1038/ni.2568

[137] Tsitsiklis A, Bangs DJ, Robey EA. CD8+ T cell responses to *Toxoplasma gondii*: Lessons from a successful parasite. Trends in Parasitology. 2019;**xx**:1-12. DOI: 10.1016/j.pt.2019.08.005

[138] Muruganandah V, Sathkumara HD, Navarro S, Kupz A. A systematic review: The role of resident memory T cells in infectious diseases and their relevance for vaccine development. Frontiers in Immunology. 2018;**9**:1574-1595. DOI: 10.3389/fimmu.2018.01574

[139] Park CO, Kupper TS. The emerging role of resident memory T cells in protective immunity and inflammatory disease. Nature Medicine. 2015;**21**: 688-697. DOI: 10.1038/nm.3883

[140] Gabriel SS, Kallies A. Tissue-resident memory T cells keep cancer dormant. Cell Research. 2019;**29**:341-342. DOI: 10.1038/s41422-019-0156-5

[141] Blanc C, Hans S, Tran T, Granier C, Saldman A, Anson M, et al. Targeting resident memory T cells for cancer immunotherapy. Frontiers in Immunology. 2018;**9**:1722. DOI: 10.3389/fimmu.2018.01722

[142] Gordon CL, Lee LN, Swadling L, Hutchings C, Zinser M, Highton AJ, et al. Induction and maintenance of CX3CR1-intermediate peripheral memory CD8+ T cells by persistent viruses and vaccines. Cell Reports. 2018;**23**:768-782. DOI: 10.1016/j.celrep.2018.03.074

[143] Chevrier S, Levine JH, Zanotelli VRT, Silina K, Schulz D, Bacac M, et al. An immune atlas of clear cell renal cell carcinoma. Cell. 2017;**169**:736-749.e18. DOI: 10.1016/j. cell.2017.04.016

# 8

# Eosinophilic Granulomatosis with Polyangiitis: The Beginning of a New Era

*Carlos Melero Moreno, Marta Corral Blanco*
*and Rocío Magdalena Díaz Campos*

## Abstract

Eosinophilic granulomatosis with polyangiitis (EGPA) is a rare type of anti-neutrophil cytoplasm antibody-associated vasculitis (AAV) with unique features, such as involvement of eosinophils in the pathogenesis, which requires different therapies from those used for other AAV. Conventional treatment includes glucocorticoids (GC) and immunosuppressants. GC are the cornerstone of the initial treatment of EGPA, but relapses are frequent. Cyclophosphamide is typically used in combination with GC for patients with life- and/or organ-threatening disease manifestations. Azathioprine and methotrexate are recommended to maintain remission after induction with cyclophosphamide or as a GC-sparing agent. Nowadays, a better comprehension of the physiopathology of EGPA has opened new therapeutic targets, such as interleukin-5, which has a key role in the refractory disease, relapses, and GC dependence, especially for asthma manifestations. Mepolizumab is the first anti-IL5 antibody approved to treat EGPA. Another anti-IL5 monoclonal antibody, reslizumab, and an anti-IL5 receptor monoclonal antibody, benralizumab, are now being investigated for EGPA.

**Keywords:** eosinophilic granulomatosis with polyangiitis, Churg-Strauss syndrome, vasculitis, eosinophilia, anti-IL5 therapy, glucocorticoids, cyclophosphamide, mepolizumab

## 1. Introduction

Eosinophilic granulomatosis with polyangiitis (EGPA), formerly Churg-Strauss syndrome, is a rare necrotizing vasculitis, with an annual incidence and prevalence of 0.9–2.4 per million [1–4] and 10.7–17.8 per million [5–8], respectively, depending on geographic regions and applied criteria. The disease is now recognized as one form of anti-neutrophil cytoplasm antibody (ANCA)-associated vasculitis (AAV) characterized by eosinophil-rich granulomatous inflammation and small to medium size vessel vasculitis associated with asthma and eosinophilia [9].

ANCA occur only in about 30–70% of patients with newly diagnosed untreated EGPA, and organ involvement can be different depending on the presence or not of ANCA [10], probably being different subgroups with specific characteristics. In this way, Matsumoto et al. [11] reported that AAV patients could be divided into three subgroups according to peripheral immune cell numbers: antibody production related, cytotoxic activity related, and neutrocytosis/lymphocytopenia. These subgroups could have different prognosis and treatment.

EGPA has been excluded from most of randomized controlled trials for AAV because of its rarity and unique features, such as involvement of eosinophils in the pathogenesis. Reliable evidence of treatment for EGPA is limited, and there are no strong recommendations for treatment of EGPA at the moment [12].

Treatment has been based on the use of glucocorticoids (GC) and immunosuppressants. Cyclophosphamide is typically used in combination with GC for patients with poor prognostic factors (assessed by the Five Factor Score). Azathioprine and methotrexate are recommended to maintain remission after induction with cyclophosphamide or as a GC-sparing agent. All these medications have many and deleterious adverse effects.

Fortunately, a better comprehension of the physiopathology of EGPA has opened new therapeutic targets, such as interleukin-5, which has a key role in the disease.

## 2. Assessing vasculitis severity

The French Vasculitis Study Group conducted two randomized controlled clinical trials to develop a score to assess the severity of vasculitis disease: the Five Factor Score (FFS) [13].

The FFS is a prognostic tool used to quantify the extent of the disease and guide therapy. It consists of five items. Age >65 years old, cardiac insufficiency, severe gastrointestinal involvement, and renal insufficiency [stabilized peak creatinine 1.7 mg/dL {150 μmol/L}] are associated with poor prognoses, each scores +1 point, while the fifth factor (ear, nose, and throat [ENT] manifestations) is associated with better outcome and its absence is scored +1 point.

## 3. Conventional therapy for EGPA

### 3.1 Systemic glucocorticoids

Glucocorticoids are the cornerstone of the initial treatment of EGPA. They act quickly against vasculitis and normalize the value of peripheral eosinophils within few days of treatment.

A multicenter retrospective study, done by Cottin et al. [14] in 2016, showed that treatment with systemic GC was associated to a decrease in peripheral eosinophilia (with a mean cell count $<1.0 \times 10^9 \, L^{-1}$ over the long-term).

The initial management of EGPA includes high doses of GC, usually 1 mg/kg/day of prednisone or its equivalent. Methylprednisolone pulses (7.5–15 mg/kg intravenously, repeated at 24 h intervals, for 3 days) can be used in the presence of life-threatening symptoms. When clinical response is obtained and inflammation reactants return to normal values, usually within 3–4 weeks, GC can be tapered slowly to the minimal effective dose or, when possible, until withdrawal. However, most patients need to maintain GC to prevent relapses of systemic manifestations and control asthma. The optimal minimal dose should be 7.5 mg/day to limit GC-induced side effects [15, 16].

In the French Vasculitis Study Group cohort [17], which included 383 EGPA patients, approximately 85% required long-term prednisone (mean dose 12.9 ± 12.5 mg/day) to control asthma, rhinitis, and/or arthralgias.

GC as monotherapy may be suitable for most EGPA patients. In a study, which included 72 EGPA patients without poor prognosis factors, 93% achieved remission with systemic GC therapy alone [18]. However, additional immunosuppression can be considered for patients with life- and/or organ-threatening disease, when the prednisone dose cannot be tapered to 7.5 mg/day after 3–4 months of therapy or for patients with recurrent disease [16, 19].

Samson et al. [20] assessed the outcomes of 118 EGPA patients (with or without FFS) enrolled in two prospective, randomized, open-label clinical trials from 1994 to 2005. Forty-four patients with poor prognosis (FFS $\geq 1$) were assigned to receive 6 or 12 cyclophosphamide (CPh) pulses plus GC, and 74 without poor prognosis factors (FFS = 0) received GC alone (with immunosuppressant [IS] adjunction when GC failed). Follow-up was done from 2005 to 2011. Twenty-nine percent achieved long-term remission, while 41% had $\geq 1$ relapse at 26 months after treatment onset. More than half of the relapses occurred when GC tapering reached <10 mg/day, especially in patients with anti-myeloperoxidase antibodies and baseline eosinophilia <3000/mm$^3$.

## 3.2 Immunosuppressants

### 3.2.1 Cyclophosphamide

Cyclophosphamide is typically used in combination with GC for patients with life- and/or organ-threatening disease manifestations (i.e., heart, gastrointestinal involvement, central nervous system, severe peripheral neuropathy, severe ocular disease, alveolar hemorrhage, and/or glomerulonephritis) [14].

In a retrospective study of 595 patients with severe necrotizing vasculitides (including EGPA), treatment had no significant impact on early death, except for patients with FFS $\geq 2$ for whom GC monotherapy showed association ($p < 0.05$). The principal cause of early death was uncontrolled vasculitis (58%), followed by infection (26%) [21]. A study of 278 patients with polyarteritis nodosa, microscopic polyangiitis, and EGPA showed that survival was significantly higher in patients with FFS > 2 treated with GC and CPh rather than GC alone [22].

Cyclophosphamide can be administered as continuous oral therapy or intravenous (IV) pulses. The doses should be adjusted according to age and renal function. Cyclophosphamide pulses are usually preferred to oral administration because of the lower cumulative dosage. The frequency of relapses, however, can be higher with pulses, and it has been shown that oral CPh can be effective when pulses have failed [15]. Sodium 2-mercaptoethanesulfonate is recommended to reduce bladder toxicity.

Regarding the duration of CPh therapy, Cohen et al. [23] conducted a prospective, multicenter trial to compare first-line treatment with systemic GC and 6 or 12 pulses of adjunctive CPh for the treatment of severe EGPA. Forty-eight patients were included, 42 (87.5%) achieved complete remission, 21 (91.3%) in the 6-pulse regimen, and 21 (84%) in the 12-pulse regimen. Severe side effects were similar in both groups. However, a too-short duration of CPh administration was associated with more relapses, so the authors concluded that a 12-pulse regimen was better to control severe EGPA than a 6-pulse regimen. Other less toxic IS, as azathioprine (AZA) or methotrexate (MTX), were not tested for maintenance so further data is needed to clarify the optimal duration of therapy.

### 3.2.2 Azathioprine and methotrexate

AZA and MTX are recommended to maintain remission after induction with CPh or as a GC-sparing agent in patients requiring long-term therapy with prednisone at doses >10 mg/day. Maintenance therapy with an IS usually begins 2–3 weeks after the last CPh pulse, or a few days after oral CPh, and continues for 12–18 months [16].

Pagnoux et al. [24] conducted a prospective, open-label, multicenter trial to evaluate the safety and efficacy of AZA and MTX in ANCA-associated vasculitis. One hundred twenty-six patients in remission with IV CPh and GC were randomly assigned to receive AZA (at a dose of 2.0 mg/kg/day) or MTX (at a dose of 0.3 mg/kg/week, progressively increased to 25 mg per week) as maintenance therapy for 12 months. Adverse events occurred in 29 AZA recipients and 35 MTX recipients. There was one death in the MTX group. Twenty-three patients who received AZA and twenty-one patients who received MTX had a relapse. The results suggested that none of the drugs were more effective at maintaining remission, but severe adverse events were more frequent in the MTX group.

## 4. New therapeutic strategies

### 4.1 Role of IL-5 in EGPA

EGPA is characterized by elevated peripheral eosinophilia with different degrees of activation. Eosinophilia is secondary to more synthesis, enhanced extravasation, and its prolonged survival in target tissues. Histological features of EGPA are small-vessel angiitis and extravascular necrotizing granulomas, usually containing eosinophilic infiltrate [25, 26].

An initial Th2-mediated immune response provokes the migration of eosinophils to tissues. IL-5, produced by TH-2 lymphocytes, plays an active role in chemotaxis, activation, degranulation, and survival of eosinophils [26]. IL-5 is not the only mediator of eosinophilic tissue infiltration; IL-4 and IL-13 are two other cytokines of Th2-mediated immune response that play an important role in tissue infiltration and degranulation of eosinophils [27, 28]. Epithelial and endothelial cells, when activated by Th2 cytokines, secrete eosinophil-specific chemokines like eotaxin 3 (CCL26), CCL17, and CCL22 that facilitate recruitment of eosinophils and effector Th2 cells in target organs, amplifying the immune response [29, 30].

A better comprehension of the physiopathology of EGPA highlights the role of eosinophils and IL-5. It has been observed that serum level of IL-5 correlates with disease activity and that it decreases with the initiation of immunosuppressive therapy [30–32].

### 4.2 Anti-IL-5 antibodies in EGPA

Interleukin-5 is well known as a key mediator in eosinophil activation. Thus, the efficacy of mepolizumab, a humanized monoclonal antibody against interleukin-5, was evaluated in EGPA patients.

Kahn et al. [33] published the first case of refractory EGPA treated with mepolizumab. The patient had many relapses despite treatment with GC, MTX, interferon alpha, CPh, IV immunoglobulin, AZA, and etoposide. Mepolizumab 750 mg IV monthly was started. After the first dose, asthma significantly improved, the eosinophil count decreased (reaching normal values), and the chest computed tomography (CT) showed complete regression of parenchymal findings. After 6 months of treatment, asthma symptoms disappeared, and chest CT did not show infiltrates, so an attempt to increase the intervals between mepolizumab infusions to 2 months was done which resulted in relapse with reappearance of asthma symptoms, interstitial lung infiltrates, and increase of peripheral eosinophilia. All parameters normalized with transient increase of prednisone and reintroduction of mepolizumab monthly infusions.

A single-center, phase 2, uncontrolled, investigator-initiated trial [34] included 10 consecutive patients with refractory or relapsing EGPA. Relapse was defined by a Birmingham Vasculitis Activity Score (BVAS) >3 despite treatment with IS plus GC at a dosage of 12.5 mg/day or higher. After stopping previous IS, the patients received nine infusions of mepolizumab, 750 mg monthly. Then it was switched to MTX maintenance therapy and a tapered dosage of GC as tolerated. Eight patients reached remission (BVAS = 0 and GC dosage <7.5 mg/day) after two or three mepolizumab infusions. One patient had a partial response (BVAS = 0 but did not achieve a GC dosage <7.5 mg/day), and another patient reached remission but was excluded owing to nonadherence. During mepolizumab treatment, no relapse occurred, the daily GC dose was reduced in all patients, and eosinophil count decreased after the first infusion. After switching mepolizumab to MTX, seven relapses occurred, over a median follow-up of 10 months. The same authors, in a later work [35], followed up these nine patients during a median of 22 months. Only three of them were still in remission at the end of the study. So, a high relapse rate after stopping mepolizumab was observed, which suggests that patients with EGPA could need a continuous treatment with mepolizumab.

An open-label pilot study [36] treated seven patients with four monthly doses of mepolizumab 750 mg IV to assess its steroid-sparing effect in GC-dependent EGPA patients. Mepolizumab allowed for safe GC reduction in all patients. The GC mean dose at baseline was 12.9 mg/day and after 12 weeks of therapy was 4.6 mg/day (64% reduction). On cessation of mepolizumab, EGPA manifestations recurred, needing steroid bursts. Mepolizumab was well tolerated, and the most frequent adverse events were headache, pruritus, and loose stools.

In 2017, a multicenter, double-blind, parallel-group, phase three trial was published [37]. It included 136 patients with relapsing or refractory EGPA, who had received treatment for at least 4 weeks and were taking a stable prednisolone or prednisone dose. They were randomized to receive 300 mg of mepolizumab ($n$ = 68) or placebo ($n$ = 68), administered subcutaneously (SC) every 4 weeks, plus standard care, for 52 weeks. Mepolizumab treatment led to significantly more accrued weeks of remission (defined as BVAS = 0 and prednisolone or predni-sone ≤4 mg/day) than placebo (28 vs. 3% of the participants had ≥24 weeks of accrued remission) and a higher percentage of participants in remission at both weeks 36 and 48 (32 vs. 3%). Remission did not occur in 47% of the participants in the mepolizumab group vs. 81% of those in the placebo group. A total of 44% of the participants in the mepolizumab group, as compared with 7% of those in the placebo group, had an average daily dose of prednisolone or prednisone of ≤4 mg/day during weeks 48 through 52. Eighteen percent of the patients receiving mepolizumab were able to discontinue prednisolone or prednisone completely, as compared with 3% receiving placebo. Also, time to first relapse was longer, and annualized relapse rate was lower in the participants in the mepolizumab group. The most commonly adverse events with mepolizumab were headache, nasopharyngitis, arthralgia, sinusitis, and upper respiratory tract infection. A post hoc analysis [38] of the results according to peripheral eosinophilia (<150 cells/μl), GC dosage (>20 mg/day), and weight (>85 kg) was done. It showed that those patients treated with mepolizumab, with peripheral eosinophilia <150 cell/μl and weight >85 kg, had greater clinical benefit (BVAS = 0 and GC dosage ≤4 mg/day) than placebo. Although no significant differences were found in patients treated with GC dosage >20 mg/day, results favored mepolizumab treatment, but it must be considered that the study include few cases ($n$ = 21).

Recently, Shiroshita et al. [39] published a case report of a 61-year-old man with refractory EGPA despite treatment with GC, CPh, and plasmapheresis who developed a diffuse alveolar hemorrhage. Rituximab and methylprednisolone pulses were administered, and remission was obtained. Then mepolizumab 100 mg SC monthly was started that kept remission until now. To our knowledge, this is the first published paper where the authors used, in an EGPA patient, the same dosage and way of administration of mepolizumab used in severe asthma.

The Food and Drug Administration (FDA) approved the use of mepolizumab in adult patients with EGPA in the United States (USA), in December 2017, based on Wechsler [5] results, being the first biological treatment approved with this indication in data sheet [40–42]. The dosage of 300 mg, three times the recommended dose in severe eosinophilic asthma, is based on observations done in asthma, but no specific dose evaluation has been done in EGPA [42].

Another anti-IL5 monoclonal antibody, reslizumab, and an anti-IL5 receptor monoclonal antibody, benralizumab, are now being investigated for EGPA (NCT02947945 and NCT03010436, respectively) [43, 44].

## 5. Conclusions

The pathogenesis and role of ANCA in EGPA are mostly unknown, although it has been reported that patients with positive ANCA usually present renal involvement (glomerulonephritis), while those with negative ANCA usually have cardiac involvement (heart failure), possibly corresponding to two different subgroups with different characteristics still to be determined which will provide information and facilitate specific treatments. GC and IS are effective in EGPA, but relapses are frequent, and there is no standard therapy based on the results of randomized clinical trials. However, there is new data that shows mepolizumab as a good treatment option due to its clinical benefit, and its use in EGPA has recently been approved in the United States.

Advances in the knowledge of EGPA pathophysiology together with the appear-ance of new drugs, such as mepolizumab, seems to be a solution to the unmet needs in this disease.

## Author details

Carlos Melero Moreno[1*], Marta Corral Blanco[2] and Rocío Magdalena Díaz Campos[2]

1 Institute for Health Research (i+12), Hospital Universitario 12 de Octubre, Madrid, Spain

2 Pneumology Service, Hospital Universitario 12 de Octubre, Madrid, Spain

*Address all correspondence to: cmelero@separ.es

## References

[1] Fujimoto S, Watts RA, Kobayashi S, Suzuki K, Jayne DR, Scott DG, et al. Comparison of the epidemiology of anti-neutrophil cytoplasmic antibody-associated vasculitis between Japan and the UK. Rheumatology. 2011;**50**:1916-1920

[2] Gonzalez-Gay MA, Garcia-Porrua C, Guerrero J, Rodriguez-Ledo P, Llorca J. The epidemiology of the primary systemic vasculitides in Northwest Spain: Implications of the Chapel Hill consensus conference definitions. Arthritis and Rheumatism. 2003;**49**:388-393

[3] Reinhold-Keller E, Herlyn K, Wagner-Bastmeyer R, Gross WL. Stable incidence of primary systemic vasculitides over five years: Results from the German vasculitis register. Arthritis and Rheumatism. 2005;**53**:93-99

[4] Mohammad AJ, Jacobsson LT, Westman KW, Sturfelt G, Segelmark M. Incidence and survival rates in Wegener's granulomatosis, microscopic polyangiitis, Churg-Strauss syndrome and polyarteritis nodosa. Rheumatology. 2009;**48**: 1560- 1565

[5] Watts RA, Lane SE, Bentham G, Scott DG. Epidemiology of systemic vasculitis: A ten-year study in the United Kingdom. Arthritis and Rheumatism; 2000;**43**:414-419

[6] Martin RM, Wilton LV, Mann RD. Prevalence of Churg-Strauss syndrome, vasculitis, eosinophilia and associated conditions: Retrospective analysis of 58 prescription-event monitoring cohort studies. Pharmacoepidemiology and Drug Safety. 1999;**8**:179-189

[7] Mahr A, Guillevin L, Poissonnet M, Ayme S. Prevalences of polyarteritis nodosa, microscopic polyangiitis, Wegener's granulomatosis, and Churg-Strauss syndrome in a French urban multiethnic population in 2000: A capture-recapture estimate. Arthritis and Rheumatism. 2004;**51**:92-99

[8] Sada KE, Amano K, Uehara R, Yamamura M, Arimura Y, Nakamura Y, et al. A nationwide survey on the epidemiology and clinical features of eosinophilic granulomatosis with polyangiitis (Churg-Strauss) in Japan. Modern Rheumatology. 2014;**24**:640-644

[9] Furuta S, Iwamoto T, Nakajima H. Update on eosinophilic granulomatosis with polyangiitis. Allergology International. 2019; pii: S1323-8930(19)30081-4. DOI: 10.1016/j.alit.2019.06.004. [Epub ahead of print]

[10] Thompson GE, Specks U. Update on the management of respiratory manifestations of the antineutrophil cytoplasmic antibodies-associated vasculitides. Clinics in Chest Medicine. 2019;**40**:573-582

[11] Matsumoto K, Suzuki K, Yoshimoto K, Seki N, Tsujimoto H, Chiba K, et al. Significant association between clinical characteristics and immune-phenotypes in patients with ANCA-associated vasculitis. Rheumatology. 2019. pii: kez327. DOI: 10.1093/rheumatology/kez327. [Epub ahead of print]

[12] Yates M, Watts RA, Bajema IM, Cid MC, Crestani B, Hauser T, et al. EULAR/ERA-EDTA recommendations for the management of ANCA-associated vasculitis. Annals of the Rheumatic Diseases. 2016;**75**:1583-1594

[13] Guillevin L, Pagnoux C, Seror R, Mahr A, Mouthon L, Toumelin PL. The five-factor score revisited. Medicine. 2011;**90**:19-27

[14] Cottin V, Bel E, Bottero P, Dalhoff K, Humbert M, Lazor R. Respiratory

manifestations of eosinophilic granulomatosis with polyangiitis (Churg-Strauss). The European Respiratory Journal. 2016;**48**:1429-1441

[15] Sinico RA, Bottero P. Churg-Strauss angiitis. Best Practice & Research. Clinical Rheumatology. 2009;**23**:355-366

[16] Groh M, Pagnoux C, Baldini C, et al. Eosinophilic granulomatosis with polyangiitis (Churg-Strauss) (EGPA) consensus task force recommendations for evaluation and management. European Journal of Internal Medicine. 2015;**26**:545-553

[17] Comarmond C, Pagnoux C, Khellaf M, Cordier JF, Hamidou M, Viallard JF, et al. Eosinophilic granulomatosis with polyangiitis (Churg-Strauss): Clinical characteristics and long-term followup of the 383 patients enrolled in the French vasculitis study group cohort. Arthritis and Rheumatism. 2013;**65**:270-281

[18] Ribi C, Cohen P, Pagnoux C. Treatment of Churg-Strauss syndrome without poor-prognosis factors: A multicenter, prospective, randomized, open-label study of seventy-two patients. Arthritis and Rheumatism. 2008;**58**:586-594

[19] Bosch X, Guilabert A, Espinosa G, et al. Treatment of antineutrophil cytoplasmic antibody associated vasculitis: A systematic review. JAMA. 2007;**298**:655-659

[20] Samson M, Puéchal X, Devilliers H, Ribi C, Cohen P, Stern M. Long-term outcomes of 118 patients with eosinophilic granulomatosis with polyangiitis (Churg-Strauss syndrome) enrolled in two prospective trials. Journal of Autoimmunity. 2013;**43**:60-69

[21] Bourgarit A, Le Toumelin P, Pagnoux C, Cohen P, Mahr A, Le Guern V, et al. Deaths occurring during the first year after treatment onset for polyarteritis nodosa, microscopic polyangiitis, and Churg-Strauss syndrome: A retrospective analysis of causes and factors predictive of mortality based on 595 patients. Medicine. 2005;**84**:323-330

[22] Gayraud M, Guillevin L, le Toumelin P, et al. Long-term followup of polyarteritis nodosa, microscopic polyangiitis, and Churg-Strauss syndrome: Analysis of four prospective trials including 278 patients. Arthritis and Rheumatism. 2001;**44**:666-675

[23] Cohen P, Pagnoux C, Mahr A, Aréne JP, Mouthon L, Le Guern V, et al. Churg-Strauss syndrome with poor-prognosis factors: A prospective multicenter trial comparing glucocorticoids and six or twelve cyclophosphamide pulses in forty-eight patients. Arthritis and Rheumatism. 2007;**57**:686-693

[24] Pagnoux C, Mahr A, Hamidou MA, Boffa JJ, Ruivard M, Ducroix JP, et al. Azathioprine or methotrexate maintenance for ANCA-associated vasculitis. The New England Journal of Medicine. 2008;**359**:2790-2803

[25] Pagnoux C, Guilpain P, Guillevin L. Churg-Strauss syndrome. Current Opinion in Rheumatology. 2007;**19**:25-32

[26] Chakraborty RK, Aeddula NR. Churg Strauss Syndrome (Allergic Granulomatosis). Treasure Island: StatPearls Publishing; 2019. StatPearls [Internet]

[27] Martínez-Moczygemba M, Huston DP. Biology of common beta receptor-signaling cytokines: IL-3, IL-5 and GM-CSF. The Journal of Allergy and Clinical Immunology. 2003;**112**:653-665

[28] Jakiela B, Szczeklik W, Sokolowska B, Mastalerz L, Sanak M,

Plutecka H, et al. Intrinsic pathway of apoptosis in peripheral blood eosinophils of Churg-Strauss syndrome. Rheumatology. 2009;**48**:1202-1207

[29] Zwerina J, Bach C, Martorana D, Jatzwauk M, Hegasy G, Moosig F, et al. Eotaxin-3 in Churg-Strauss syndrome: A clinical and immunogenetic study. Rheumatology. 2011;**50**:1823-1827

[30] Polzer K, Karonitsch T, Neumann T, Eger G, Haberler C, Soleiman A, et al. Eotaxin-3 is involved in Churg-Strauss syndrome—A serum marker closely correlating with disease activity. Rheumatology. 2008;**47**:804-808

[31] Jakiela B, Sanak M, Szczeklik W, Sokolowska B, Plutecka H, Mastalerz L, et al. Both Th2 and Th17 responses are involved in the pathogenesis of Churg-Strauss syndrome. Clinical and Experimental Rheumatology. 2011;**29**:S23-S34

[32] Dallos T, Heiland GR, Strehl J, Karonitsch T, Gross WL, Moosig F, et al. CCL17/thymus and activation-related chemokine in Churg-Strauss syndrome. Arthritis and Rheumatism. 2010;**62**:3496-3503

[33] Kahn JE, Grandpeix-Guyodo C, Marroun I, Catherinot E, Mellot F, Roufosse F, et al. Sustained response to mepolizumab in refractory Churg-Strauss syndrome. The Journal of Allergy and Clinical Immunology. 2010;**125**:267-270

[34] Moosig F, Gross WL, Herrmann K, Bremer JP, Hellmich B. Targeting interleukin-5 in refractory and relapsing Churg-Strauss syndrome. Annals of Internal Medicine. 2011;**155**:341-343

[35] Herrmann K, Gross WL, Moosig F. Extended follow-up after stopping mepolizmab in relapsing/refractory Churg-Strauss syndrome. Clinical and Experimental Rheumatology. 2012;**30**(Suppl. 70): S62-S65

[36] Kim S, Marigowda G, Oren E, Israel E, Wechsler ME. Mepolizumab as a steroid-sparing treatment option with Churg-Strauss syndrome. The Journal of Allergy and Clinical Immunology. 2010;**125**:1336-1343

[37] Wechsler ME, Akuthota P, Jayne D, Khoury P, Klion A, Langford CA, et al. Mepolizumab or placebo for eosinophilic granulomatosis with polyangiitis. The New England Journal of Medicine. 2017;**376**:1921-1932

[38] Steinfeld J, Bradford ES, Brown J, Mallet S, Yancey SW, Akuthota P, et al. Evaluation of clinical benefit from treatment with mepolizumab for patients with eosinophilic granulomatosis with polyangiitis. The Journal of Allergy and Clinical Immunology. 2019;**143**:2170-2177

[39] Shiroshita A, Nakashima K, Motojima S, Aoshima M. Refractory diffuse alveolar hemorrhage caused by eosinophilic granulomatosis with polyangiitis in the absence of elevated biomarkers treated successfully by rituximab and mepolizumab: A case report. Respiratory Medicine Case Reports. 2019;**26**:112-114

[40] Faverio P, Bonaiti G, Bini F, Vaghi A, Pesci A. Mepolizumab as the first targeted treatment for eosinophilic granulomatosis with polyangiitis: A review of current evidence and potential place in therapy. Therapeutics and Clinical Risk Management. 2018;**14**:2385-2396

[41] GSK achieves approval for Nucala (mepolizumab) for the treatment of eosinophilic granulomatosis with polyangiitis (EGPA) for adults in the U.S. [news release]. GlaxoSmithKline plc. 12 December 2017

[42] Raffray L, Guillevin L. Treatment of eosinophilic granulomatosis with polyangiitis: A review. Drugs. 2018;**78**:809-821

[43] U.S. National Library of Medicine. Reslizumab in the treatment of eosinophilic granulomatosis with polyangiitis (EGPA) study. [Internet]. ClinicalTrials.gov identifier: NCT02947945. Available from: https://clinicaltrials.gov/ct2/show/NCT02947945

[44] U.S. National Library of Medicine. Benralizumab in the treatment of eosinophilic granulomatosis with polyangiitis (EGPA) study. [Internet]. ClinicalTrials.gov identifier: NCT03010436. [cited 2019 Aug 29]. Available from: https://clinicaltrials.gov/ct2/show/NCT03010436

# 9

# Eosinophilic Cholangitis

*Gilles Jadd Hoilat, Judie Noemie Hoilat,*
*Mohamad Fekredeen Ayas, Sana Riaz and Divey Manocha*

## Abstract

A variety of benign etiologies of biliary stricture may initially be mistaken for hilar cholangiocarcinoma. Consequently, many patients undergo surgery for a benign disease that could have been treated medically. Eosinophilic cholangitis (EC) is an uncommon, benign, self-limiting disease that should be considered when approaching a case of obstructive jaundice since it causes biliary stricture formation. Transmural eosinophilic infiltration of the biliary tree is characteristic of EC. It may initially be indistinguishable from hilar cholangiocarcinoma. We worked on a case of a patient who was referred to our hospital for jaundice and abdominal mass investigation with the provisional diagnosis of cholangiocarcinoma. During the workup, the index of suspicion for malignancy remained high as the typical laboratory and radiological findings for benign causes of biliary stricture were not present. Hence, the patient underwent left hepatectomy with caudate lobe resection and received a retrograde diagnosis of EC. The case demonstrates that EC could present in the elderly with cardinal signs of cancer and absence of the typical findings of EC which was not previously reported. Furthermore, this disorder has been reported to respond well to steroid therapy, hence, diagnostic criteria for EC would provide another treatment option for elderly and/or those who are not fit for surgery.

**Keywords:** bile duct diseases, cholangitis, constriction, pathologic, stricture

## 1. Introduction

While approaching a patient with jaundice, it is important to understand the different types and approach towards jaundice in order to reach the correct diagnosis. Similarly, when approaching a biliary stricture, one must consider benign as well as malignant etiologies since they can be clinically identical. Eosinophilic cholangitis (EC) is a rare benign disorder of the biliary tract which can cause biliary obstruction.

This is the first book that has a specific chapter for a very rare disease, eosinophilic cholangitis. In this chapter, we will briefly discuss the approach towards jaundice before jumping to the main topic of eosinophilic cholangitis. We hope that you will find the information provided informative.

## 2. Approach to jaundice

Jaundice (i.e., icterus) is the buildup of bilirubin; a waste product stemmed from the metabolism of aging/destruction of red blood cells (RBCs), causing a yellowish discoloration in tissues that are filled with elastic collagen, such as skin, sclera, and mucus membranes, etc. [1].

Let us take some cases here to further understand how jaundice can present.

## 2.1 Case-1

A 14-year-old (y/o) African-American male presented to the emergency department (ED) with severe abdominal pain, swelling of both hands and jaundice. Family history includes two uncles that suffer from "blood problems." Blood tests showed normal alkaline phosphatase (ALP), aspartate aminotransferase (AST), alanine aminotransferase (ALT), bilirubin was 3.2 mg/dL (2.8 indirect). On peripheral blood smear, sickling was found. Hemoglobin electrophoresis confirmed SS hemoglobin and patient was diagnosed with sickle cell anemia (SCA).

## 2.2 Case-2

A 42-year-old Caucasian male presented to the office with 2 months of jaundice and abdominal pain. The patient had a blood transfusion in 1988 at the age of 15.

| Type of jaundice | Differential diagnosis |
|---|---|
| Pre-hepatic (hemolytic) | • Excess aged/destroyed RBCs (e.g., hemolysis, blood transfusion)<br>• Decreased hepatic uptake (e.g., portosystemic shunt, drugs)<br>• Decreased conjugation (e.g., Gilbert's syndrome) |
| Hepatic (hepatocellular) | • Excretion defect (Dubin-Johnson syndrome, Rotor syndrome)<br>• Viral hepatitis<br>• Hepatic steatosis<br>• Alcoholic hepatitis<br>• Non-alcoholic steatohepatitis<br>• Autoimmune hepatitis<br>• Ischemic hepatitis<br>• Drug-induced hepatitis<br>• Hemochromatosis<br>• Wilson's disease |
| Post-hepatic (obstructive) | • Biliary tract disease (primary sclerosing cholangitis, primary biliary cirrhosis, eosinophilic cholangitis, etc.)<br>• Biliary tract obstruction (gallstones, cholangiocarcinoma, pancreatic or liver cancer, pancreatic pseudocyst, etc.) |

**Table 1.**
*Types of Jaundice [2, 3].*

| Lab findings | AST + ALT | ALP | Conjugated bilirubin (CB) | Unconjugated bilirubin (UCB) | Total bilirubin | Conjugated bilirubin in urine |
|---|---|---|---|---|---|---|
| Pre-hepatic (hemolytic) | Normal | Normal | Normal | Normal/↑ | Normal/↑ | Negative |
| Hepatic (hepatocellular) | ↑ | ↑ | ↑ | ↑ | ↑ | Positive |
| Post-hepatic (obstructive) | ↑ | ↑ | ↑ | Normal | ↑ | Positive |

**Table 2.**
*Lab findings depending on type of jaundice [4].*

| Clinical findings | Urine color | Stool color | Large spleen |
|---|---|---|---|
| Pre-hepatic (hemolytic) | Normal | Brown | Positive |
| Hepatic (hepatocellular) | Dark (combination of CB + urobilinogen) | Slightly pale | Positive |
| Post-hepatic (obstructive) | Dark (CB) | Pale | Negative |

**Table 3.**
*Clinical findings depending on type of jaundice [4].*

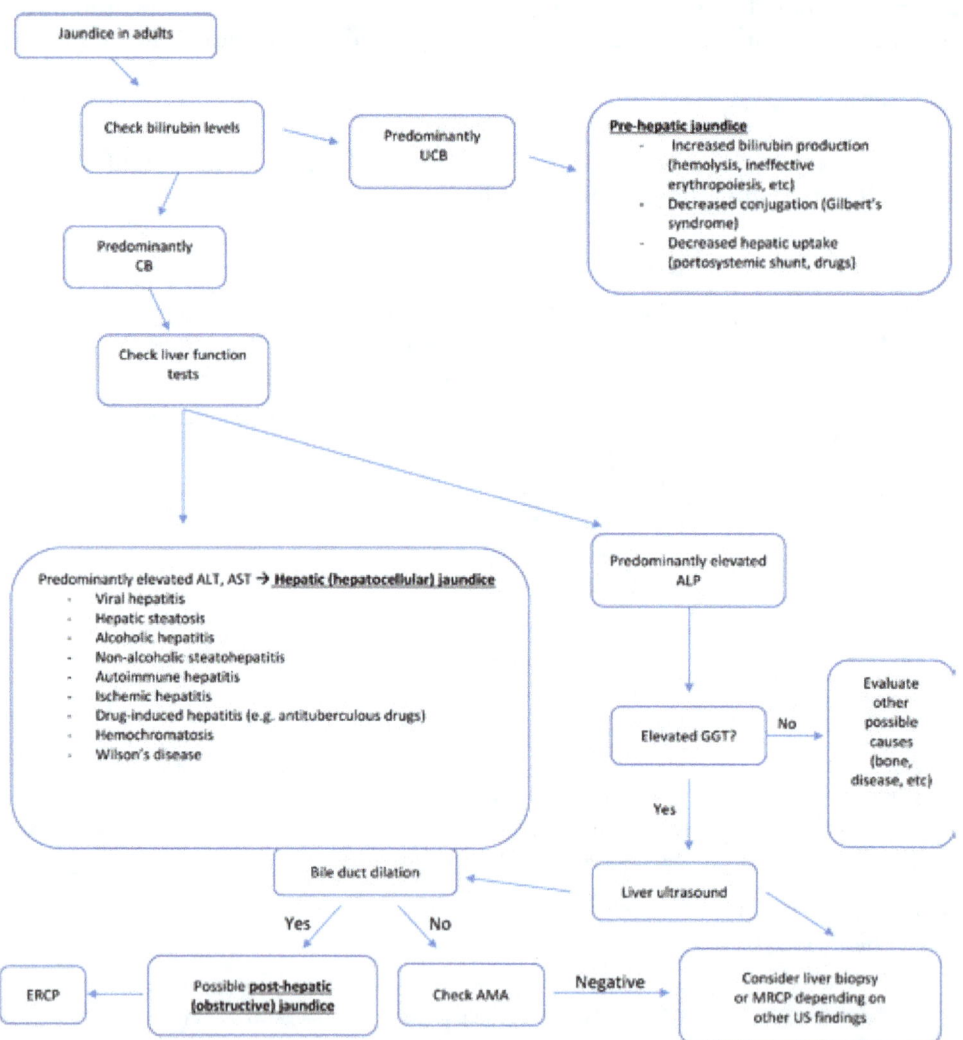

**Figure 1.**
*Approach to Jaundice.*

Physical exam showed typical signs of cirrhosis. Labs showed an ALP of 200, ALT 2810, AST 2670 U/L, normal gamma-glutamyl transferase (GGT), bilirubin of 3.3 mg/dL (2 direct, 1.3 indirect), and normal iron and copper levels. Patient was positive for hepatitis C, attributed to his previous blood transfusion. Alpha feto-protein (AFP) levels were elevated and patient was scheduled for a liver ultrasound (US) and biopsy to rule out hepatocellular carcinoma (HCC).

## 2.3 Case-3

A 39-year-old Caucasian female with a body mass index (BMI) of 36 and a history of hamishoto's thyroiditis, presented to the ED with worsening itching and jaundice. Patient's thyroid function tests were within normal range. Cholesterol was 310 mg/dL, ALP 318, ALT 24, AST 21, and GGT 1120 U/L. Liver US showed no signs of bile duct dilation. Anti-mitochondrial antibody (AMA) titers were elevated. Patient was diagnosed with primary biliary cholangitis (PBC) and was started on ursodiol.

Now what do we take from these three different cases, all of whom presented or were seen to have jaundice? To understand the different presentations of jaundice, let us classify it.

The causes of jaundice can be classified in different ways such as pre-hepatic (hemolytic), hepatic (hepatocellular), and post-hepatic (obstructive) (see **Table 1**). Now, we can differentiate between them in many laboratory and clinical findings (see **Tables 2** and **3**) and know how to approach it (see **Figure 1**).

Understanding the classification, differentiating lab results and approach towards jaundice is important. **Figure 1** can help you as a guide in term of what to do and what to expect. It is helpful to keep it in mind as we go through the chapter.

## 3. Approach to eosinophilic cholangitis

### 3.1 Introduction

Now that we have established the approach towards obstructive jaundice. We will dig deeper into eosinophilic cholangitis.

EC is an uncommon, benign, self-limiting cause of biliary structure characterized by transmural eosinophilic infiltration of the biliary tree which may result in obstructive jaundice. The severity and prognosis vary considerably and may affect part or the entire biliary tree mimicking malignancy [5].

### 3.2 Pathogenesis

The exact pathogenesis is poorly understood.

The cause of eosinophilic cholangitis is unknown. In some reports, hypereosinophilic syndrome (HES) has been mentioned as possible cause. The diagnosis of hypereosinophilic syndrome is based on the following criteria [6]:

1. Sustained eosinophilia (more than 1500 eosinophils per cubic millimeter) for more than 6 months.

2. The absence of other causes of eosinophilia, including parasitic infections and allergies.

3. Signs and symptoms of organ involvement.

Since all reported cases do not appear to have completely met the criteria for HES, the relationship between eosinophilic cholangitis and HES is uncertain.

An allergic mechanism is thought to play a key role in the development of eosinophilic cholangitis, hence the name. In most reported cases, there was an increased level of IgE, interleukin 5, or eosinophilic cationic protein. The latter is one of the major cationic granules released by activated eosinophils and is the most widely used clinical biomarker of eosinophil in atopic diseases. Furthermore, it has been it has been demonstrated that eosinophils produce transforming growth factor-beta, a cytokine known to stimulate fibrosis, a devastating effect that may leave liver transplantation as the only cure [7, 8].

### 3.3 Clinical presentation

Nash et al. conducted a study where they collected around 23 cases of EC revealing that this disease [9]:

- Slightly more prevalent in men than women (1,6:1).

- The most common presenting symptoms were abdominal pain followed by jaundice.

- Around 69.6% of patients demonstrated peripheral eosinophilia and 30.4% had normal eosinophilic count.

One of the challenges that accompanies eosinophilic cholangitis is the fact that it can present with a multitude of nonspecific signs and symptoms that makes it hard to differentiate from malignancy such as:

- Abdominal mass

- Abdominal pain

- Jaundice

- Generalized fatigue

- Nausea and vomiting

- Weight loss

At this point, it can be anything and a more in-depth investigation is required. So where do we go from there?

### 3.4 Investigations

The issue with eosinophilic cholangitis is that it mimics malignancy very closely so what are the options that we have that can help differentiate it from cancer?

Normal routine labs, taking into account the presenting symptoms should be done.

- CBC with differential to look at the eosinophilic count.

- A liver function test:

  o Bilirubin (total and direct) may be elevated.

  o ALT and AST may or may not be increased.

○ ALP and GGT are usually increased like any other diseases involving the biliary tree.

○ Amylase and lipase to rule out a pancreatic cause.

○ Since eosinophilic cholangitis can mimic cholangiocarcinoma, tumors markers such as carcinoembryonic antigen (CEA) and carbohydrate antigen 19-9 (CA19-9) can be ordered and surprisingly may be elevated making the diagnosis even more challenging.

Again, looking at the laboratory investigation, it is still hard to pinpoint the diagnosis, the next step would be to move on into imaging modalities.

## 3.5 Imaging modalities

There are many available imaging modalities that are helpful in visualizing and evaluating the biliary system. Noninvasive imaging modalities can demonstrate common nonspecific findings of EC such as bile duct wall thickening (segmental or diffuse) on US (see **Figure 2**) and contrast enhanced CT and MRCP with or

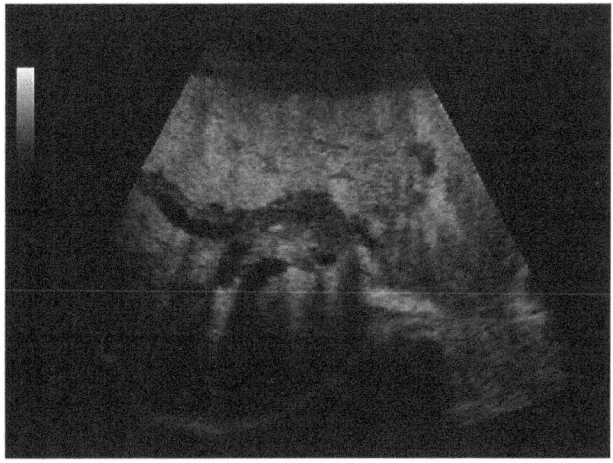

**Figure 2.**
*This contrast enhanced ultrasound (CEUS) shows thickened wall of intrahepatic bile ducts (from hilar to peripheral) with dilation, and the lesion was well enhanced.*

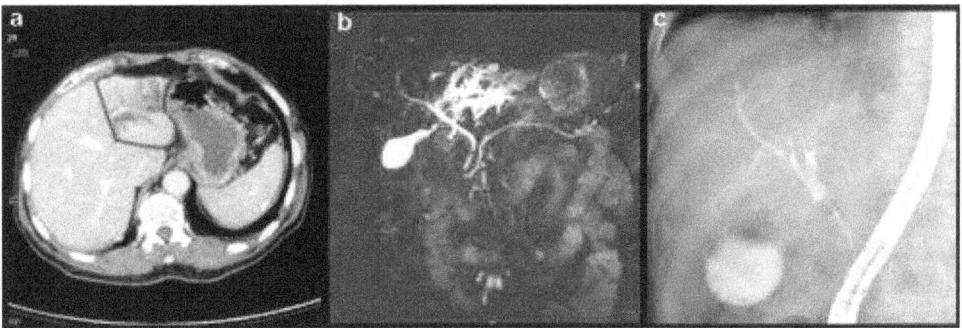

**Figure 3.**
*(a) Computed tomography scan (CT scan) of abdomen and pelvis; (b) magnetic resonance cholangiopancreatography (MRCP); (c) endoscopic retrograde cholangiopancreatography showing a focal dilation of the biliary tree to the left lobe through the suggestion of subtle ill-defined enhancing mass lesion at the level of liver hilum.*

without biliary dilation (see **Figure 3**). These findings can also be seen in malignant processes, hence the need to obtain a brush cytology and tissue biopsy by means of performing invasive imaging modalities such as ERCP.

While MRCP is useful in demonstrating an irregular narrowing of the bile duct, ERCP and percutaneous transhepatic cholangiography (PTC) provide additional information such as irregularities of the common bile duct and the intrahepatic ducts as well as the length and site of biliary stricture.

ERCP with brush biopsy, PET-CT (see **Figure 4**) and an endoscopic guided fine needle aspiration (EUS guided FNA) are also used to try to differentiate a benign from a malignant cause of biliary tree dilation. As you can see, the CT scan shows an ill-defined enhancing mass lesion at the level of liver hilum suggesting cholangiocarcinoma.

ERCP with brush biopsy may not show malignant cells.

EUS-guided FNA may show a background of mixed inflammation including many eosinophils.

Sometimes the diagnosis can be made, and targeted treatment can be started but most of the time, the index of suspicion for malignancy remains high.

### 3.6 Proposed diagnostic criteria

Matsumoto et al. revealed a characteristic feature of EC that  helped rule out malignancy: staining of a parenchymal echo in the bile duct wall on

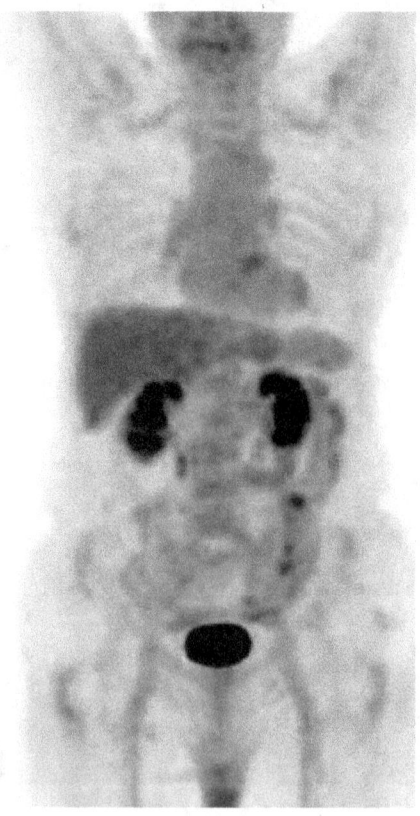

**Figure 4.**
*This positron emission tomography-computed tomography (PET-CT) reveals a soft tissue lesion within the main left biliary duct but does not show any fluorodeoxyglucose (FDG) activity. This still does not exclude cholangiocarcinoma.*

contrast-enhanced ultrasound (CEUS). However, they suggested the following requirements to accurately diagnose EC [6]:

1. Thickening of the biliary wall or narrowing of the biliary tree;

2. Eosinophilic infiltration on histopathology;

3. Regression of the stricture or resolution of other biliary abnormalities in the absence of treatment or subsequent steroid therapy.

### 3.7 Treatment

Even though EC is a self-limiting disease, it has a variable course, making precise treatment recommendations difficult. The challenge remains to exclude malignancy, which is not always possible with various imaging modalities and biopsies. Hence, mandatory surgical intervention is an effective and definitive measure of treating EC if there is diagnostic uncertainty.

According to the literature, two cases of EC described a stricture in the common hepatic duct that regressed spontaneously without any medical intervention within 3 weeks, but most of the published cases of EC were treated surgically and received a retrograde diagnosis (see **Figure 5**) [10].

Seow-En et al. suggested that the best option to simultaneously treat a stricture, exclude malignancy, and attain a definite diagnosis of EC is surgical intervention. They also described the advantages of surgery over medical therapy, indicating that medical treatment does not eradicate the chance of recurrence and that it could put patients at risk of complications of repeated steroid therapy [11].

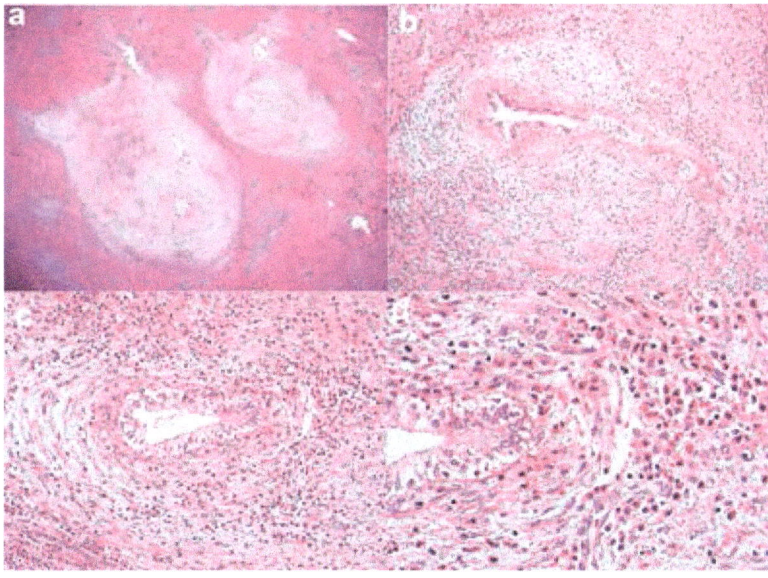

**Figure 5.**
*(a) Severe degree of periductal onion skin fibrosis (hematoxylin and eosin stain displaying 2× magnification). (b and c) The inflammatory infiltrates around the partially damaged bile duct are mostly eosinophilic cells (hematoxylin and eosin stain displaying 10× magnification). (d) The eosinophilic count exceeds 40 cells per HPF (hematoxylin and eosin stain displaying 40× magnification).*

A diagnostic trial of oral corticosteroid can be tried to see if any resolution occurs, however the dose and duration of treatment are yet to be determined due to the poor understanding of the diseased natural course.

## 4. Conclusion

In conclusion, EC is an uncommon, benign, and self-limiting cause of biliary stricture. Although this disease has a good response to corticosteroid therapy, it often mimics cholangiocarcinoma which makes reaching a definite diagnosis by clinical and radiological findings difficult. Hence most cases are treated surgically and receive a retrograde diagnosis.

## Author details

Gilles Jadd Hoilat[1], Judie Noemie Hoilat[2], Mohamad Fekredeen Ayas[3], Sana Riaz and Divey Manocha[1*]

1 State University of New York Upstate Medical University, Syracuse, United States of America

2 Alfaisal University College of Medicine, Riyadh, Saudi Arabia

3 Ascension St. John Hospital, Detroit, United States of America

*Address all correspondence to: manochad@upstate.edu

# References

[1] Rao D. Differential Diagnosis in Surgical Diseases. 1st ed. New Delhi: Jaypee Brothers Medical Pub.; 2010

[2] Goljan E. Rapid Review Pathology. 4th ed. Philadelphia, PA: Elsevier Saunders; 2013

[3] Limdi J. Evaluation of abnormal liver function tests. Postgraduate Medical Journal. 2003;**79**(932):307-312

[4] Goljan E. Rapid Review Pathology. 2nd ed. Philadelphia, PA: Mosby Elsevier; 2007

[5] Hoilat J, Hoilat G, AlQahtani S, Alhussaini H, Alabbad S. A typical presentation of a rare disease: Eosinophilic cholangitis posing as a cancer. American Journal of Case Reports. 2018;**19**:76-81

[6] Matsumoto N. A case of eosinophilic cholangitis: Imaging findings of contrast-enhanced ultrasonography, cholangioscopy, and intraductal ultrasonography. World Journal of Gastroenterology. 2007;**13**(13):1995

[7] Miura F, Asano T, Amano H, Yoshida M, Toyota N, Wada K, et al. Resected case of eosinophilic cholangiopathy presenting with secondary sclerosing cholangitis. World Journal of Gastroenterology. 2009;**15**(11):1394

[8] Fang S, Fan T, Fu H, Chen C, Hwang C, Hung T, et al. A novel cell-penetrating peptide derived from human eosinophil cationic protein. PLoS ONE. 2013;**8**(3):e57318

[9] Shukla S, Kharat P, Kumar K. Clinicopathological study on patients presenting with obstructive jaundice. International Surgery Journal. 2018;**5**(2):705

[10] Nashed C, Sakpal S, Shusharina V, Chamberlain R. Eosinophilic cholangitis and cholangiopathy: A sheep in wolves clothing. HPB Surgery. 2010;**2010**:1-7

[11] Seow-En I, Chiow AK, Tan SS, Poh WT. Eosinophilic cholangiopathy: The diagnostic dilemma of a recurrent biliary stricture. Should surgery be offered for all? BMJ Case Reports. 2014;**2014**. pii: bcr2013202225

# 10

# Eosinophilic Phenotype: The Lesson from Research Models to Severe Asthma

*Guida Giuseppe and Antonelli Andrea*

## Abstract

Eosinophilic airway inflammation is a hallmark in the pathophysiological and clinical definition of asthma. In the last decades, asthma evolved in the recognition of different phenotypes identified by natural history, clinical and physiological characteristics, and the underlying immune mechanisms. Among these phenotypes, many have been associated with eosinophilic-driven inflammation. This is the case of either early-onset allergic Th2 asthma or late-onset persistent eosinophilic asthma. Both animal models and analysis from human samples have contributed to elucidate the role of eosinophils in the asthmatic inflammatory response and the synergic role of Th2 cytokines. In severe asthma, high numbers of eosinophils can persist despite treatment with inhaled and oral corticosteroids leading to the definition of severe refractory eosinophilic asthma. The combined role of IL-4-, IL-13- and IL-5-associated pathways has focused the view over the T2-type endotypes, wherein a specific biological pathway explains the observable properties of different phenotypes and the identifiable biomarkers can predict response to monoclonal antibodies directed against a selected immune target. In the era of precision medicine and personalized therapy, both the identification of Th2 molecules and eosinophils as targets and biomarkers have become the best clue for treating and monitoring severe asthma.

**Keywords:** severe asthma, eosinophilic phenotypes, T2-type inflammation, eosinophilic refractory asthma, anti-IL5 treatment

## 1. Introduction

Asthma and chronic rhinosinusitis (CRS) are chronic inflammatory disorders involving the lower and upper airways. According to the definition by Global Initiative for Asthma (GINA) documents, asthma is a heterogeneous disease characterized by chronic airway inflammation associated with a history of respiratory symptoms such as wheeze, shortness of breath, chest tightness and cough and evidence of variable expiratory airflow limitation [1]. Airway inflammation is usually present and persists even when symptoms are absent or lung function is normal.

In the last decades, the role of chronic airway inflammation has been central in the definition of asthma that was recognized as a chronic inflammatory disorder in which many cells and cellular mediators play a role and result in the characteristic pathophysiological changes [2]. The inflammation involves all the airways from the main bronchi to the peripheral small airways. A characteristic pattern of inflammation has been described in asthma involving inflammatory cells mainly mast cells, eosinophils, T lymphocytes, dendritic cells, macrophages and neutrophils, which release mediators that induce symptoms. Both animal models and analysis from human samples have contributed to elucidate the type of inflammation involved in asthma [3]. The most common phenotype of asthma is characterized by eosinophilic airway inflammation and the role of eosinophils as a key player in the pathophysiology of asthma is well documented. Eosinophils emerged as leading cells from the first post-mortem studies of asthmatic lungs, passing through the finding of increased in number and activation status of eosinophils in asthmatic airways [4] and of increased eosinophil surrogates as fractional exhaled nitric oxide (FENO) [5]. Nowadays, the focus is on the definition of the forms of uncontrolled or severe eosinophilic asthma in which airways, sputum and blood eosinophils are consistently increased and represent a biomarker of the eosinophilic endotype of asthma and a guide for biologic target therapies [6, 7].

## 2. Eosinophils and allergic asthma

Allergen challenge models have been conceived to reproduce many features of clinical asthma [8]. Actually, atopy, which is the production of allergen-specific IgE antibodies, is a predisposing factor for asthma development, and birth cohort studies have shown that sensitization to allergens such as house dust mite, cat and dog dander and Aspergillus is independent risk factors for wheezing in children [9]. Moreover, exposure to allergens is one of the most recognized environmental factors that trigger asthma symptoms. The term allergic asthma has been used to define the presence of sensitization to environmental allergens and the clinical correlation between exposure and symptoms, both indoor and outdoor allergens being well-known triggers of asthma exacerbations [10].

Both allergen challenged animal models of asthma and allergic asthma in humans are associated with a T-lymphocyte CD4+ Th2-polarized response as the main feature of airway inflammation. The allergic response is characterized by immediate and late inflammatory responses in which Th2 cells govern the inflammatory cell recruitment and activation by the release of the signature cytokines IL-4, IL-5 and IL-13 as well as IgE antibody synthesis.

### 2.1 Mouse models of allergic asthma

In acute allergen challenged mouse models of asthma, after the sensitization period (usually 14–21 days), the animal is challenged with the allergen via the airway and this causes many key features of clinical asthma. The analysis of bronchoalveolar lavage (BAL) and bioptic samples of airway walls has supported the hypothesis that asthma is a Th2-mediated disease. A dominating influx of eosinophils has been demonstrated and related to the development of AHR [11]. Moreover, the adoptive transfer of Th2 cells into recipient mice was able to reproduce airway eosinophilia, mucus hypersecretion and AHR after allergen inhalation [12].

However, some of these effects resulted in transient changes and do not involve structural changes. Through chronic allergen exposure in mice, allergen-dependent sensitization, Th2-dependent allergic inflammation, eosinophilic influx into the airway mucosa, mucus overproduction and AHR have been reproduced [11, 13]. Generally, acute and chronically treated mice had similar early and late asthmatic responses; however, the acute model had higher levels of eosinophilia, whereas the chronic model showed hyperresponsiveness to lower doses of methacholine and had higher total IgE. On the other hand, many of the lesions observed in chronic human asthma, such as chronic inflammation of the airway wall and airway remodeling changes, are absent.

Moreover, transgenic mice that overexpress the Th2 cytokines—IL-4, IL-5, IL-13 and IL-9—in the airway epithelium exhibit the same inflammatory features. IL5 is a Th2 cytokine essential for differentiation, maturation and survival of eosinophils. A key role in allergen-induced inflammatory responses has been shown in murine IL-5-deficient model chronically challenged with an allergen in which the eosinophilia, lung damage and airway hyperreactivity were abolished. The reconstitution of IL-5 production using recombinant vaccinia virus that expressed IL-5 restored eosinophilia and airway dysfunction [14]. Using a clinically relevant model of chronic allergic asthma in mice, Kumar RK et al. showed that anti–IL-5 inhibited inflammation in terms of accumulation of eosinophils in the tracheal epithelium and inflammatory cells in the lamina propria, but had no effect on airway responsiveness to methacholine [15].

Many studies have demonstrated the significant role of IL/4IL-13 pathway in asthma. Through the agonization of IL-4R, both IL4 and IL13 activate a tyrosine kinase-dependent signal that after phosphorylation of STAT6 regulates the transcription of Th2-involved genes. Models of IL-4−/− mice were protected from the development of AHR and aspects of remodeling, while the administration of soluble IL-4 receptor reduced inflammation and mucus hypersecretion, but had no effect on AHR [8] Similarly, soluble IL-13 suppressed pulmonary inflammation but had a limited effect on AHR [15].

Limitations evidenced in mouse models are that inflammation is not restricted to the conducting airways, but extended to vascular and parenchymal parts of the lung; moreover, some of the clues of asthma inflammation such as the large increases in airway smooth muscle and MC infiltration are not generally observed.

## 2.2 Human models of allergic asthma

In humans, the role of Th2 cytokines and eosinophils in allergic asthma comes from many experimental data that in part differ from the mice models.

Sensitizations to environmental allergens in allergic subjects are documented by positive skin prick test reactions and elevated allergen-specific IgE serum levels. Activation of FcεRI on mast cells and basophils by allergen-bound IgE induces the release of preformed vasoactive mediators, which rapidly elicit edema of the bronchial mucosa, mucus production and smooth muscle constriction. This mechanism is confirmed by the increased numbers of cells expressing the high-affinity receptor for IgE (FcεRI) in allergic asthmatic tissues [16].

Biopsies from bronchial mucosa show CD4+ cell infiltrates and enhanced expression of Th2-type cytokines and chemokines. IL-4 and IL-5 mRNA were localized in activated T cells (CD3+), mast cells (tryptase +) and activated eosinophils (EG2+) both in BAL and bronchial biopsies from mild atopic asthmatic patients [17], and the number of activated CD4+ T cells and IL-5 mRNA positive cells is increased in asthmatic airways following antigen challenge. This skewed cytokine involvement is reflected by the expression of the transcriptional regulators GATA-3 (GATA binding protein 3) after segmental allergen challenge in asthmatics [18]. GATA-3 is a transcriptor factor that finds its binding site in the IL-5 promoter and induces Th2 cytokine gene expression by biasing Th1/Th2 balance. The increase in GATA-3 expression in the asthmatic subjects correlated significantly with IL-5 expression and AHR [19]. In summary, CD4+ Th2 cells are believed to initiate and perpetuate the inflammatory response in allergic asthma.

IL-5 expression is increased 18–48 h after allergen challenge in BAL samples in mite-associated bronchial asthma when they were stimulated with Dermatophagoides farinae [20]. The levels of IL-5 mRNA-positive cells and IL-5 correlate with the number of eosinophils infiltrating the bronchial mucosa and BAL of asthmatic subjects, with pulmonary function and symptom severity [21]. Biopsies from the respiratory mucosa of allergic asthmatics show the enhanced expression of other Th2-type cytokines and chemokines such as IL-4, IL-6, IL-9, IL-10 and IL-13. Allergen challenge induces in patients with asthma IL13 and IL4 release in BAL and sputum eosinophils that positively correlate with IL-13 expression in asthmatic bronchial submucosa [22]. IL13 is thus involved in the regulation of allergen-induced late-phase inflammatory responses. IL-13, indeed, can modulate the production of IgE through the isotype class switching of B cells; therefore, it is involved in the early phase of allergic reactions.

### 2.3 Recruitment of eosinophils in allergic asthma

Eosinophils are recruited from progenitors after allergen exposure. Levels of Eo progenitors arise in the peripheral blood after seasonal allergen exposure, during controlled exacerbations of atopic asthma and after single allergen challenge to the airways in atopic asthmatics and animal models. Trafficking of these cells from the bone marrow, where they are produced, to the airways was also demonstrated. In fact, these CD34+ CD45+ progenitors express the IL-5 receptor alpha and are recruited by IL5 and GM-CSF produced in asthmatic airways, subsequently acquiring an activating form that reaches the inflamed airways [23]. Eosinophilopoiesis develops after 24 h from allergen challenges and is followed by the accumulation of eosinophils in the airways.

### 2.4 Eosinophils in different phases of allergic asthma

The sensitization phase is supposed to be determined by the differentiation of Th naive cells into Th2 lymphocytes. Dendritic cells (DCs) in response to allergen stimulation drive a Th2-oriented response. DC subsets have been described to respond to various stimuli coming from the inflammatory milieu generated after the allergenic encounter. Myeloid CD1c + DCs respond to thymic stromal lymphopoietin (TSLP) produced by the epithelium after allergen encounter by activating allergen-specific memory CD4+ cells [24]. Eosinophils also contribute to the initiation phase of Th2 response by suppressing the Th1/Th17 pathway.

The main role of eosinophils in asthmatic response is yet related to the effector phase of the inflammatory response. After allergen challenge, asthmatics generally develop immediate bronchoconstriction, the so-called early asthmatic response, which is maximized within 30 min and resolves between 1 and 3 h. A proportion of subjects develop a second, delayed bronchoconstrictor response, named the late asthmatic response, which is characterized by prolonged AHR and pronounced airway eosinophilia [25]. So it can be assumed that in isolated early responders a significant or sustained eosinophilic response does not develop. On the other hand, the so-called dual responders develop a sustained IL-5-dependent eosinophilic response in terms of both bone marrow recruitment and sputum accumulation. This response is accompanied by increases in circulating eosinophils, greater increases of activated eosinophils in the airways, and the development of airway hyperresponsiveness [26].

Recruited eosinophils in the airways release a variety of toxic products, oxygen radicals, granule-associated cytotoxic proteins and membrane-derived proinflammatory mediators that damage the bronchial epithelium and increase AHR.

IL-5 is the most important constituent increasing eosinophil survival, recruitment, degranulation and lung injury following inhalation of antigen, as demonstrated in a segmental antigen lung challenge model [20], and the levels of eosinophils and their cationic proteins in the BAL fluid following allergen challenge correlate with the magnitude of the late phase response. Moreover, a positive correlation between the percentage of BAL eosinophils and the ECP was demonstrated at baseline but not after 4–6 h after allergen inhalation, thus suggesting that eosinophil recruitment and activation seem to follow different temporal kinetics [27].

The effect of IL-5 on eosinophils is demonstrated by the finding of increased expression of the alpha chain of IL-5R mRNA in the bronchial biopsies of atopic and nonatopic asthmatic subjects; the membrane-bound aIL-5R is coexpressed with EG2 in the eosinophils within the bronchial mucosa of asthmatics and inversely correlated with FEV1 [28].

## 2.5 Eosinophilic chemokines in allergic asthma

IL-5 acts as chemotactic factors for eosinophils, promoting eosinophil-endothelial adhesion by inducing the expression of VCAM-1 on endothelial cells. In turn, VCAM-1 may bind to integrins on the eosinophils leading to the migration of eosinophils to sites of airway inflammation. Blood eosinophils stimulated with IL-5 adhere to VCAM-1 via the integrins $\alpha4\beta1$ and $\alpha M\beta2$ that are the major eosinophil integrin-mediating cell adhesion [29]. Eosinophils obtained from BAL after segmental antigen challenge have both $\beta1$ and $\beta2$ integrins in a high-activity conformation and adhere to VCAM-1 to a higher degree than blood eosinophils [30]. It seems, therefore, that blood eosinophils are primed by IL-5 or P-selectin (expressed by platelets) to an integrin activation status and are consequently arrested in vessels of inflamed bronchi and move into lung tissue. It is remarkable that the administration of anti–IL-5 can lower $\beta2$ integrin activation [31]. IL-5 not only has got the ability to prime eosinophils for subsequent activation but also enhances their survival at sites of allergic inflammation.

The role of other chemokines in allergic asthma is sustained by different pieces of evidence. Eotaxin and regulated on activation, normal T-cell expressed and secreted (RANTES) act on eosinophils inducing chemotaxis as well as specifically activation. In human challenges with the HDM allergen, the peak of eosinophils immunopositive for eotaxin, RANTES and IL-5 occurs at 7 h after allergen inhalation, but persisting eosinophilic airway inflammation and AHR remained for 7 days after allergen inhalation [32].

These chemokines are released by several cell types in the lung: endothelial cells, epithelial cells, fibroblasts, DCs and smooth muscle cells. Eotaxin creates a chemotactic gradient so that eosinophils pass the endothelium of the blood vessels and migrate to the site of inflammation [33]. Eotaxin has the potential to mobilize eosinophils and their progenitors from bone marrow and this effect is potentiating with that of IL5. Second, in atopic asthmatic patients, high concentrations of eotaxin in BAL fluid are detected as well as an increased expression of eotaxin mRNA and protein in the epithelium and submucosa of their airways. In the airways of allergic asthmatics, eotaxin is in sufficient concentrations to exert chemotactic activity on eosinophils in vitro and this effect is enhanced by IL-5 [34].

RANTES is also found in high concentrations in the sera in allergic asthma, as well as monocyte chemoattractant protein-1 and -3 (MCP). These chemokines play a role in ongoing lung inflammation, lung leukocyte infiltration, bronchial hyper-responsiveness and the recruitment of eosinophils.

Eotaxins and RANTES bind to the CCR3 receptor expressed on Th2 cells, eosinophils and basophils. Eosinophils in CCR3R knockout mice reach the blood vessels and the endothelium but fail to migrate into lung tissue. Indeed, these mice are protected from AHR after allergen challenges [35]. After antigen challenge, the percentage of CCR3+ eosinophils is downregulated on BAL eosinophils compared with peripheral blood eosinophils, while other chemokine receptors like CCR4, CCR9 and CXCR3 do not, being predominantly involved in activation of eosinophil effector responses [36].

The relationships between the levels of eosinophilic chemokines and AHR or bronchoconstriction are not documented in the same way. Some data suggest that mediators released by cells other than eosinophils, similar to MCs or basophils, can contribute to AHR. In addition, chemokine receptors might be involved in the activation of airway eosinophils for degranulation or prolonged survival. Even if antagonists derived from peptides and small molecules exist to block the chemokine receptor CCR3, the in vivo effect on airway inflammation is not sufficiently proved [33].

Once activated, eosinophils may produce effector molecules like eosinophil major basic protein and eosinophil-derived neurotoxin and degranulate at the site of injury contributing to tissue damage in the asthmatic lung. These molecules have cytotoxic effects on respiratory epithelium, facilitate the entry of other toxic molecules and trigger the degranulation of mast cells and basophils. In asthmatic airways, eosinophils also take part in respiratory-burst–oxidase reactions and generate large amounts of cysteinyl leukotrienes that contribute to increase vascular permeability, mucus secretion and smooth muscle contraction [37].

## 2.6 Local eosinophilopoiesis

It has been proposed that CD34+ IL-5Ra+ progenitors after mobilization from the BM during allergen challenge are able to undergo in situ differentiation at the site of allergic inflammation. Actually, CD34+45+IL-5Rα+ progenitors are increased in BAL in mouse models after allergen challenge and precede an increase in BAL eosinophils through a local differentiation via an IL-5-dependent mechanism [38]. Moreover, the CD34+ eosinophil committed pool is maintained within the airways via autocrine IL-5 release and IL-5-induced upregulation of IL-5R. CD34+/IL-5Rα mRNA+ cell number is increased in the airways of asthmatic subjects and related to asthma severity [39]. Surprisingly, eosinophilic precursors persist in the sputum of severe asthmatics that are prednisone resistant after anti-IL-5 treatment [40] and it has been documented that anti-CCR3 strategies do not suppress circulating and airway eosinophils in moderate-to-severe asthmatics. Consequently, it can be hypothesized that blocking local differentiation and expansion of CD34+/IL-5Rα+ cells may reduce eosinophilic inflammation in the airway in asthma.

## 2.7 Other mechanisms of eosinophil activity into allergic asthmatic airways

Allergic inflammation is locally perpetuated in the airway by the cross-talk between eosinophils and other resident cells. MCs are activated by MPB and stem cell factor (SCF), both released by eosinophils, contributing, by their direct effects on mast cells, to the perpetuation of allergic inflammation [41].

Eosinophils can also affect fibroblast properties, modulating the process of tissue remodeling. First, eosinophils are the main source in asthma of transforming growth factor-beta (TGF-β) that induces proliferation and regulates fibroblast function as well as controls the production of proteins of the extracellular matrix (ECM). In turn, tumor necrosis factor-α (TNF-α) derived from mast cells enhances TGF-β synthesis from eosinophils as well as fibroblasts promote survival of MCs and eosinophils by releasing SCF and granulocyte–macrophage-colony stimulating factor (GM-CSF) [42]. Anti-IL-5 humanized monoclonal antibody has been shown to decrease the deposition of many ECM proteins such as collagen III in the RBM of mild atopic asthmatics as well as the number of eosinophils and the degree of TGF-α in the BAL fluid [43].

In addition, eosinophils express basic fibroblast growth factor (β-FGF) and VEGF in the submucosa of asthmatic subjects and release many pro-angiogenic cytokines such as IL-8, IL-6, TGF-β and GM-CSF.

The effect on T-cell immune modulation of eosinophils is more controversial. Cytokine produced by eosinophils may directly influence T-cell selection by DCs determining T-cell tolerance or activation. One example is the induction by IFN-γ of indoleamine 2,3-dioxygenase (IDO) in eosinophils that in turn converts tryptophan (TRYP) to kynurenine (KYN) inducing apoptosis in Th1 cells, while Th2 cells are spared from KYN-induced apoptosis by IL-4 [44].

## 3. Eosinophils in nonallergic asthma

The increase of the number of activated Th2 lymphocytes and eosinophils, as well as IL-5 levels, in both BAL fluid and bronchial biopsies from intrinsic asthmatics, has been extensively reported [45]. No difference between atopic and intrinsic asthmatics have been observed in studies examining the expression of high-affinity IgE receptor, IL-5 and IL-4 mRNA and protein expression in bronchial biopsies [16]. Actually, total serum IgE levels have been noted to be increased in the serum of patients with intrinsic asthma. This reflects the increases in Iå and Cå RNA+ cells in the bronchial mucosa and provides evidence for a local IgE synthesis even in the absence of a known antigen or allergen trigger.

Eosinophilic infiltration in nonallergic asthma can be even much more than in allergic asthma and this fact is reflected by the finding of a larger amount of RANTES in the bronchoalveolar lavage fluid of patients with nonallergic asthma compared with patients with allergic asthma [46].

Attempts to differentiate the inflammatory cascade between allergic and nonallergic asthma have proposed a different signal in the Th2 pathway of nonallergic asthma attributed to reduced signal transducer and activator of transcription 6 (STAT6) expression and consequently reduced IL-4R signaling in nonallergic asthma [47]. Another peculiar finding was the increased expression of GM-CSF receptor alpha expression in the macrophages detected in mucosa and BAL. Peripheral blood eosinophilia is present both in allergic and nonallergic asthma, in some studies being higher in the former compared to the latter group [48].

## 4. The eosinophilic phenotype of asthma

Different attempts have been found in order to identify an eosinophilic phenotype of asthma. Eosinophilic asthma is reported to account for approximately 50–60% of the total asthma population. The definition of eosinophilic asthma implies that eosinophils are the dominant cells responsible for the pathophysiological changes of the disease. The pathogenic role of eosinophils in these patients is demonstrated by their increased number and status of activation in the airways, and consequently, they are detected in sputum, bronchoalveolar lavage, or bronchial mucosa or submucosa. These findings may be persistent and associated with severe or uncontrolled asthma [7].

Eosinophils may be demonstrated in the airways in the bronchial mucosa or submucosa or in the lumen (in the bronchial wash, BAL, or sputum). Bronchial biopsy is not routinely used as it is an invasive procedure and practicable only far from exacerbations to avoid dangerous complications and the quantification of eosinophils in BAL is not standardized and generally reflects samples of the peripheral airways.

Sputum examination is currently the most comprehensive and noninvasive method for measuring airway inflammation, processing and analysis being standardized and reliability, validity, and responsiveness proven [49].

The definition of "eosinophilic asthma" implies the existence of noneosinophilic asthma. A large cohort of patients with mild-to-moderate asthma in longitudinal studies resulted in approximately 50% of them with the absence of eosinophilic airway inflammation. The cellular pattern in noneosinophilic asthma may result in either predominant neutrophilic inflammation or normal sputum cell count. Within eosinophilic asthma, eosinophilia may result in persistent (22%) or on at least 1 occasion (intermittent eosinophilia, 31%) under multiple sputum examinations [50]. Sputum inflammatory granulocytes may identify phenotypic subgroups of differing pathology and clinical characteristics within asthmatics. Within the Severe Asthma Research Program (SARP), which included a population of severe and nonsevere patients with and without corticosteroid treatment, the stratification in four groups by granulocyte % in sputum showed significant clinical differences. Patients were divided combined for stratification by granulocytes in <2%Eos + <40%Neu, <2%Eos + ≥ 40%Neu, ≥2%Eos + <40% Neu, and ≥ 2%Eos + ≥40%Neu. In this study, eosinophilic asthma, indicated by ≥2%Eos, accounted for 31% of patients, those being with combined increased sputum eosinophils and neutrophils the most severe patients in terms of lowest lung function measures, worse asthma control, greatest symptoms and use of healthcare resources [51]. In another retrospective series of 508 asthmatics, the proportion of patients with raised sputum eosinophil counts ≥3% was 42% independent of the exclusion of steroid-treated patients. Eosinophilic phenotype exhibited higher atopy, levels of IgE, bronchial hyperresponsiveness to methacholine, FENO levels and lower asthma control, while the mixed granulocytic phenotype, with both eosinophilic and neutrophilic inflammation, had the lowest lung function and the highest degree of bronchial hyperresponsiveness to methacholine [52].

In most mild-to-moderate asthma patients untreated with steroids, sputum eosinophilia >2% was significantly and inversely associated with PC20 methacholine identifying 69% of the asthma group [53]. Sputum eosinophils correlate, in addition, with symptom score and FEV% and, as previously reported, are increased by exposure to common allergens. The association between asthma exacerbations and sputum eosinophilia is suggested by different pieces of evidence. First, sputum eosinophil count is able to predict asthma deterioration after cessation of ICSs treatment in mild-to-moderate asthma, while it is decreased by treatment with corticosteroids [54]. Sputum eosinophilia may be a good additional predictor of FEV1, PC20 methacholine or quality of life of response to inhaled steroids [55].

Consequently, a clinical strategy, based on re-administration of ICSs when a change in sputum eosinophil percentage by using the 0.8% threshold was reached, could lower the rates of asthma deteriorations and the number of individuals treated with ICSs by 48%. In addition, an increase in sputum eosinophils is detected up to 3 months before the development of a clinical exacerbation [56]. The usefulness of sputum cell count to improve treatment has been shown by Green et al. that showed the efficacy of reducing exacerbations when treatment was guided according to the sputum eosinophils (to achieve a sputum eosinophil count of less than 3%) [54]. A different study used sputum cell counts to guide corticosteroid therapy to keep eosinophils <2% in moderate-to-severe asthma resulting in the sputum strategy group lower number and milder exacerbations (overall risk of exacerbations by 49%, it reduced the number of severe exacerbations) that were prevalently noneosinophilic [57].

Management of asthma-inhaled corticosteroid treatment based on sputum eosinophil levels has been the object of a Cochrane review that concluded that actually the risk of exacerbations is significantly reduced compared to that based on clinical symptoms with or without lung function, as well as the rate and severity of exacerbations defined by requirement for use of oral corticosteroids and hospitalizations [58]. Sputum eosinophilia may, therefore, be considered a modifiable risk factor to reduce exacerbations. Small studies in selected populations have suggested increasing ICS dose independent of the level of symptom control.

In this contest, the eosinophilic subtype of asthma may be defined as symptomatic asthma in the presence of airway eosinophilia and that is characterized generally by a good response to glucocorticosteroids.

## 5. Eosinophilic refractory severe asthma

When eosinophilic inflammation in asthma leads to uncontrolled disease, the patient is at risk of exacerbations. In a proportion of patients, asthma becomes difficult to be treated despite the adequate use of high-dose corticosteroid treatment. Once the management of modifiable factors such as incorrect inhaler technique, poor adherence, smoking or comorbidities is optimized but asthma remains still uncontrolled, the diagnosis of severe asthma can be formulated [59].

In a subgroup of patients with severe asthma, eosinophilic inflammation is still active despite the high-dose ICS treatment or oral corticosteroid intake. The use of sputum cell counts was thus defined as a marker allowing the identification of a subgroup of subjects with severe eosinophilic asthma who were at risk of more frequent asthma exacerbations [60].

In patients with severe eosinophilic asthma, sputum eosinophils may be suppressed by using increasing doses of inhaled steroids reducing the number of subsequent exacerbations [54, 57]. Yet, the persistence of airway eosinophilia in these subjects reflects a failure of usually adequate doses of corticosteroid to suppress inflammation [61]. Corticosteroid insensitivity is therefore intrinsic in the definition of severe asthma resulting in persistent lack of control despite corticosteroid therapy or worsening of asthma control on reduction or discontinuation of corticosteroid therapy [62]. A majority of severe asthmatics are corticosteroid dependent, refractory or insensitive and require oral corticosteroids (OCS) in addition to ICS to maintain some degree of asthma control. Only a small portion of severe asthmatics can be considered completely "corticosteroid unresponsive" or resistant [63]. The proportion of asthmatics with corticosteroid insensitivity is confirmed from the fact that one-third of the current SARP cohort were on regular OCS, with over half needing more than three bursts of OCS in the previous year [64].

A dose-response relationship between the use of OCS in asthmatic patients and the risk of many adverse events has been documented. Long-term exposure to OCS leads to increased risk of osteoporosis, arterial hypertension, diabetes, metabolic syndrome, cataracts, gastrointestinal bleeding and neuropsychiatric diseases such as depression [65]. The negative effect of systemic corticosteroid is associated not only to its maintenance or use but also to cumulative prescriptions of OCS burst [66].

In the global strategy for asthma management and prevention (GINA) 2019 update, sputum eosinophilia ≥2% is presented as a criteria to identify patients with severe asthma with refractory type 2 inflammation despite high-dose ICS or daily OCS treatment [1, 59].

Type 2 high asthma was initially used to identify the eosinophilic phenotype of asthma. The current concept of type 2 asthma includes a phenotype, characterized by the release of signature cytokines like interleukin IL-4, IL-5 and IL-13 from cells of both the innate and the adaptive immune systems. Th2 cells and type 2 innate lymphoid cells (ILC2s) are primarily responsible for the production of high levels of T2 cytokines in the airways. The demonstration of this cytokine pathway from cellular to molecular and transcriptomic levels represents the signature for type 2 (T2) asthma [67]. The importance of identifying different phenotypes of asthma has been addressed by hypothesis-based and unbiased analyses that showed different characteristics of asthma phenotype in terms of severity, functional and clinical features, comorbidities, prognosis and response to treatment [68].

### 5.1 Severe eosinophilic asthma in cluster analysis

Asthma phenotyping has involved biased and unbiased approaches with the aim of grouping clinical, physiological and genetic characteristics.

In the TENOR study (the epidemiological and natural history of asthma: outcome and treatment regiments), a severe allergic asthma phenotype emerged as a high-risk group of patients for severe exacerbations with early-onset, IgE and allergen sensitization [69]. The existence of this population was confirmed in the cluster analysis by Haldar P and coworkers who found an early-onset atopic asthma cluster in which a concordance between symptom expression and eosinophilic airway inflammation is present and a symptom-based approach to therapy titration may be sufficient. On the other side, a marked discordant cluster with late-onset active predominant eosinophilic inflammation emerged as a refractory phenotype of severe asthma [70].

The predominance of sputum eosinophilia in the inflammatory patterns of severe asthmatic subphenotypes is confirmed in the unsupervised hierarchical cluster analysis of the Severe Asthma Research Program cohort where cluster 4 of severe asthmatics was associated to atopic disease and reversible severe reductions in pulmonary function, while cluster 5 was characterized mainly by later-onset disease and airflow limitations that remain with a FEV1 < 80% predicted [71].

The expansion of this analysis using a supervised learning approach that included blood, bronchoscopic, exhaled nitric oxide and clinical data gave a further focus on severe asthma phenotypes. Therefore, while cluster 4 resembled that previously described with early-onset allergic asthma with low lung function and eosinophilic inflammation, the eosinophilic refractory asthma could be further split into cluster 5, characterized by late-onset severe asthma with nasal polyps and eosinophilia and cluster 6 with persistent inflammation in blood and bronchoalveolar lavage fluid, increased FENO levels and exacerbations despite high systemic corticosteroid use and side effects. Consequently, cluster 5 was characterized as more prone to respond to corticosteroid treatment, even if rapidly deteriorated after discontinuation (corticosteroid dependent), while cluster 6 was characterized to be corticosteroid complete insensitivity [72].

### 5.2 Blood eosinophilia as a biomarker of severe eosinophilic asthma

The question of whether blood eosinophilia may be considered, in this contest, a surrogate marker of airway eosinophilia, is debated. The measurement of eosinophil counts in blood is inexpensive and widely available. However, blood eosinophilia is nonspecific for asthma and often asthmatic patients have normal levels of eosinophils. In asthmatics with increased blood eosinophilia, there exists a direct correlation with symptom scores and an inverse correlation with FEV1 in both children and adults, independently of atopy [73].

Blood eosinophilic counts have been reported to exhibit a moderate-to-good correlation with sputum eosinophils in asthma in large cohorts of asthmatics. A high blood eosinophil count >220/mm$^3$ resulted in good predictors of sputum eosinophilia ≥3% as revealed by an AUC of ROC curves of 79% that yielded 77% sensitivity and 70% specificity and an independent factors associated with the presence of sputum eosinophilic inflammation in multiple logistic regression models [52]. Other studies confirmed that blood eosinophils are an accurate biomarker of eosinophilic airway inflammation comparing two independent cohorts, mild-to-moderate asthma versus moderate-to-severe asthma. The authors used a cut-off point of ≥0.27 × 10$^9$/L blood eosinophils that were able to differentiate eosinophilic inflammation of ≥3% with a sensitivity of 78% and specificity of 91% [74].

In a multiple clinical variable analysis within the SARP cohort, the sensitivity and specificity of blood eosinophil counts of greater than 300/mL to detect an "eosinophil phenotype" based on sputum eosinophil counts of greater than 2% were 59% and 65%, respectively. This means that a blood eosinophil count of less than 300/L yields a 41% false-negative that has yet a sputum eosinophil percentage of greater than 2%, and likewise, many subjects with sputum eosinophil count of less than 2% would also be misclassified with a false-positive rate of 35%. Therefore, although statistically significant, the AUC of the ROC curve for predicting sputum eosinophil percentages of less than 2% or 2% and greater shows fair-to-poor accuracy and positive predictive values. These results are not improved when the cut-off of sputum eosinophil counts is more than 3% or whether the analysis is restricted to subjects with severe asthma only [51]. The stratification of SARP subjects based on blood eosinophil counts of less than 300 or 300/mL and greater showed significant differences only in methacholine bronchial hyperresponsiveness (log PC20), FEV1 percent predicted and FEV1/FVC ratio, neither in any variable related to overall asthma health care use or frequency and severity of exacerbations. This not-enthusiastic result has been confirmed both in patients with mild-to-moderate or in those with severe asthma who entered a clinical trial for mepolizumab for severe eosinophilic asthma [6].

In a study that evaluated 75 uncontrolled asthmatic patients, a significant positive relationship between the percentage of sputum eosinophils and the percentage of blood eosinophils (r = 0.3647; p = 0.0013) was demonstrated. An important limits of this study were the cut-off point of blood eosinophils of 2% of WBC and again the low accuracy of ROC curves [75].

Increasing the peripheral blood eosinophil cut-off percentage (2.7% or 0.26 × 10$^9$/L) yielded a significant higher sensitivity and specificity and AUC as a diagnostic biomarker of sputum eosinophilia (≥3%) in a population of uncontrolled asthmatics [76] suggesting that blood eosinophils can be used in the clinic for detecting airway eosinophilia in uncontrolled asthma. These data are confirmed when looking at the population selected for treatment with reslizumab, another anti-IL-5 mAb, in which blood eosinophil counts of greater than 400/mL might be able to improve the prediction of sputum eosinophil counts of greater than 3% [77].

A systematic review and meta-analysis estimated the diagnostic accuracy of markers for airway eosinophilia in patients with asthma. Looking at the 14 studies that investigated blood eosinophils as a predictor marker, an overall modest ability to distinguish between patients with or without airway eosinophilia was reported with a summary estimate of AUC of 0.78 [78]. To be noticed that among the different studies, five different definitions of airway eosinophilia had been used, but either eosinophils ≥2% or 3% was used and this did not affect the accuracy of the test. Moreover, a subanalysis of the study showed the forest plots for blood eosinophilia in detecting sputum eosinophilia in subgroup populations of asthmatics. Smoking habit, steroid-treated or untreated and asthma severity revealed a considerable variability of positive thresholds of the marker. In severe asthma, only groups with the cut-point between 275 and 315 μL gave the highest sensibility and specificity [79]. As the most robust clinical value of sputum eosinophilia is tailoring inhaled corticosteroids and reducing the frequency of asthma exacerbations, it is expected that blood eosinophilia to replace induced sputum in this context should yield a sensitivity and specificity of at least 90%, so that only a small portion of patients will be misclassified. One of the most evident limits in the role of blood eosinophilia as a biomarker comes for the cross-sectional nature of the study populations. Significant variability of blood eosinophil count in the same patient over time and according to treatment status must be taken into account.

### 5.3 Treatment of severe eosinophilic asthma

Asthma guidelines are recommending the use of sputum eosinophil count in severe asthma. The international ERS/ATS guidelines on the definition, evaluation and treatment of severe asthma addressed the phenotypic management of severe asthma and evaluated the utility use of sputum eosinophilia to guide treatment. The document suggested that treatment guided by clinical criteria and sputum eosinophil counts should be performed in centers with experience in this procedure and in selected patients, allowing avoidance of inappropriate escalation of treatment and waste of resources [62]. In the global strategy for asthma management and prevention (GINA) 2019 update, this concept is reinforced by claiming that treatment guided by sputum eosinophil count has the best benefits in patients with moderate-to-severe asthma requiring secondary care [1]. Within step 5 of treatment scale, adults with persistent symptoms or exacerbations despite high-dose ICS or ICS/LABA are advised to adjust treatment based on sputum eosinophilia >3%.

When a refractory or underline type 2 inflammation is proven in severe asthma, add-on biologic type 2 target treatment must be considered for patients with exacerbations or poor symptom control [1, 59]. Actually, sputum eosinophil count also provides an effective method to identify patients who will benefit from targeted therapy with anti–IL-5 monoclonal antibodies (mAbs). In patients with refractory eosinophilic asthma that had a sputum eosinophilia >3% DCC, despite high dose of inhaled corticosteroids, and at least 2 exacerbations in the last 2 years, with the need to make a short course of systemic corticosteroids, mepolizumab therapy reduces exacerbations and improves AQLQ scores [80]. Other studies confirmed the efficacy of anti-IL-5 mAb therapy in patients with asthma who had consistently increased eosinophil counts in sputum of greater than 2.5–3% on at least two occasions [81] .

Yet, the measurement of eosinophils in sputum or airway fluids may not truly reflect the contributions of airway tissue eosinophils. Actually, a study was assessed to understand whether induced sputum has the ability to distinguish the eosinophilic and noneosinophilic phenotypes compared to bronchial biopsies in moderate and severe asthma. This study showed that among patients with severe asthma could identify a BrEos+ group with high mucosal eosinophils and a BrEos– group. Even if there was no a correlation between sputum eosinophil count and eosinophils found in the bronchial mucosa, there was a significant correlation between the number of asthma exacerbations reported by the subjects with severe asthma during the year preceding the study and the percentage of sputum eosinophils [82]. This result is reflected by the fact that on one hand mepolizumab depleted <50% of bronchial tissue and bone marrow eosinophils in spite of its effect in reducing blood, BAL fluid and sputum eosinophils abolishing established airway eosinophil infiltration [83]. Among the explanation to this phenomenon, it can be supposed that eosinophils in the airway lumen may be in a different state of activation than in the bronchial mucosa or may reflect greater concentrations of intraluminal chemokines such as eotaxin and RANTES or epithelial activation.

Another possible consequence of the supposed partial effect of mepolizumab over all the aspects of eosinophilic inflammation is that FEV1, symptoms and FENO levels were not affected [80]. On one hand, this means that these therapeutic strategies may not be sufficient to reverse remodeling changes of severe asthma even if mepolizumab has been shown to decrease the deposition of tenascin, lumican and collagen III in the basal membrane of mild atopic asthmatics as well as the degree of TGF-β in the bronchoalveolar lavage fluid [43]. Accordingly, lung function was not expected to be positively modified by anti-IL-5 treatments in severe asthma and a meta-analysis of nine randomized, placebo-controlled, clinical trials including mepolizumab or reslizumab reported a mild absolute difference of FEV1 in favor of the anti-IL-5 treatment compared to placebo [84].

On the other hand, the persistently high level of FENO can guess, in a proportion of eosinophilic refractory severe asthmatics, that the IL-5 pathway is not in these patients the predominant. This fact can explain why targeting the type 2 phenotype on the IL4/IL13 pathway with dupilumab, a humanized MoAb to IL4-Ra, gave partially different results. When type 2 severe asthmatics with sputum eosinophilia >3% had been enrolled to be treated with dupilumab, the endpoints consisting of improvement of control (ACQ), symptoms and FEV1 were reached. These clinical and functional results were coupled with decreasing FENO, eotaxin 3 and IgE levels [85].

Another question is whether blood eosinophils are a good predictor of response to mepolizumab in patients with severe eosinophilic asthma. The DREAM study identified a blood eosinophil count of 300/mL or greater as a high predictive biomarker of response to mepolizumab [86].

In systemic corticosteroid severe asthma with persistent blood eosinophilia, at least 150 cells, the goal of reducing >75% of oral corticosteroid dose was reached in more than 40% of patients, confirming the role of persistent blood eosinophilia as predictor marker [87].

Benralizumab binds with high affinity to the alpha-chain of human IL-5R, blocking its activation and transduction and determining a neutralizing activity. Moreover, it is able to induce antibody-dependent cell-mediated cytotoxicity (ADCC) on NK cells that release cytotoxic mediators and cause eosinophil apoptosis [88]. A significant clinical efficacy in terms of reduction of annual exacerbations, improvement of FEV1 and steroid-sparing effect was demonstrated in the clinical trials [89]. A threshold of >300 cells per mcl represents a useful marker for quantifying the advantage of this treatment in patients with steroid-dependent asthma. It has been supposed that benralizumab results in a complete depletion of eosinophils in the airway lumen and this can in part explain why in the registrative studies pre-bronchodilator FEV1 improved in the treatment groups. Actually, benralizumab is highly selective on eosinophil and basophil protein and gene-related immune signaling pathways [90] and not only reaches almost complete eosinophil eliminations at plasma levels but also determines the reduction of blood eosinophil precursors [91].

## 6. Conclusions

The definition of eosinophilic asthma engages different models according to different contests [92]. However, a single common thread can be glimpsed in the ability of eosinophils to catch biological and clinical features that are crucial in each contest. Mouse and human allergic asthma models teach us that as the eosinophilic cascade can be dominant after acute exposition to triggers but only within the chronic stimulation, it contributes to deeper structural changes of the airways [11, 17]. The role of eosinophils in different phases of allergic asthma as well as the involving of Th2 cells, cytokines including IL5, IL4 and IL13 and chemokines has been smartly showed in the majority of the experimental studies. In addition, the mechanisms leading to AHR or persistent inflammation imply the need of sharing of different pathways of the Th2 cascade and the cross-talk between eosinophils and other immune cells [41]. The contribution of either IL-5–independent ways or the regulation of local or systemic eosinophilopoiesis has been addressed [40]. In real life, these phenomena can explain the ability of eosinophilic inflammation to be controlled by corticosteroid treatments, and, under certain circumstances, it becomes insensitive to this treatment.

Accordingly, in the context of severe asthma, eosinophilic airway inflammation becomes exceptionally deregulated and needs a biological approach to be controlled. The eosinophilic phenotype of asthma is currently defined by sputum examination that reveals eosinophilic airway inflammation. Generally, eosinophilic subtype of asthma may be defined as symptomatic asthma in the presence of airway eosinophilia and that is characterized by a good response to glucocorticosteroids. The efficacy of reducing exacerbations when corticosteroid treatment was guided according to the sputum eosinophils has addressed the point of eosinophilic target therapy in a subgroup of patients who encounter worse asthma control, higher use of healthcare resources, higher risk of exacerbations and the need of high-dose ICS or systemic corticosteroid treatment to be controlled. Continuous or bust oral corticosteroid exposure is associated to significant adverse effects that significantly impact on the patients' outcome [66], highlighting the urgent need of sparing corti-costeroid approaches. Even if limits in accuracy have been evidenced, blood eosinophils can be used in the clinic for detecting airway eosinophilia in uncontrolled severe asthma [78] and as eligibility criteria for anti–IL-5 target therapy. Therefore, new add-on therapies for severe asthma have showed to reduce both asthma exacerbation rate compared to standard of care and daily OCS use. Five biologicals have been now approved for severe eosinophilic asthma and can be applied depending on asthma phenotype and endotype [93]. As a consequence, the precision medicine and personalized therapy have become the best clue for treatment and monitoring the response by identification of suitable biomarkers in patients with more severe and refractory forms of asthma [94].

## Author details

Guida Giuseppe* and Antonelli Andrea
Allergy and Pneumology Unit, A.S.O Santa Croce and Carle, Cuneo, Italy

*Address all correspondence to: giuseppe.alesgui@gmail.com

## References

[1] Asthma G initiative for. Global Initiative for Asthma 2019. Glob Strateg Asthma Manag Prev. 2019

[2] Global Initiative for Asthma. Global Strategy for Asthma Management and Prevention. Global Initiative for Asthma. 2014

[3] Holgate ST. Pathogenesis of asthma. Clinical and Experimental Allergy: Journal of the British Society for Allergy and Clinical Immunology. 2008;38(6):872-897

[4] Bousquet J, Chanez P, Lacoste JY, Barneon G, Ghavanian N, Enander I, et al. Eosinophilic inflammation in asthma [see comments]. The New England Journal of Medicine. 1990;323:1033-1039

[5] Berry MA, Shaw DE, Green RH, Brightling CE, Wardlaw AJ, Pavord ID. The use of exhaled nitric oxide concentration to identify eosinophilic airway inflammation: An observational study in adults with asthma. Clinical and Experimental Allergy. 2005;35(9):1175-1179

[6] Nair P. What is an "eosinophilic phenotype" of asthma? Journal of Allergy and Clinical Immunology. 2013;132:81-83

[7] Aleman F, Lim HF, Nair P. Eosinophilic Endotype of Asthma. Immunology and Allergy Clinics of North America; 2016;36(3):559-568

[8] Nials AT, Uddin S. Mouse models of allergic asthma: Acute and chronic allergen challenge. DMM: Disease Models and Mechanisms. 2008;1:213-220

[9] Wahn U, Lau S, Bergmann R, Kulig M, Forster J, Bergmann K, et al. Indoor allergen exposure is a risk factor for sensitization during the first three years of life. The Journal of Allergy and Clinical Immunology. 1997;99(6 Pt 1):763-769

[10] Schatz M, Rosenwasser L. The allergic asthma phenotype. The Journal of Allergy and Clinical Immunology. In Practice. 2014;2(6):645-648

[11] Fernandez-Rodriguez S, Ford WR, Broadley KJ, Kidd EJ. Establishing the phenotype in novel acute and chronic murine models of allergic asthma. International Immunopharmacology. 2008;8:756-763

[12] Cohn L, Tepper JS, Bottomly K. IL-4-independent induction of airway hyperresponsiveness by Th2, but not Th1, cells. Journal of Immunology. 1998;161:3813-3816

[13] Ulrich K, Hincks JS, Walsh R, Wetterstrand EMC, Fidock MD, Sreckovic S, et al. Anti-inflammatory modulation of chronic airway inflammation in the murine house dust mite model. Pulmonary Pharmacology & Therapeutics. 2008;21:637-647

[14] Foster PS, Hogan SP, Ramsay AJ, Matthaei KI, Young IG. Interleukin 5 deficiency abolishes eosinophilia, airways hyperreactivity, and lung damage in a mouse asthma model. The Journal of Experimental Medicine. 1996;183:195-201

[15] Kumar RK, Herbert C, Webb DC, Li L, Foster PS. Effects of anticytokine therapy in a mouse model of chronic asthma. American Journal of Respiratory and Critical Care Medicine. 2004;170(10):1043-1048

[16] Humbert M, Durham SR, Ying S, Kimmitt P, Barkans J, Assoufi B, et al. IL-4 and IL-5 mRNA and protein in bronchial biopsies from patients with atopic and nonatopic asthma:

Evidence against "intrinsic" asthma being a distinct immunopathologic entity. American Journal of Respiratory and Critical Care Medicine. 1996;**154**(5):1497-1504

[17] Ying S, Durham SR, Corrigan CJ, Hamid Q, Kay AB. Phenotype of cells expressing mRNA for TH2-type (interleukin 4 and interleukin 5) and TH1-type (interleukin 2 and interferon gamma) cytokines in bronchoalveolar lavage and bronchial biopsies from atopic asthmatic and normal control subjects. American Journal of Respiratory Cell and Molecular Biology. 1995;**12**(5):477-487

[18] Erpenbeck VJ, Hagenberg A, Krentel H, Discher M, Braun A, Hohlfeld JM, et al. Regulation of GATA- 3, c-maf and T-bet mRNA expression in bronchoalveolar lavage cells and bronchial biopsies after segmental allergen challenge. International Archives of Allergy and Immunology. 2006;**139**(4):306-316

[19] Nakamura Y, Ghaffar O, Olivenstein R, Taha RA, Soussi- Gounni A, Zhang DH, et al. Gene expression of the GATA-3 transcription factor is increased in atopic asthma. The Journal of Allergy and Clinical Immunology. 1999;**103**:215-222

[20] Ohnishi T, Sur S, Collins DS, Fish JE, Gleich GJ, Peters SP. Eosinophil survival activity identified as interleukin-5 is associated with eosinophil recruitment and degranulation and lung injury twenty-four hours after segmental antigen lung challenge. The Journal of Allergy and Clinical Immunology. 1993;**92**:607-615

[21] Sur S, Gleich GJ, Swansonb MC, Bartemesb KR, Broide DH. Eosinophilic inflammation is associated with elevation of interleukin-5 in the airways of patients with spontaneous symptomatic asthma. The Journal of Allergy and Clinical Immunology. 1995;**96**:661-668

[22] Huang SK, Xiao HQ, Kleine-Tebbe J, Paciotti G, Marsh DG, Lichtenstein LM, et al. IL-13 expression at the sites of allergen challenge in patients with asthma. Journal of Immunology. 1995;**155**(5):2688-2694

[23] Denburg JA. Bone marrow in atopy and asthma: Hematopoietic mechanisms in allergic inflammation. Immunology Today. 1999;**20**:111-113

[24] Melum GR, Farkas L, Scheel C, Van Dieren B, Gran E, Liu YJ, et al. A thymic stromal lymphopoietin-responsive dendritic cell subset mediates allergic responses in the upper airway mucosa. The Journal of Allergy and Clinical Immunology. 2014;**134**(3):613.e7-621.e7

[25] Weersink EJM, Postma DS, Aalbers R, de Monchy JGR. Early and late asthmatic reaction after allergen challenge. Respiratory Medicine. 1994;**88**:103-114

[26] Dorman SC, Sehmi R, Gauvreau GM, Watson RM, Foley R, Jones GL, et al. Kinetics of bone marrow eosinophilopoiesis and associated cytokines after allergen inhalation. American Journal of Respiratory and Critical Care Medicine. 2004;**169**(5):565-572

[27] Oddera S, Silvestri M, Penna R, Galeazzi G, Crimi E, Rossi GA. Airway eosinophilic inflammation and bronchial hyperresponsiveness after allergen inhalation challenge in asthma. Lung. 1998;**176**(4):237-247

[28] Kotsimbos ATC, Hamid Q. IL-5 and IL-5 receptor in asthma. Memórias do Instituto Oswaldo Cruz. 1997;**92** (Suppl 2):75-91

[29] Barthel SR, Annis DS, Mosher DF, Johansson MW. Differential engagement of modules 1 and 4 of vascular cell adhesion molecule-1 (CD106) by integrins $\alpha4\beta1$ (CD49d/29) and $\alpha M\beta2$ (CD11b/18) of eosinophils.

The Journal of Biological Chemistry. 2006;**281**(43):32175-32187

[30] Johansson MW, Gunderson KA, Kelly EAB, Denlinger LC, Jarjour NN, Mosher DF. Anti-IL-5 attenuates activation and surface density of β2-integrins on circulating eosinophils after segmental antigen challenge. Clinical and Experimental Allergy. 2013;**43**(3):292-303

[31] Johansson MW, Mosher DF. Integrin activation states and eosinophil recruitment in asthma. Frontiers in Pharmacology. 2013;**4**:33

[32] Cauvreau GM, Watson RM, O'Byrne PM. Kinetics of allergen-induced airway eosinophilic cytokine production and airway inflammation. American Journal of Respiratory and Critical Care Medicine. 1999;**160**(2):640-647

[33] Elsner J, Escher SE, Forssmann U. Chemokine receptor antagonists: A novel therapeutic approach in allergic diseases. Allergy: European Journal of Allergy and Clinical Immunology. 2004;**59**:1243-1258

[34] Lamkhioued B, Renzi PM, Abi-Younes S, Garcia-Zepada EA, Allakhverdi Z, Ghaffar O, et al. Increased expression of eotaxin in bronchoalveolar lavage and airways of asthmatics contributes to the chemotaxis of eosinophils to the site of inflammation. Journal of Immunology [Internet]. 1997;**159**(9):4593-4601. Available from: http://www.ncbi.nlm.nih.gov/pubmed/9379061

[35] Humbles AA, Lu B, Friend DS, Okinaga S, Lora J, Al-garawi A, et al. The murine CCR3 receptor regulates both the role of eosinophils and mast cells in allergen-induced airway inflammation and hyperresponsiveness. Proceedings of the National Academy of Sciences of the United States of America. 2002;**99**(3):1479-1484

[36] Liu LY, Jarjour NN, Busse WW, Kelly EAB. Chemokine receptor expression on human eosinophils from peripheral blood and bronchoalveolar lavage fluid after segmental antigen challenge. The Journal of Allergy and Clinical Immunology. 2003;**112**(3):556-562

[37] Rothenberg ME. Eosinophilia. New England Journal of Medicine. 28 May 1998;**338**(22):1592-1600

[38] Southam DS, Widmer N, Ellis R, Hirota JA, Inman MD, Sehmi R. Increased eosinophil-lineage committed progenitors in the lung of allergen-challenged mice. The Journal of Allergy and Clinical Immunology. 2005;**115**:95-102

[39] Robinson DS, Damia R, Zeibecoglou K, Molet S, North J, Yamada T, et al. CD34+/interleukin-5Rα messenger RNA + cells in the bronchial mucosa in asthma: Potential airway eosinophil progenitors. American Journal of Respiratory Cell and Molecular Biology. 1999;**20**(1):9-13

[40] Sehmi R, Smith SG, Kjarsgaard M, Radford K, Boulet LP, Lemiere C, et al. Role of local eosinophilopoietic processes in the development of airway eosinophilia in prednisone-dependent severe asthma. Clinical and Experimental Allergy. 2016;**46**(6):793-802

[41] Munitz A, Levi-Schaffer F. Eosinophils: "New" roles for "old" cells. Allergy: European Journal of Allergy and Clinical Immunology. 2004;**59**:268-275

[42] Guida G, Riccio AM. Immune induction of airway remodeling. Seminars in Immunology. 2019;**46**:101346

[43] Flood-Page P, Menzies-Gow A, Phipps S, Ying S, Wangoo A, Ludwig MS, et al. Anti-IL-5 treatment

reduces deposition of ECM proteins in the bronchial subepithelial basement membrane of mild atopic asthmatics. The Journal of Clinical Investigation. 2003;112(7):1029-1236

[44] Adamko DJ, Odemuyiwa SO, Vethanayagam D, Moqbel R. The rise of the phoenix: The expanding role of the eosinophil in health and disease. Allergy: European Journal of Allergy and Clinical Immunology. 2005;60:13-22

[45] Bentley AM, Durham SR, Kay AB. Comparison of the immunopathology of extrinsic, intrinsic and occupational asthma. Journal of Investigational Allergology & Clinical Immunology. 1994;4(5):222-232

[46] Ying S, Meng Q, Zeibecoglou K, Robinson DS, Macfarlane A, Humbert M, et al. Eosinophil chemotactic chemokines (eotaxin, eotaxin-2, RANTES, monocyte chemoattractant protein-3 (MCP-3), and MCP-4), and C-C chemokine receptor 3 expression in bronchial biopsies from atopic and nonatopic (intrinsic) asthmatics. Journal of Immunology. 1999;163(11):6321-6329

[47] Christodoulopoulos P, Cameron L, Nakamura Y, Lemière C, Muro S, Dugas M, et al. TH2 cytokine-associated transcription factors in atopic and nonatopic asthma: Evidence for differential signal transducer and activator of transcription 6 expression. The Journal of Allergy and Clinical Immunology. 2001;107(4):586-591

[48] Zoratti E, Havstad S, Wegienka G, Nicholas C, Bobbitt KR, Woodcroft KJ, et al. Differentiating asthma phenotypes in young adults through polyclonal cytokine profiles. Annals of Allergy, Asthma & Immunology. 2014;113(1):25-30

[49] Vignola AM, Rennar SI, Hargreave FE, Fah JV, Bonsignore MR,

Djukanović R, et al. Standardised methodology of sputum induction and processing. Future directions. The European Respiratory Journal, Supplement. 2002;37:51s-55s

[50] McGrath KW, Icitovic N, Boushey HA, Lazarus SC, Sutherland ER, Chinchilli VM, et al. A large subgroup of mild-to-moderate asthma is persistently noneosinophilic. American Journal of Respiratory and Critical Care Medicine. 2012;185(6):612-619

[51] Hastie AT, Moore WC, Li H, Rector BM, Ortega VE, Pascual RM, et al. Biomarker surrogates do not accurately predict sputum eosinophil and neutrophil percentages in asthmatic subjects. The Journal of Allergy and Clinical Immunology. 2013;132(1):72-80

[52] Schleich FN, Manise M, Sele J, Henket M, Seidel L, Louis R. Distribution of sputum cellular phenotype in a large asthma cohort: Predicting factors for eosinophilic vs neutrophilic inflammation. BMC Pulmonary Medicine. 2013;13(1):11

[53] Louis R, Sele J, Henket M, Cataldo D, Bettiol J, Seiden L, et al. Sputum eosinophil count in a large population of patients with mild to moderate steroid-naive asthma: Distribution and relationship with methacholine bronchial hyperresponsiveness. Allergy: European Journal of Allergy & Clinical Immunology. 2002;57(10):907-912

[54] Green RH, Brightling CE, McKenna S, Hargadon B, Parker D, Bradding P, et al. Asthma exacerbations and sputum eosinophil counts: A randomised controlled trial. Lancet. 2002;360(9347):1715-1721

[55] Meijer RJ, Postma DS, Kauffman HF, Arends LR, Koëter GH, Kerstjens HAM. Accuracy of eosinophils and eosinophil cationic protein to

predict steroid improvement in asthma. Clinical and Experimental Allergy. 2002;**32**(7):1096-1103

[56] Deykin A, Lazarus SC, Fahy JV, Wechsler ME, Boushey HA, Chinchilli VM, et al. Sputum eosinophil counts predict asthma control after discontinuation of inhaled corticosteroids. The Journal of Allergy and Clinical Immunology. 2005;**115**(4):720-727

[57] Jayaram L, Pizzichini MM, Cook RJ, Boulet LP, Lemière C, Pizzichini E, et al. Determining asthma treatment by monitoring sputum cell counts: Effect on exacerbations. The European Respiratory Journal. 2006;**27**(3):483-494

[58] Petsky HL, Li A, Chang AB. Tailored interventions based on sputum eosinophils versus clinical symptoms for asthma in children and adults. Cochrane Database of Systematic Reviews. 2017;**8**:CD005603

[59] Darcey J, Qualtrough A. Difficult-to-treat & severe asthma in adolescent and adult patients - diagnosis and management. Global Initiative for Asthma [Internet]. 2019;**214**(10):493-509. DOI: 10.1038/sj.bdj.2013.482

[60] Buhl R, Humbert M, Bjermer L, Chanez P, Heaney LG, Pavord I, et al. Severe eosinophilic asthma: A roadmap to consensus. Europeaen Respiratory Journal. 2017;**49**:1700634

[61] Chakir J, Hamid Q, Bossé M, Boulet LP, Laviolette M. Bronchial inflammation in corticosteroid-sensitive and corticosteroid-resistant asthma at baseline and on oral corticosteroid treatment. Clinical and Experimental Allergy. 2002;**32**(4):578-582

[62] Chung KF, Wenzel SE, Brozek JL, Bush A, Castro M, Sterk PJ, et al. International ERS/ATS guidelines on definition, evaluation and treatment of severe asthma. The European Respiratory Journal. 2014;**43**(2):343-373

[63] Bossley CJ, Saglani S, Kavanagh C, Payne DNR, Wilson N, Tsartsali L, et al. Corticosteroid responsiveness and clinical characteristics in childhood difficult asthma. The European Respiratory Journal. 2009;**34**(5):1052-1059

[64] Moore WC, Bleecker ER, Curran-Everett D, Erzurum SC, Ameredes BT, Bacharier L, et al. Characterization of the severe asthma phenotype by the National Heart, Lung, and Blood Institute's Severe Asthma Research Program. The Journal of Allergy and Clinical Immunology. 2007;**119**(2):405-413

[65] Fardet L, Flahault A, Kettaneh A, Tiev KP, Généreau T, Tolédano C, et al. Corticosteroid-induced clinical adverse events: Frequency, risk factors and patient's opinion. The British Journal of Dermatology. 2007;**157**(1):142-148

[66] Sullivan PW, Ghushchyan VH, Globe G, Schatz M. Oral corticosteroid exposure and adverse effects in asthmatic patients. The Journal of Allergy and Clinical Immunology. 2018;**141**(1):110-116.e7

[67] Pavord ID, Afzalnia S, Menzies-Gow A, Heaney LG. The current and future role of biomarkers in type 2 cytokine-mediated asthma management. Clinical and Experimental Allergy. 2017;**47**:148-160

[68] Wenzel SE. Asthma phenotypes: The evolution from clinical to molecular approaches. Nature Medicine. 2012;**18**:716-725

[69] Chipps BE, Zeiger RS, Borish L, Wenzel SE, Yegin A, Lou HM, et al. Key findings and clinical implications from the Epidemiology and Natural History of Asthma: Outcomes and Treatment Regimens (TENOR) study. The Journal of Allergy and Clinical Immunology. 2012;**130**(2)

[70] Haldar P, Pavord ID, Shaw DE, Berry MA, Thomas M, Brightling CE, et al. Cluster analysis and clinical asthma phenotypes. American Journal of Respiratory and Critical Care Medicine. 2008;178(3):218-224

[71] Moore WC, Meyers DA, Wenzel SE, Teague WG, Li H, Li X, et al. Identification of asthma phenotypes using cluster analysis in the severe asthma research program. American Journal of Respiratory and Critical Care Medicine. 2010;181(4):315-323

[72] Wu W, Bleecker E, Moore W, Busse WW, Castro M, Chung KF, et al. Unsupervised phenotyping of severe asthma research program participants using expanded lung data. The Journal of Allergy and Clinical Immunology. 2014;133(5):1280-1288

[73] Ulrik CS. Peripheral eosinophil counts as a marker of disease activity in intrinsic and extrinsic asthma. Clinical and Experimental Allergy. 1995;25(9):820-827

[74] Wagener AH, De Nijs SB, Lutter R, Sousa AR, Weersink EJM, Bel EH, et al. External validation of blood eosinophils, FENO and serum periostin as surrogates for sputum eosinophils in asthma. Thorax. 2015;70(2):115-120

[75] Gao J, Wu F. Association between fractional exhaled nitric oxide, sputum induction and peripheral blood eosinophil in uncontrolled asthma. Allergy, Asthma & Clinical Immunology. 2018;14:21

[76] Zhang XY, Simpson JL, Powell H, Yang IA, Upham JW, Reynolds PN, et al. Full blood count parameters for the detection of asthma inflammatory phenotypes. Clinical and Experimental Allergy. 2014;44(9):1137-1145

[77] Castro M, Mathur S, Hargreave F, Boulet LP, Xie F, Young J, et al. Reslizumab for poorly controlled, eosinophilic asthma: A randomized, placebo-controlled study. American Journal of Respiratory and Critical Care Medicine. 2011;184(10):1125-1132

[78] Korevaar DA, Westerhof GA, Wang J, Cohen JF, Spijker R, Sterk PJ, et al. Diagnostic accuracy of minimally invasive markers for detection of airway eosinophilia in asthma: A systematic review and meta-analysis. The Lancet Respiratory Medicine. 2015;3(4):290-300

[79] Westerhof GA, Korevaar DA, Amelink M, De Nijs SB, De Groot JC, Wang J, et al. Biomarkers to identify sputum eosinophilia in different adult asthma phenotypes. The European Respiratory Journal. 2015;44(Supll 58):P2053

[80] Haldar P, Brightling CE, Hargadon B, Gupta S, Monteiro W, Sousa A, et al. Mepolizumab and exacerbations of refractory eosinophilic asthma. The New England Journal of Medicine. 2009;360(10):973-984

[81] Nair P, Pizzichini MMM, Kjarsgaard M, Inman MD, Efthimiadis A, Pizzichini E, et al. Mepolizumab for prednisone-dependent asthma with sputum eosinophilia. The New England Journal of Medicine. 2009;360(10):985-993

[82] Lemière C, Ernst P, Olivenstein R, Yamauchi Y, Govindaraju K, Ludwig MS, et al. Airway inflammation assessed by invasive and noninvasive means in severe asthma: Eosinophilic and noneosinophilic phenotypes. The Journal of Allergy and Clinical Immunology. 2006;118(5):1033-1039

[83] Flood-Page PT, Menzies-Gow AN, Kay AB, Robinson DS. Eosinophil's role remains uncertain as anti-interleukin-5 only partially depletes numbers in asthmatic airway. American Journal of Respiratory and Critical Care Medicine. 2003;167(2):199-204

[84] Henriksen DP, Bodtger U, Sidenius K, Maltbaek N, Pedersen L, Madsen H, et al. Efficacy, adverse events, and inter-drug comparison of mepolizumab and reslizumab anti-IL-5 treatments of severe asthma—A systematic review and meta-analysis. European Clinical Respiratory Journal. 2018;**5**(1):1536097

[85] Wenzel S, Ford L, Pearlman D, Spector S, Sher L, Skobieranda F, et al. Dupilumab in persistent asthma with elevated eosinophil levels. The New England Journal of Medicine. 2013;**368**(26):2455-2466

[86] Pavord ID, Korn S, Howarth P, Bleecker ER, Buhl R, Keene ON, et al. Mepolizumab for severe eosinophilic asthma (DREAM): A multicentre, double-blind, placebo-controlled trial. Lancet. 2012;**380**(9842):651-659

[87] Bel EH, Wenzel SE, Thompson PJ, Prazma CM, Keene ON, Yancey SW, et al. Oral glucocorticoid-sparing effect of mepolizumab in eosinophilic asthma. The New England Journal of Medicine. 2014;**371**:1189-1197

[88] Pelaia C, Calabrese C, Vatrella A, Busceti MT, Garofalo E, Lombardo N, et al. Benralizumab: From the basic mechanism of action to the potential use in the biological therapy of severe eosinophilic asthma. BioMed Research International. 2018;**2018**:4839230

[89] Menzella F, Biava M, Bagnasco D, Galeone C, Simonazzi A, Ruggiero P, et al. Efficacy and steroid-sparing effect of benralizumab: Has it an advantage over its competitors? Drugs in Context. 2019;**8**:212580

[90] Sridhar S, Liu H, Pham TH, Damera G, Newbold P. Modulation of blood inflammatory markers by benralizumab in patients with eosinophilic airway diseases. Respiratory Research. 2019;**20**(1):14

[91] Matera MG, Calzetta L, Rinaldi B, Cazzola M. Pharmacokinetic/pharmacodynamic drug evaluation of benralizumab for the treatment of asthma. Expert Opinion on Drug Metabolism & Toxicology. 2017;**13**(9):1007-1013

[92] Coumou H, Bel EH. Improving the diagnosis of eosinophilic asthma. Expert Review of Respiratory Medicine. 2016;**10**(10):1093-1103

[93] Agache I, Jessica Beltran J, Akdis C, Akdis M, Canelo-Aybar C, Canonica W, et al. Efficacy and safety of treatment with biologicals (benralizumab, dupilumab, mepolizumab, omalizumab and reslizumab) for severe eosinophilic asthma. Allergy. 8 February 2020. DOI: 10.1111/all.14221

[94] Chung KF. Asthma phenotyping: A necessity for improved therapeutic precision and new targeted therapies. Journal of Internal Medicine. 2016;**279**(2):192-204

# 11

# Immune-Mediated Inflammation: Human T CD4 Helper Lymphocyte Diversity and Plasticity in Health and Disease

*Rodolfo Alberto Külliker Frers, Matilde Otero-Losada, María Inés Herrera, Sabrina Porta, Vanesa Cosentino, Eduardo Kerzberg, Lucas Udovin and Francisco Capani*

## Abstract

The CD4+ T helper (Th) cells have a critical role in organizing the adaptive immune response. The emerging cells of the differentiation after the immune synapse produce helper T cell subpopulations that activate, suppress, or regulate the immune response upon interaction with varying immune cells. There are two main Th cell functional categories: the "effector cells" and the "regulatory T cells." Classic T helper lymphocytes can also be distinguished by their lineage according to the developmental microenvironment, the expression of cell adhesion-homing receptors, the profile of cytokines they are exposed to, and the involved transcription factors. Traditionally, the CD4+ and CD8+ phenotypes have been considered as helper and cytotoxic/suppressor T lymphocytes, respectively. Currently, the distinction is little rigorous. The immune response is exceedingly complex beyond the classic Th1 and Th2 effector cells' involvement, and other populations of helper T lymphocytes like the Th17, Tfh, Th22, and Th9 lymphocytes have been phenotypically characterized. These lymphocytes also participate in the pathogenesis of several immune-mediated inflammatory disorders. Here, we revisit and discuss the essential aspects of the state of the art regarding phenotypic diversity and plasticity of TCD4 cells in the T lymphocyte repertoire frame and their potential implication in human inflammatory diseases.

**Keywords:** CD4+ subsets, inflammation, health, disease, plasticity, diversity, CD+, Th17

## 1. Introduction

The CD4+ T cells play a key role in triggering various immunological effector and regulatory functions, promoting or attenuating inflammation.

Such a diverse repertoire includes the early activation during immune synapses in the ganglion, activation of cytotoxic T cells, full activation of macrophages effector functions, maturation of B cells into plasma cells and memory B cells, antibody production by B cells, immunoglobulin isotype switching, recruitment of PMNs, and eosinophil and basophil inflammation [1]. The Th cells promote the amplification of inflammatory leukocytes effector activity in a broad spectrum of scenarios which under physiological conditions determinate protective and tolerogenic immune response. Failure in T effector and/or dysregulated regulatory functions could aid immune disorders, including immunodeficiency, autoimmunity, and cancer [2–5].

Helper T cells assist in B cells' differentiation into antibodies-producing plasma B cells in a concerted cellular-humoral immune response. This process is triggered by specific cytokines and ligand-receptor interactions [6].

The effector T cell phenotype is driven by a specific transcriptional factor, a distinctive array of cell surface molecules, and a specific profile of cytokines, which along with microenvironmental specific conditions enable T cell subset within an arm of the immune system [7].

The Jak/Stat (Janus kinase/signal transducer and activator of transcription) pathways [8] and a specific Stat associated with one of the four main transcriptional "signature" factors, T-bet (T-box transcription factor), GATA-3, RORγt (retinoic acid receptor-related orphan receptor gamma), and Foxp3 (forkhead-box/winged-helix transcription factor P3), are essential for Th differentiation [9].

Each differentiation pathway requires specific transcription factors: T-bet and STAT-4 for Th1 and GATA 3 and STAT 6 for Th2 cells and RORyt for TH17 and Foxp3 cells for regulatory T cells (Treg) [10–13].

The T lymphocytes present a remarkable phenotypic, functional, and anatomical diversity. The T cell lineages are extraordinarily diverse and present a very broad functional repertoire (**Table 1**) bearing innate [14] and adaptive immunogenic or tolerogenic immune properties [15, 16]. According to the greater complexity and heterogeneity of subsets of T cells, reconsidering the pathogenicity of inflammatory diseases beyond the "classical Th1/Th2 paradigm", Th17 effector cells and T-regulatory lymphocytes (Treg) would be appropriate. Relative increases in the number of Th9 lymphocytes, follicular helper T cells (Tfh), and Th22 subsets have been described, and even NK and NKT cells contribute to the pathogenesis of immune-mediated inflammatory diseases [17]. These helper T-cell subtypes trigger specific responses upon different tissue environments by expressing a unique set of cytokines and chemokine receptors (**Figure 1**).

The T cells, like the CD1d-restricted natural killer T cells (iNKT) and gamma delta T cells, and other "unconventional" T cell subsets with invariant TCRs (T-cell receptors) exhibit several characteristics that place them at the border between the innate immune system and the adaptive immune system, influencing subsequent challenges by the same antigen. Although "unconventional" T cells provide rapidly available protection and contribute to the adaptive immune system, they have no ordinary helper properties [18].

The natural killer NK (large granular lymphocytes) and NKT (T cells) cells contribute to the pathogenesis of immune-mediated inflammatory diseases (IMIDs). A

| CD4 T cell | Th1, Th2, Th3 (iTreg), Th9, Th17, Th22, ThF, nTreg, and Tr1 |
| --- | --- |
| CD8 T cell | Tc1, Tc2, Tc9, and Tc17 |
| Gamma delta T cell | Tγδ1 and Tγδ2 |
| Natural killer T cell | NKT and NK cells |

*h, helper; c, cytotoxic; reg, regulatory; n, natural; i, induced*

**Table 1.**
*Representative T cell types.*

large increase in these infiltrating innate immune cells has been observed in IMIDs lesions and also in blood as reported for moderate to severe skin psoriasis. In addition, NKT cells might display different cytokine profiles [19, 20].

Gamma delta T cells express a distinctive surface TCR which, unlike TCRαβ, is made up of one γ (gamma) chain and one δ (delta) chain. These cells are abundant in the mucosa and do not require antigen processing and major histocompatibility complex (MHC) presentation of peptide epitopes [21].

Gamma delta T cells, often tissue-specific, are abundant in the epithelia, orches-trating immune responses in inflammation, tumor surveillance, infectious disease, and autoimmunity.

Gamma delta 1 (Tγδ1) and gamma delta 2 (Tγδ2) cells were defined as a CD3+ cell subtype expressing γδ TCR [22]. Phenotypic analysis of gated CD3+ Tγδ1-positive cells has revealed that nearly 75% of them are CD4⁻ CD8⁻ (glycoprotein cluster of differentiation). Gamma delta T cells may be regarded as a rapidly available response to pathogens triggering the innate and adaptive immune system and a memory phenotype. Besides,

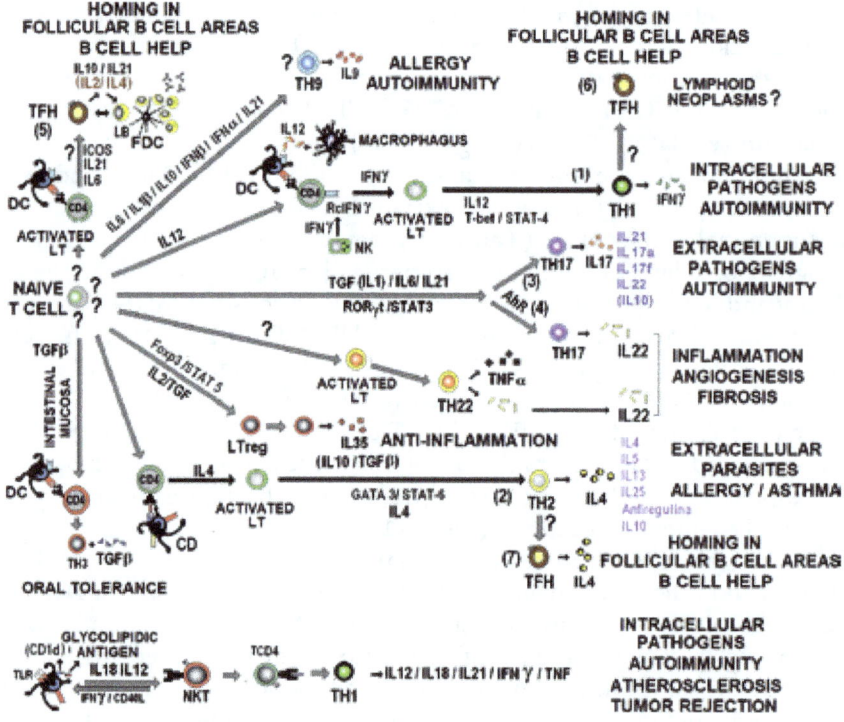

**Figure 1.**
*Schematic representation of T lymphocyte differentiation. The T lymphocyte differentiation progresses upon the presence of IL12, IFNγ, and other signals provided by the antigen-presenting cells. Each differentiation pathway requires specific transcription factors, e.g., T-bet and STAT-4 for Th1 and GATA 3 and STAT 6 for Th2 cells, retinoid-related retinoid receptor orphan receptor (ROR t) for TH17, and FOXP3 cells for regulatory T cells (Treg). The production of IL12 and IL18 by the immune system cells triggers the early release of IFNγ, which influences the natural and adaptive immune response. According to the current differentiation model, a new subpopulation known as Th17 or Th IL17, which originates from virgin T helper cells might comprise a separate lineage from Th1/Th2. The differentiation of Th17 requires the presence of several factors in humans. The IL-23 might be an essential requirement for the development of effector cells. The IL21 might amplify the differentiation to Th17. The effector cells may eventually differentiate upon the participation of the aryl hydrocarbon receptor AhR, a cytoplasmic receptor that translocates to the nucleus. Although RORγt and AhR are highly expressed in the cells, it is unknown whether the AhR is preferentially found in Th17 cells producing IL22. The relationship between the Th17 cells producing IL22 and the recently identified Th22 effectors is not clear. The Th22 subpopulation typically secretes IL22 and TNFα but not IFNγ, IL4, or IL17. The secretion profile includes growth factors and chemokines involved in angiogenesis and fibrosis. TFH, follicular helper T lymphocyte; DC, dendritic cell.*

they show potent antigen-presenting properties upon translocation to the ganglion. However, the various subsets may also be considered part of the innate immunity where a restricted TCR may be used as a pattern recognition receptor, indicating the importance of these lymphocytes in immunity and tissue monitoring of pathogens [21].

In particular situations, T CD8 cells can exert helper functions and vice versa, regardless of the existing heterogeneity of CD4 and CD8 T cells. Two functionally distinctive T lymphocytes subpopulations having effector or regulatory properties were considered [23]. Currently, the traditional distinction between the CD4 phenotype as a T helper and the CD8 phenotype as a cytotoxic/suppressor T lymphocyte is relative. Both CD4+ lymphocytes with cytotoxic properties and CD8+ lymphocytes presenting a secretory profile of cytokines have been identified [24], both unable to recognize the antigen in its soluble form.

Like CD4 (+) T cells, under particular conditions, also CD8 (+) T cells express different types of interleukins or gain suppressive activity [2]. Certainly, neither the heterogeneity of T cells nor the relative cytotoxic capacity of CD8 and CD4 cells is limited to the mentioned phenotypes. Regarding CD8+ T cells, the proliferative response prevails over its cytotoxic potential against cells infected by viruses, tumors, and allogeneic cells in different situations.

Recent studies have shown differences in the effector function of memory cells depending on their localization. While memory cells in the secondary lymphoid organs are generally non-cytotoxic, the cells in peripheral tissues show intense cytolytic activity. These observations follow the concept developed by Sallusto et al. [25], stating that centrally located memory cells expressing CCR7 occupy secondary lymphoid organs, whereas effector cells lacking CCR7 remain peripheral.

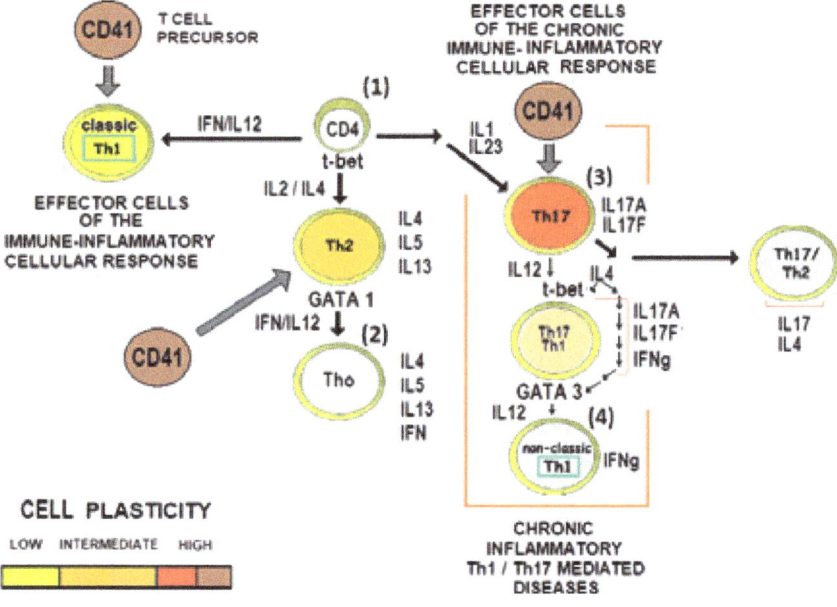

**Figure 2.**
*T helper cell plasticity in inflammation. (1) Human Th1 cells originating from virgin CD41 cells in response to the coordinated activity of IFN and IL-12 induce stable expression of the transcription factor T-bet. (2) Human Th2 cells also originate from naive CD41 cells in response to the combined activity of IL-2 and IL-4, which induce stable expression of the GATA3 transcription factor. In the presence of IL-12, T-bet is upregulated in Th2 cells, which change to produce IFN (Tho). Human Th17 cells originate from a small subset of native CD41 cells present in the newborn thymus with receptors IL-23R, IL-1RI, and CCR6 and differentiate into mature Th17 cells in response to the combined activity of IL-1b and IL-23 in vitro. (3) In the presence of IL-12, the expression of T-bet is upregulated in Th17 cells, which change to the production of IFNγ. (4) In the presence of IL-4, GATA3 expression is upregulated in Th17/Th1 cells, which progress to nonclassical Th1 cells producing IFNγ.*

No doubt that the immediate availability of effector memory cells upon infection in peripheral tissue is critical to the rapid control of pathogens. Centrally located memory cells represent a precursor T population with the ability to acquire effector properties after antigen-directed expansion.

Virgin T cells are the most homogeneous subpopulation of T lymphocytes. After activation in immunological synapses, lymphocytes differentiate into effector and memory cells with a broad phenotypic repertoire. Their properties may obey to different maturation programs, localization, and particularities in the antigenic presentation. Likewise, CD4 T cells of different lineage show phenotypic plasticity [26], eventually shifting into another T cell subset (**Figure 2**).

## 2. T-helper cell subtypes 1 and 2

The Th1 and Th2 are the most studied subtypes of helper T cells [27]. They can be distinguished by their characteristic cytokine secretion profile, Th1 classically producing IFNγ and Th2 producing IL4 and IL5, among other cytokines. Following CD4 lymphocyte characterization, different studies have found similitudes for the CD8 subpopulations called Tc1 (or type I) and Tc2 (or type II) [28]. At first sight, IL12 and IL4 appear critically involved in the differentiation to type I and II cells of the CD4 and CD8 subtypes, though the scenario is not that simple. Whereas IL21 suppresses type I differentiation and promotes type II differentiation, IL18 blocks IL4-mediated suppression of type II differentiation and promotes IL12 receptor expression and type I differentiation. Collectively, different experimental outcomes seem to support the existence of factors that stabilize, retard, or reverse Th1/Th2 polarization [27]. Likewise, as variations in the secretion profile of cytokines do not respond to the prototypical type I and II dichotomy, some authors have postulated that Th1/Th2 polarization is artefactual and may not resemble the in vivo situation [29].

Recently, transcription factors associated with lymphocyte differentiation like T-bet associated with the induction of Th1 differentiation have been characterized [30]. Certainly, TCD4 cells lacking T-bet are unable to produce IFNg but release large amounts of Th2 cytokines IL4 and IL5. Transcription factor T-bet induces the expression of the IL12 receptor and transactivates the IFNg gene. The IL12 derived from dendritic cells and macrophages triggers the release of IL12, which induces STAT 4 activation in developing Th1 cells by increasing IFNg level and IL18 receptor expression [31].

Dendritic cells are also involved in Th2 differentiation. Histamine acting on H1 and H2 receptors in dendritic cells downregulates IL12 expression and stimulates IL10 release, which with the participation of specific transcription factors (GATA-3 and STAT-6) promotes Th2 differentiation [32].

## 3. Follicular helper T lymphocyte

Described over a decade ago, T helper lymphocytes with follicle-positive tropism (ThF) differ from the classic Th1 and Th2 lymphocytes by expressing an array of factors essential to interact with follicular B lymphocytes [33]. The differentiation markers include CXCR5, CD25, CD69, CD95, CD57 (only in humans), OX40 (CD134), and CD40L (CD154). The homing pattern and functional characteristics of ThF have been the subject of intense investigation. The ThF interacts with B lymphocytes and modify the type of humoral response inducing long-lived memory B cells that release high-affinity antibodies [34].

Curiously, ThF cells dysfunction may induce systemic autoimmunity. The ThF cells comprise a TCD4+ subpopulation restricted to the B areas of the lymphatic organs, critically involved in the events following the interaction of dendritic cells with the virgin T lymphocytes in the secondary lymphatic organ T zone [35]. The development of follicular homing capacity by activated T cell helper is the first event in the generation of ThF cells. Virgin T cells expressing CD62L and CCR7 enter the secondary lymphatic organs in the T paracortical lymphoid region, and T-lymphocyte activation induces sub-sensitivity to lymphoid chemokines along with an increase in follicular chemokines CXCL13 (also known as B cell-attracting chemokine BCA-1 or B lymphocyte chemoattractant BLC) [36].

Activated ThF and lymphoblast B lymphocytes express the CXCR5 receptor, which confers follicle-positive tropism, and the stroma and dendritic follicular cells express the ligand CXCL13. Follicular dendritic cells supply proliferative, antiapoptotic signals, and ThF lymphocytes undergo changes increasing antigenic specificity and promote the differentiation of lymphoblasts into plasma cells or B lymphocytes with memory. The antigen-dependent T-B interaction is critical in triggering the humoral immune response [37]. The T-B collaboration is essential to generating short-lived plasma cells and inducing the germinal center where they trigger isotype change and somatic hypermutation, yielding high-affinity long-lived plasma cells and memory cells [38].

Regarding ThF relationship with Th1, Th2, and Th17 subpopulations, some authors mention that ThF cells produce IL4, IFNγ, and IL17, respectively, associated with them [39].

## 4. T helper subtype 9 (Th9) cells

Certain inflammatory conditions give rise to the T helper subtype 9 (Th9) cells of unknown functional contribution to the immune response [40, 41]. The in vitro development of effector cells specific to constituents of oligodendrocytes (myelin oligodendrocyte glycoprotein) Th17, Th1, Th2, and Th9 allowed evaluating the encephalitogenic activity in adoptive transfer. All Th1, Th17, and Th9 subpopulations but not Th2 successfully induced experimental allergic encephalitis [23]. The Th9 cells might express varied chemokine patterns involved in different immune responses. Their effector function balanced by regulatory T cells induces regulatory activity restoring homeostasis. This recently described Th9 subset of helper lymphocytes may escalate chronic inflammation under certain conditions independently from Th1, Th2, Th17, and regulatory T cells [42].

## 5. T helper subtype 22 cells

Another LT helper subpopulation, the Th22, has been recently identified in epidermic infiltrates in a variety of inflammatory skin disorders, including psoriasis [43]. They secrete IL22 and TNFα but not IFNg, IL4, or IL17, and their clones derived from psoriatic patients are stable in culture, exhibiting a distinctive transcription profile compared with the already mentioned subpopulations. Secretion profile includes fibroblast growth factors and chemokines potentially involved in angiogenesis and fibrosis [44].

## 6. T helper subtype 17 cells

Differentiation of Th17 cells, like Th1 and Th2 cells, requires the co-participation of CD28 and ICOS after the initial stimulus derived from antigenic recognition via the TCR complex (TCR, CD3, ζ chains) for differentiation from virgin CD4+ T cells [45]. Ivanov and colleagues suggested that the nuclear receptor ROR gamma T is the key transcriptional factor [46] in the differentiation of the Th17 lineage. The Th17 cells producing IL17 induce inflammatory responses [47].

Differentiation to Th17 requires IL6, TGFβ, and IL23 [48], whereas IL1 and TNFα might be involved in Th17 maturation. According to this model, IL27, another member of the IL12 family, programs the TCD4+ cells to differentiate to Th1 inducing the expression of IL12Rβ2. The IL12 is required for the differentiation of the programmed cells into Th1 cells producing IFNγ. In turn, IL23, a member of the IL12 family [49], triggers the proliferation of Th1 cells from memory cells and induces the development of inflammatory Th17 cells [50]. Conversely, IL27 inhibits differentiation to Th17 cells by an unknown mechanism suppressing inflammation. The relative amount of IL6 and TGFβ in the cellular microenvironment is crucial to the severity of inflammation [51].

The proinflammatory cytokine IL-17, originally named IL-17A, has been the subject of intense research since its discovery in 1993 [52]. Interest in this cytokine increased considerably when its production by a specific subset of CD4 + T cells, the so-called Th17 cells [53], was reported. Nevertheless, Th17 lymphocytes can change their phenotype to Th1 or Th2 cells depending on the dominant cytokines [2, 54]. **Figure 2** illustrates how this plasticity can influence arthritis and cardiovascular risk.

Other immune cells subsets can also synthesize and express IL-17, including CD8 + T cells (CD8 + IL17 T-cell, or Tc17). Differentiation of CD8 (+) T cells depend on the antigen, co-stimulatory molecules, cytokines, and transcription factors inducing them to progress to Tc1, Tc2, Tc9, Tc17, or TCD8 [55].

Since Th17 hyperactivation is responsible for the Th17/Treg imbalance in certain pathologies, IL-17A might be considered a potential therapeutic target in modulating Th1 activity enhancing the regulatory response [56].

## 7. Regulatory T cells

Following Th3 cell identification and characterization based on their functions in the intestinal mucosa, many studies investigated the phenotypic characteristics of conventional Treg cells in different tissues and pathological situations. The Th3 cells (CD4+ TGFβ +) and the Foxp3+ can be induced by oral tolerance, and the TGFβ released by iTreg prevents experimental colitis [57]. Though regarded as separate lineages, the induced Treg (iTreg) and Th3 cells are substantially superimposed.

Regulatory T cells and maintenance of self-tolerance rely on natural Treg cells, typically expressing CD4, CD25, and Foxp3. They develop in the thymus and recognize specific autoantigens [58].

The Treg-induced cells (iTreg), another subset of Treg cells, are also generated in the periphery during an active immune response. In fact, CD4 + CD25− cells in the periphery can be converted, in the presence of TGFβ and IL10 into CD25 + CD4 + Foxp3 + cells. The iTreg cells induced by IL-10 are called Tr1 cells and if induced by TGFβ are called Th3. One subpopulation of nTreg expresses activation markers suggesting that it comprises autoreactive Tregs continuously activated by tissue autoantigens.

Three suppression mechanisms, not fully elucidated, have been proposed to explain the inhibitory actions of Treg cells on activated T cells. These are the contact-dependent inhibition between Treg and effector cells, the consumption and limitation of growth factors like IL-2, and the inhibition of LT effectors by the production of soluble inhibitory cytokines (TGFβ, IL-10, and IL-35) and CTL4 ligands of the Treg which interacts with the CPA molecules [59].

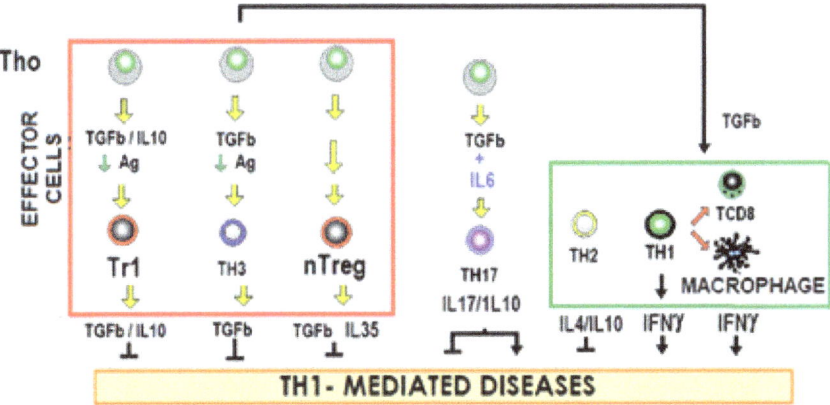

**Figure 3.**
*Modulation of T lymphocyte function by TGFβ factor and its importance in Th1-mediated diseases. TGFb released by different types of regulatory cells modulates the inflammatory activity of all effector cells, Th1 cells included.*

The T-regulatory activity (Treg) is pathologically low in both psoriasis and atherosclerosis [60]. The activity of pathogenic T cells is regulated by Treg cells activity via IL-10 and TGFβ [61]. The TGFβ inhibits Th1, and Th2 differentiation favors Th1 and Th17 hyperactivity [62] in both pathologies [60]. The increase in TGFβ [63] was reported inversely correlated with cardiovascular and psoriatic severity.

The critical role of TGFβ and Treg cells was evidenced by the finding that TGFβ-deficient mice developed multiple inflammatory diseases [64–66].

Both nTreg cells and Tr1-induced cells are able to produce IL10. The relevance of IL10 was evidenced by the specific blocking experiments of lymphocyte IL-10 triggering protection against inflammatory processes. The Tr1 cells expressing IL-10 require the presence of TGFα [67]. Regarding Th2-mediated counterregulation, the Th2 produces anti-inflammatory IL-4, IL-5, and IL-13 which decrease Th1 cells activity. The proinflammatory, metabolic, and systemic mechanisms that operate in the pathogenesis of psoriatic disease may explain the accelerated atherosclerotic process in these patients (**Figure 3**). Serum level of proinflammatory cytokines can increase cell-mediated immunity, which upon decreased regulatory Th2 activity and Treg level promote endothelial infiltration of inflammatory cells and plaque formation [68].

## 8. Conclusions

The heterogeneity of the T cells in general and TCD4 helper, in particular, may reflect divergent pathways in response to epigenetic factors or different stages of a unique differentiation pathway. Adhesion molecules, e.g., LFA1 and ICAM, CCR and CXCR chemokine receptors, and activation molecules, among others of undetermined function, reflect the transition.

The heterogeneity may obey to a programmed developmental process or to microenvironmental stimulation. Immunosuppressive or stimulatory signals like cytokines seem crucially involved though both may participate. This information is expected to shed light on the possible pathogenic role of Th cells in human inflammatory diseases beyond the Th1/Th2 paradigm.

The relationships between the classic Th1/ Th2 and the more recently defined Th17/iTreg/ Tfh/Th9 cells and effector-regulatory cell interactions need clarification regarding their pathogenic role in human inflammatory diseases.

## Author details

Rodolfo Alberto Kölliker Frers[1,2], Matilde Otero-Losada[1*], María Inés Herrera[1,3], Sabrina Porta[2], Vanesa Cosentino[2], Eduardo Kerzberg[2], Lucas Udovin[1] and Francisco Capani[1,3]

1 Institute of Cardiological Research, University of Buenos Aires, National Research Council, ININCA, UBA-CONICET, Buenos Aires, Argentina

2 Hospital Ramos Mejía, Buenos Aires, Argentina

3 Pontifical Catholic University of Argentina, Buenos Aires, Argentina

*Address all correspondence to: molly1063@gmail.com

# References

[1] Gagliani N, Huber S. Basic aspects of T helper cell differentiation. Methods in Molecular Biology. 2017;**1514**:19-30. DOI: 10.1007/978-1-4939-6548-9_2

[2] Cosmi L, Maggi L, Santarlasci V, Liotta F, et al. T helper cells plasticity in inflammation. Cytometry Part A. 2014;**85**:36-42. DOI: 10.1002/cyto.a.22348

[3] Dong C. Helper T cells and cancer-associated inflammation: A new direction for immunotherapy? Journal of Interferon & Cytokine Research. 2017;**37**:383-385. DOI: 10.1089/jir.2017.0012

[4] Qiu H, Wu H, Chan V, Lau CS, et al. Transcriptional and epigenetic regulation of follicular T-helper cells and their role in autoimmunity. Autoimmunity. 2017;**50**:71-81. DOI: 10.1080/08916934.2017.1284821

[5] Shamriz O, Patel K, Marsh RA, Bleesing J, et al. Hypogammaglobulinemia with decreased class-switched B-cells and dysregulated T-follicular-helper cells in IPEX syndrome. Clinical Immunology. 2018;**197**:219-223. DOI: 10.1016/j. clim.2018.10.005

[6] Shinomiya N, Kuratsuji T, Yata J. Cell Immunol the role of T cells in immunoglobulin class switching of specific antibody production system in vitro in humans. Cellular Immunology. 1989;**118**:239-249. DOI: 10.1016/0008-8749(89)90375-4

[7] Caza T, Landas S. Functional and phenotypic plasticity of CD4(+) T cell subsets. BioMed Research International. 2015;**2015**:521957. DOI: 10.1155/2015/521957

[8] Shi Z, Jiang W, Wang M, Wang X, et al. Inhibition of JAK/STAT pathway restrains TSLP-activated dendritic cells mediated inflammatory T helper type 2 cell response in allergic rhinitis. Molecular and Cellular Biochemistry. 2017;**430**:161-169. DOI: 10.1007/s11010-017-2963-7

[9] Nogueira LG, Santos RH, Fiorelli AI, Mairena EC, et al. Myocardial gene expression of T-bet, GATA-3, Ror-γt, FoxP3, and hallmark cytokines in chronic Chagas disease cardiomyopathy: An essentially unopposed TH1-type response. Mediators of Inflammation. 2014;**2014**:914326. DOI: 10.1155/2014/914326

[10] Ivanov II, McKenzie BS, Zhou L, Tadokoro CE, et al. The orphan nuclear receptor RORgamma T directs the differentiation program of proinflammatory IL-17+ T helper cells. Cell. 2006;**126**:1121-1133. DOI: 10.1016/j.cell.2006.07.035

[11] Levine AG, Mendoza A, Hemmers S, Moltedo B, et al. Stability and function of regulatory T cells expressing the transcription factor T-bet. Nature. 2017;**546**(7658):421-425. DOI: 10.1038/nature22360

[12] Miyara M, Yoshioka Y, Kitoh A, Shima T, et al. Functional delineation and differentiation dynamics of human CD4+ T cells expressing the FoxP3 transcription factor. Immunity. 2009;**30**:899-911. DOI: 10.1016/j.immuni.2009.03.019

[13] Tindemans I, Serafini N, Di Santo JP, Hendriks RW. GATA-3 function in innate and adaptive immunity. Immunity. 2014;**41**:191-206. DOI: 10.1016/j.immuni.2014.06.006

[14] Schäfer C, Ascui G, Ribeiro CH, López M, et al. Innate immune cells for immunotherapy of autoimmune and cancer disorders. International Reviews of Immunology. 2017;**36**:315-337. DOI: 10.1080/08830185.2017.1365145

[15] Hall BM. CD4+ CD25+ T regulatory cells in transplantation tolerance: 25 years on. Transplantation. 2016;**100**:2533-2547. DOI: 10.1097/TP.0000000000001436

[16] Schülke S. Induction of Interleukin-10 producing dendritic cells As a tool to suppress allergen-specific T helper 2 responses. Frontiers in Immunology. 2018;**9**:455. DOI: 10.3389/fimmu.2018.00455

[17] Moser B, Eberl M. Gamma delta T cells: Novel initiators of adaptive immunity. Immunological Reviews. 2007;**215**:89. DOI: 10.1111/j.1600-065X.2006.00472.x

[18] Lee YJ, Starrett GJ, Lee ST, Yang R, et al. Lineage-specific effector signatures of invariant NKT cells are shared amongst γδ T, innate lymphoid, and Th cells. Journal of Immunology. 2016;**197**:1460-1470. DOI: 10.4049/jimmunol.1600643

[19] Kadowaki N, Antonenko S, Ho S, Rissoan MC, et al. Distinct cytokine profiles of neonatal natural killer T cells after expansion with subsets of dendritic cells. The Journal of Experimental Medicine. 2001;**193**:1221. DOI: 10.1084/jem.193.10.1221

[20] Zhou D, Mattner J, Cantu C 3rd, Schrantz N, et al. Lysosomal glycosphingolipid recognition by NKT cells. Science. 2004;**306**:1786. DOI: 10.1126/science.1103440

[21] Morita CT, Mariuzza RA, Brenner MB. Antigen recognition by human gamma delta T cells: Pattern recognition by the adaptive immune system. Springer Seminars in Immunopathology. 2000;**22**:191-217

[22] Nielsen MM, Witherden DA, Havran WL. γδ T cells in homeostasis and host defence of epithelial barrier tissues. Nature Reviews. Immunology. 2017;**17**:733-745. DOI: 10.1038/nri.2017.101

[23] Jäger A, Dardalhon V, Sobel RA, Bettelli E, et al. Th1, Th17, and Th9 effector cells induce experimental autoimmune encephalomyelitis with different pathological phenotypes. Journal of Immunology. 2009;**183**:7169. DOI: 10.4049/jimmunol.0901906

[24] Aandahl EM, Sandberg JK, Beckerman KP, Tasken K, et al. CD7 is a differentiation marker that identifies multiple CD8 T cell effector subsets. Journal of Immunology. 2003;**170**:2349. DOI: 10.4049/jimmunol.170.5.2349

[25] Sallusto F, Lenig D, Forster R, Lipp M, et al. Two subsets of memory T lymphocytes with distinct homing potentials and effector functions. Nature. 1999;**401**(6754):708-712. DOI: 10.1038/44385

[26] Zhou L, Chong MM, Littman DR. Plasticity of CD4+ T cell lineage differentiation. Immunity. 2009;**30**:646. DOI: 10.1016/j.immuni.2009.05.001

[27] Zhang Y, Zhang Y, Gu W, He L, et al. Th1/Th2 cell's function in immune system. Advances in Experimental Medicine and Biology. 2014;**841**:45-65. DOI: 10.1007/978-94-017-9487-9_3

[28] Cerwenka A, Carter LL, Reome JB, Swain SL, et al. In vivo persistence of CD8 polarized T cell subsets producing type 1 or type 2 cytokines. Journal of Immunology. 1998;**161**:97-105

[29] Sekiya T, Yoshimura A. In vitro Th differentiation protocol. Methods in Molecular Biology. 2016;**1344**:183-191. DOI: 10.1007/978-1-4939-2966-5_10

[30] Kallies A, Good-Jacobson KL. Transcription factor T-bet orchestrates lineage development and function in the immune system. Trends in Immunology. 2017;**38**:287-297. DOI: 10.1016/j.it.2017.02.003

[31] Kaplan MH, Wurster AL, Grusby MJ. A signal transducer and activator of

transcription (Stat) 4-independent pathway for the development of T helper type 1 cells. The Journal of Experimental Medicine. 1998;**188**:1191-1196. DOI: 10.1084/jem.188.6.1191

[32] Zhu J, Yamane H, Cote-Sierra J, Guo L, et al. GATA-3 promotes Th2 responses through three different mechanisms: Induction of Th2 cytokine production, selective growth of Th2 cells and inhibition of Th1 cell-specific factors. Cell Research. 2006;**16**:3-10. DOI: 10.1038/sj.cr.7310002

[33] Yu D, Batten M, Mackay CR, King C. Lineage specification and heterogeneity of T follicular helper cells. Current Opinion in Immunology. 2009;**21**(6):619. DOI: 10.1016/j.coi.2009.09.013

[34] Laurent C, Fazilleau N, Brousset P. A novel subset of T-helper cells: Follicular T-helper cells and their markers. Haematologica. 2010;**95**:356. DOI: 10.3324/haematol.2009.019133

[35] Sauma D, Espejo P, Ramirez A, Fierro A, et al. Differential regulation of Notch ligands in dendritic cells upon interaction with T helper cells. Scandinavian Journal of Immunology. 2011;**74**:62-70. DOI: 10.1111/j.1365-3083.2011.02541.x

[36] Havenar-Daughton C, Lindqvist M, Heit A, Wu JE, et al. CXCL13 is a plasma biomarker of germinal center activity. Proceedings of the National Academy of Sciences of the United States of America. 2016;**113**:2702-2707. DOI: 10.1073/pnas.1520112113

[37] Papa I, Saliba D, Ponzoni M, Bustamante S, et al. TFH-derived dopamine accelerates productive synapses in germinal centres. Nature. 2017;**547**(7663):318-323. DOI: 10.1038/nature23013

[38] Eisen HN. Affinity enhancement of antibodies: How low-affinity antibodies produced early in immune responses are followed by high-affinity antibodies later and in memory B-cell responses. Cancer Immunology Research. 2014;**2**:381-392. DOI: 10.1158/2326-6066.CIR-14-0029

[39] Morita R, Schmitt N, Bentebibel SE, Ranganathan R, et al. Human blood CXCR5(+)CD4(+) T cells are counterparts of T follicular cells and contain specific subsets that differentially support antibody secretion. Immunity. 2011;**34**:108-121. DOI: 10.1016/j.immuni.2010.12.012

[40] Chen H, Zhang L, Wang P, Su H, et al. mTORC2 controls Th9 polarization and allergic airway inflammation. Allergy. 2017;**72**:1510-1520. DOI: 10.1111/all.13152

[41] Li Y, Yu Q, Zhang Z, Wang J, et al. TH9 cell differentiation, transcriptional control and function in inflammation, autoimmune diseases and cancer. Oncotarget. 2016;**7**:71001-71012. DOI: 10.18632/oncotarget.11681

[42] Li J, Chen S, Xiao X, Zhao Y, et al. IL-9 and Th9 cells in health and diseases-from tolerance to immunopathology. Cytokine & Growth Factor Reviews. 2017;**37**:47-55. DOI: 10.1016/j.cytogfr.2017.07.004

[43] Eyerich S, Eyerich K, Pennino D, Carbone T, et al. Th22 cells represent a distinct human T cell subset involved in epidermal immunity and remodeling. The Journal of Clinical Investigation. 2009;**119**:3573. DOI: 10.1172/JCI40202

[44] Nikoopour E, Bellemore SM, Singh B. IL-22, cell regeneration and autoimmunity. Cytokine. 2015;**74**:35-42. DOI: 10.1016/j.cyto.2014.09.007

[45] Louten J, Boniface K, de Waal Malefyt R. Development and function of TH17 cells in health and disease. The Journal of Allergy and Clinical

Immunology.      2009;**123**:1004-1011.
DOI: 10.1016/j.jaci.2009.04.003

[46] Han L, Yang J, Wang X, Wu Q , et al. The E3 deubiquitinase USP17 is a positive regulator of retinoic acid-related orphan nuclear receptor γt (RORγt) in Th17 cells. The Journal of Biological    Chemistry.    2014;**289**: 25546-25555.    DOI:    10.1074/jbc. M114.565291

[47] Beringer A, Noack M, Miossec P. IL-17 in chronic inflammation: From discovery to targeting. Trends in Molecular Medicine. 2016;**22**:230-241. DOI: 10.1016/j.molmed.2016.01.001

[48]    Langrish    CL,    Chen    Y, Blumenschein WM, Mattson J, et al. IL23 drives a pathogenic T cell population that induces autoimmune inflammation. Journal of Experimental Medicine. 2005;**201**:233. DOI: 10.1084/ jem.20041257

[49] Bending D, De la Peña H, Veldhoen M, Phillips JM, et al. Highly purified Th17 cells from BDC2.5NOD mice convert into Th1-like cells in NOD/ SCID recipient mice. The Journal of Clinical    Investigation.    2009;**119**: 565-572. DOI: 10.1172/JCI37865

[50] Park H, Li Z, Yang XO, Chang SH, et al. A distinct lineage of CD4 T cells regulates tissue inflammation by producing interleukin 17. Nature Immunology.    2005;**6**:1133.    DOI: 10.1038/ni1261

[51] Bettelli E, Carrier Y, Gao W, Korn T, et al. Reciprocal developmental pathways for the generation of pathogenic effector TH17 and regulatory T cells. Nature. 2006;**441**:235. DOI: 10.1038/nature04753

[52] Rouvier E, Luciani MF, Mattei MG, Denizot F, et al. CTLA-8, cloned from an activated T cell, bearing AU-rich messenger RNA instability sequences, and homologous to a herpesvirus saimiri gene. Journal of Immunology. 1993;**150**:5445-5456

[53] O'Connor W Jr, Esplugues E, Huber S. The role of TH17-associated cytokines in health and disease. Journal of    Immunology    Research. 2014;**2014**:936270. DOI: 10.1155/2014/ 936270

[54] Basdeo SA, Cluxton D, Sulaimani J, Moran B, et al. Ex-Th17 (nonclassical Th1) cells are functionally distinct from classical Th1 and Th17 cells and are not constrained by regulatory T cells. Journal    of    Immunology.    2017;**198**: 2249-2259.    DOI:    10.4049/ jimmunol.1600737

[55] Srenathan U, Steel K, Taams LS. IL-17+ CD8+ T cells: Differentiation, phenotype and role in inflammatory disease.    Immunology    Letters. 2016;**178**:20-26.    DOI:    10.1016/j. imlet.2016.05.001

[56] Kagami S, Rizzo HL, Lee JJ, Koguchi Y, et al. Circulating Th17, Th22, and Th1 cells are increased in psoriasis. The Journal of Investigative Dermatology. 2010;**130**:1373-1383. DOI: 10.1038/jid.2009.399

[57] Lee CR, Kwak Y, Yang T, Han JH, et al. Myeloid-derived suppressor cells are controlled by regulatory T cells via TGF-β during murine colitis. Cell Reports.    2016;**17**:3219-3232.    DOI: 10.1016/j.celrep.2016.11.062

[58] Stephens GL, Shevach EM. Foxp3+ regulatory T cells: Selfishness under scrutiny. Immunity. 2007;**27**:417-419. DOI: 10.1016/j.immuni.2007.08.008

[59] Collison LW, Workman CJ, Kuo TT, Boyd K, et al. The inhibitory cytokine IL-35 contributes to regulatory T-cell    function.    Nature. 2007;**450**:566-569.    DOI:    10.1038/ nature06306

[60]    Armstrong    AW,    Voyles    SV, Armstrong EJ, Fuller EN, et al. A tale of two plaques: Convergent mechanisms

of T-cell-mediated inflammation in psoriasis and atherosclerosis. Experimental Dermatology. 2011;**20**:544-549.       DOI: 10.1111/j.1600-0625.2011.01308.x

[61] Sakaguchi S, Yamaguchi T, Nomura T, Ono M. Regulatory T cells and immune tolerance. Cell. 2008;**33**:775-787.    DOI: 10.1016/j.cell.2008.05.009

[62] Gojova A, Brun V, Esposito B, Cottrez F, et al. Specific abrogation of transforming growth factor-{beta} signaling in T cells alters atherosclerotic lesion size and composition in mice. Blood.    2003;**102**:4052-4058.    DOI: 10.1182/blood-2003-05-1729

[63] Nickoloff BJ, Nestle FO. Recent insights into the immunopathogenesis of psoriasis provide new therapeutic opportunities. The Journal of Clinical Investigation.    2004;**113**:1664-1675. DOI: 10.1172/JCI22147

[64] Grainger DJ, Mosedale DE, Metcalfe JC, Bottinger EP. Dietary fat and reduced levels of TGFbeta1 act synergistically to promote activation of the   vascular   endothelium   and formation of lipid lesions. Journal of Cell Science. 2000;**113**:2355-2361

[65]   Mallat   Z,   Gojova   A, Marchiol-Fournigault C, Esposito B, et al.    Inhibition   of   transforming growth    factor-beta    signaling accelerates atherosclerosis and induces an unstable plaque phenotype in mice. Circulation          Research. 2001;**89**:930-934.    DOI:    10.1161/ hh2201.099415

[66]   Nakamura   K,   Kitani   A, Strober W. Cell contact-dependent immunosuppression   by   CD4   (+) CD25(+) regulatory T cells is mediated by cell surface-bound transforming growth factor beta. The Journal of Experimental   Medicine.   2001;**194**: 629-644. DOI: 10.1084/jem.194.5.629

[67]   Maynard   CL, Harrington   LE, Janowski   KM,   Oliver   JR,   et al. Regulatory   T   cells   expressing interleukin 10 develop from Foxp3+ and Foxp3− precursor cells in the absence of interleukin 10. Nature Immunology.   2007;**8**:931-941.   DOI: 10.1038/ni1504

[68] Nestle FO, Kaplan DH, Barker J. Mechanisms of disease: Psoriasis. The New England Journal of Medicine. 2009;**361**:496-509.    DOI:    10.1056/ NEJMra0804595

# 12

# Eosinophilic Disorders: Extrinsic and Intrinsic Immune Response, New Diagnostic Perspectives and Therapeutic Alternatives

*Maria-de-Lourdes Irigoyen-Coria,*

*Vilma-Carolina Bekker-Mendez,*

*Maria-Isabel Leyva-Carmona, Cecilia Rosel-Pech,*

*Samuel Moreno-Olivares and David Solis-Hernandez*

## Abstract

Eosinophils are immune response cells located in the peripheral blood, bone marrow, and lymph nodes, among others; an increase in the number of eosinophils in the peripheral blood above $5000/mm^3$ is associated with conditions ranging from infections (bacterial and parasitic) and allergy (asthma, rhinitis, or drugs), even neoplasms. Various study groups have classified them according to their etiology, thus facilitating their diagnosis and treatment. The WHO divides them as primary and secondary and also considers the number of eosinophils/$mm^3$ and the involvement of white organs, while others have divided them into intrinsic and extrinsic. The former include mutations in the pluripotential hematopoietic cells, which lead to chronic myeloid leukemias with clonal expansion of eosinophils and extrinsic ones where the changes are related to a TH2 response activated by different cytosines such as IL-5. Current treatments are specifically aimed at modifying the clonal expansion of eosinophils with corticosteroids, hydroxyurea, interferon (peg) alpha, imatinib, among others, and bone marrow transplantation, while in extrinsic alterations corticosteroids and IL inhibitors are used −5 (mepolizumab).

**Keywords:** eosinophilia, hypereosinophilic syndrome, interleukin-5, diagnosis, treatment

## 1. Introduction

### 1.1 Characteristics: morphological, physiological, origin, immunological regulation, and distribution of eosinophil

Eosinophils are leukocytes (white cells) found in the peripheral blood, hematopoietic, lymphatic organs, the bone marrow, spleen, and thymus, and can migrate to connective tissues and digestive tract; they are part of the group of leukocytes called granulocytes, along with basophils and neutrophils. They were described by P. Ehrlich in 1879 calling them eosinophils because their acidic granules in the cytoplasm were stained by their affinity dye aniline-eosin giving them the form of red-orange ammunition observed by optical microscopy: They are rounded cells from 8 to 15 μm in diameter, with a bilobed core with a fine nuclear bridge joining both lobes [1].

Identification and quantification.

Methodology: Manual count in Neubauer chamber and automatic hematology analyzer using impedance and colorimetry and flow cytometry CD16 (FcYRIII-CD16). Under normal conditions peripheral blood eosinophils represent 1–5% of total leukocytes, with an upper limit of 0.4 × 109 L,, the absolute eosinophilic count (AEC) of 350–500/mm$^3$ and in children is greater than 0.75 × 109 L, increasing the number of eosinophils (eosinophilia) to more than 3–5 times which is indicative of an activity of infectious, parasitic, allergic, and eosinophilic and hypereosinophilic disorders [1–5].

They originate in the bone marrow, by a process of maturation and differentiation that lasts approximately 8 days (hematopoiesis) from a pluripotential precursor cell (stem cell) differentiating itself as myeloid granulocytic line, under the influence of IL-3, IL-4 - granulocytic colony stimulation factor (GM-CSF) of eotaxin; evolving toward a mixed eosinophil-basophilic precursor and then differentiating toward eosinophils by action of IL-3, GM-CSF, and especially IL-5, they have a survival of 6–12 hours before moving to tissues where they remain between 2 and 5 days; once there is a stimulus, they respond by exercising their multiple functions regulated by T lymphocytes (**Figure 1**) [1, 2, 6].

The text begins with: Its main functions are the defense against parasites, helminths, nematodes, participate in allergic responses, inflammatory processes, restoration, and tissue repair; since they have specific chemotactic receptors on their membrane, eotaxin, cytokines (IL-3 -IL-5 and GM-CSF), eosinophil chemotactic factor of anaphylaxis (ECF-A); and nonspecific such as f MLP (from the wall of bacteria), complement activation products (C3a, C5a, C6, and C7), platelet-activating factor (PAF), leukotrienes (LTB 4 and LTD 4), histamine and IL-8. Diapedesis is mainly performed by integrins to adhere to the vascular endothelium

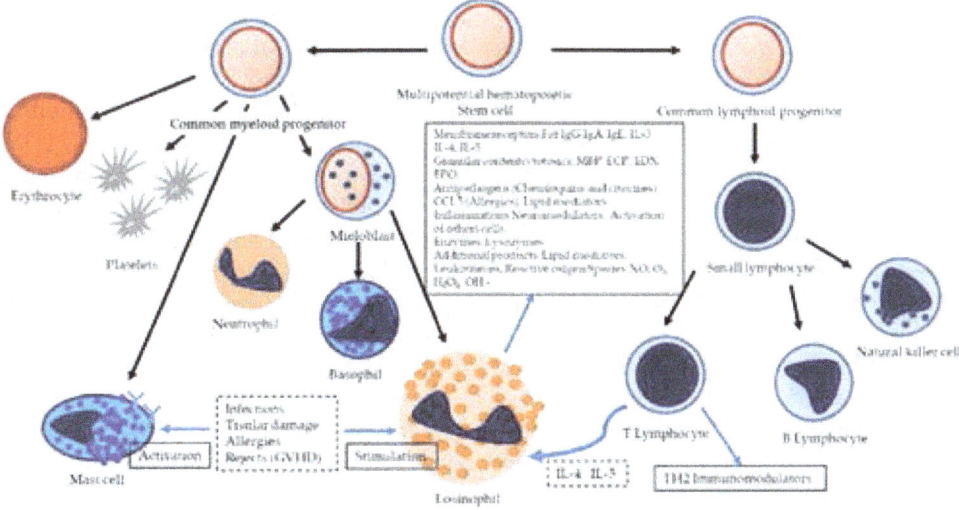

**Figure 1.**
*Scheme representing hematopoiesis, origin of eosinophil and its main functions associated with eosinophilic disorders. Molecules expressed on its surface (FcεRI-CD23-IgE). CCR4, CD88,H4R. Adhesion molecules: CD11b, CD11c, CD62L, and chemokines that attract eosinophils from blood to tissues [3, 7].*

(e.g., LFA-1-ICAM-1, the VLA-VCAM-1) and other multiple antibody receptors: IgA (Fc α R1-CD89), (FcεRIII-CD23-IgE), (FcYεRI-degranulation), (FcYRI-CD64-IgG1, IgG3 respiratory burst induction of microbial death), (FcYA-CD32-Ig G1-degranulation), (FcYRIIB-CD32-IgG1-No Phagocytosis, inhibition of cellular activity) (**Figure 1**) [2, 6, 8].

Granular content: Eosinophil mature contains in its cytoplasm primary granules rich in phospholipase A, rich in crystalline proteins of Charcot-Leyden-specific secondary granules containing the major or main basic protein (MBP), the eosinophilic peroxidase (EPO), eosinophilic protein (ECP)), and eosinophil-derived neurotoxin (EDN) that also appears in basophils and neutrophils; its response capacity is less than 1 hour, small granules containing arylsulfatase B and acid phosphatase and five lipid bodies main source of arachidonic acid, can be presenting cells, proliferation of T lymphocytes and basophils are capable of deliberating more than 35 cytokines, chemokines, and growth factors (**Figure 1**) [5, 9].

## 2. Diseases and classification

The severity of eosinophilia has been arbitrarily divided into mild (AEC from the upper limit of normal to 1500/mm$^3$), moderate (AEC 1500–5000/mm$^3$), and severe (AEC >5000/mm$^3$).

The classification of eosinophilic diseases was revised in 2008 and reaffirmed in 2016. In 2017 its diagnosis, risk stratification (prognosis), and management (treatment) proposed by the World Health Organization were covered [10].

Eosinophilic diseases can be classified in two types: primary, intrinsic hematology due to clonal disorders, and secondary, extrinsic or reactive disorders to an external cause that cause damage to different organs. Primary eosinophilias or clonal disorders can be diagnosed by studying the blood and bone marrow by the following methods: standard cytogenetics, molecular biology with monoclonal antibodies, flow cytometry, in situ hybridization, and evaluation of T cell clonality.

The major category of primary diseases corresponds to myeloid/lymphoid neoplasms with eosinophilia and rearrangements PDGFRA, PDGFRB, or FGR1; with PCMiJAK2 and MPN, a subtype of chronic eosinophilic leukemia or not specified by CEL-NOS, there is another lymphoid-eosinophilic variant of aberrant T cell clone.

The modern definition of hypereosinophilic syndrome (HES) is a vestige of the historical criteria outlined by Chusid and colleagues in 1975: The absolute eosinophil count is >1500/mm$^3$ for more than 6 months, and tissue damage is present [10, 11].

The Working Conference on Eosinophil Disorders and Syndromes proposed a new terminology for eosinophilic syndromes. Hypereosinophilia (HE) for persistent and marked eosinophilia (AEC >1500/mm$^3$) in turn, HE subtypes were divided into a hereditary (familiar) variant (HEfa); HE of undetermined significance (HEus), primary (clonal-neoplastic), HE produced by clonal/neoplastic eosinophils (HEn), and secondary (reactive) (HEr) can be considered a provisional diagnosis until a primary or secondary cause of eosinophilia is ascertained [12].

To have to a better understanding of the pathogenetic aspects of eosinophilia, other classifications of eosinophilic diseases were generated according to the site of eosinophilic infiltration associated with organ damage and dysfunction. The primary cause of eosinophilia located within the eosinophils (and/or eosinophil precursors) themselves or in other cells, similar to allergic diseases, can be divided in IgE-mediated (extrinsic) and non-IgE-mediated (intrinsic) diseases; the terms extrinsic and intrinsic eosinophilic disorders indicate whether the primary cause of eosinophilia is inside or outside the eosinophil lineage [11].

## 2.1 Eosinophilic intrinsic disorders

Chronic eosinophilic leukemias belong to a special group of chronic myeloid leukemias, in which eosinophil differentiation is dominant, resulting in blood eosinophil counts of greater than 1500/mm$^3$. However, other lineages are also affected, because the disease is the result of a mutation in a pluripotent hematopoietic stem cell. The chromosomal translocations related to breakpoints on chromosome 8p11 result in fibroblast growth factor receptor 1 fusion genes with increased kinase activity causing the so-called 8p11 syndrome. The increase in tyrosine kinase activity is caused by gene 1 and the growth factor, and this leukemia has a worse prognosis, which transforms chronic leukemia to an acute, 1–2 years. Another type of cause may be the increase in tyrosine kinase by fusion of the platelet growth factor alpha receptor genes (PDGFRA). PDGFRA is fused by the Fip1-like 1 (FIP1L1) gene as a result of a 4q12.9 chromosome damage. This is both in eosinophils and in other hematopoietic lineages such as neutrophils, monocytes, lymphocytes, and mast cells. This type of leukemia is pluripotent hematopoietic stem cell which responds to the tyrosine kinase inhibitor (imatinib) [10, 11].

Mutations in multipotent myeloid stem cells: In the chronic myeloid leukemias with eosinophilia, eosinophils are part of the clone. This is because eosinophil differentiation is often not as prominent as other myeloid cells, such as monocytes, which also show increased differentiation. Chromosomal translocations related to breakpoints on chromosome 5q33 are common and represent the basis for the formation of platelet-derived growth factor receptor b (PDGFRB) fusion genes; this result increases the tyrosine kinase activity. There are patients with positive Philadelphia chromosome who can develop chronic leukemia with eosinophilia due to two factors: fusion by breakpoint cluster region-Abelson (ABL) and fusion of transcription gene 6 (ETV6). Marked eosinophilia often associated with a cytogenetic evolution and other accelerated phases of ABL can occur during an acute transformation; ABL may be fused with the transcription factor E26 by means of variant ETV6 triggering chronic leukemia [10].

Myelodysplastic syndromes: During hematopoiesis there may be an inefficient process in the differentiation of stem cell by mutations, malignant clones producing myelodysplastic syndromes that lead to myeloproliferative diseases such as polycythemia vera, essential thrombocythemia, and agnogenic myeloid metaplasia. The exact molecular genetic abnormalities resulting in eosinophilia in these disorders remain to be determined [10, 11].

## 2.2 Eosinophilic extrinsic disorders

T cell-mediated eosinophilias: The common diseases are allergic rhinoconjunctivitis, bronchial asthma, drug allergic, eosinophilic esophagitis, and atopic dermatitis. Eosinophilia and IgE production due to the polarization of TH2 cells whose causes are extrinsic or external by stimulation of environmental immunogens or chemical compounds, which are presented by APC-MHC, stimulating the release of pro-inflammatory cytokines (IL4, IL5, and IL13), induce the increase in eosinophils of IgE survival, high affinity receptors with PKC activation, cross-linking and signaling for histamine release, as well as vasoactive amines that produce inflamma-tory processes and organ damage [10, 11].

Infectious diseases: TH2 inflammatory responses are induced by helminths; these responses are characterized by IgE antibody production and eosinophilia; both have been implicated in mediating protective immunity to the parasites. In contrast, there is little doubt that eosinophils contribute to tissue damage and therefore to the pathogenesis of these infections.

Viral infections are not common; however, when virus-specific T cells are generated in a TH2 environment, they can also release IL-5 and therefore trigger eosinophilia. In chronic rhinosinusitis, eosinophilia is related to fungal infections with certain molds (e.g., Alternaria) which is present in the nasal and paranasal cavities [5, 10, 11].

Autoimmune diseases: Because these diseases are often associated with a TH1-associated inflammatory response, eosinophilia is not frequent, but in systemic sclerosis, levels of major basic protein and extracellular major basic protein depositions were observed in skin and lung tissues. In primary biliary cirrhosis, eosinophilia is a distinctive feature that might be useful in the diagnosis of the disease [10, 11, 13].

Graft-versus-host diseases: When an allogeneic bone marrow transplant is carried out and there are differences in MHC molecule polymorphism, these can be recognized by the immune system, and responses can be made against the allo-antigens, producing graft-versus- host-disease (GVHDs), carrying out a reaction antigen antibody, cellular or cytotoxic that produces lysis and destruction in specific organs (skin, liver, and gastrointestinal tract mainly).

Drug-induced diseases: Hypersensitivity drug reactions may present in some cases increased eosinophils. The manifestations range from maculopapular rashes of the skin to severe life-threatening drug reactions with eosinophilia and systemic symptoms (DRESS). Drugs and their metabolites can produce hypersensitivity by means of mechanisms mediated by APC-MHC TCR pi concept, generating TH2 polarity or TH1 with memory T cells [10, 11, 13].

There are other subgroups of this syndrome as episodic angioedema and hereditary eosinophilia. Where there is evidence of mechanism mediated by IL-5-producing T cells [5].

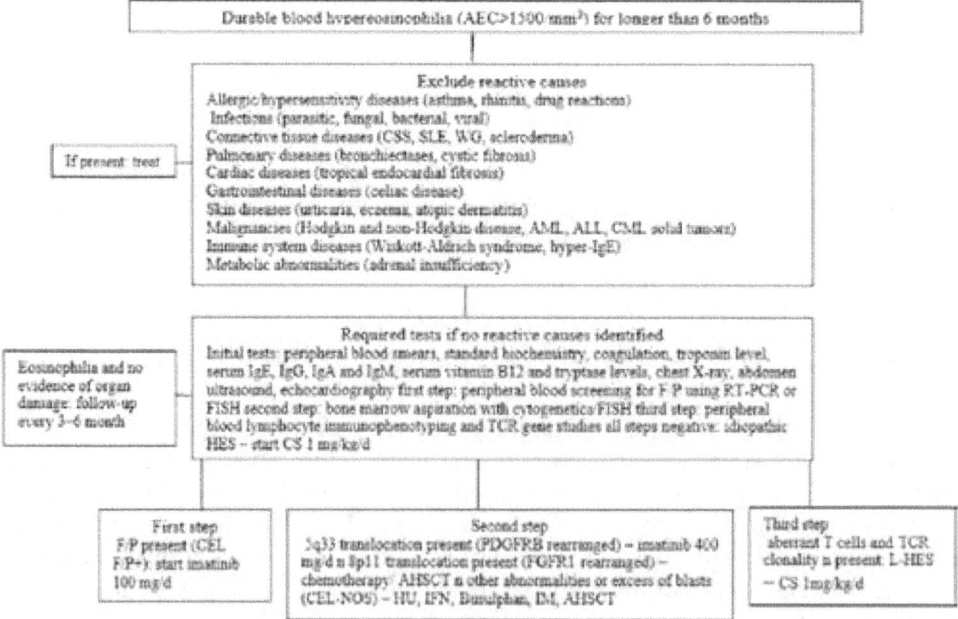

**Figure 2.**
*Diagnostic algorithm for patients with hypereosinophilia. Due to the fact that eosinophilia can occur in different pathologies, an exclusion of the unlikely causes for hypereosinophilia is performed, in addition to a three-step follow-up treatment with imatinib due to mutation processes that is considered. Laboratory tests would be at the discretion of the doctor according to the medical history and the search according to the type of response to the genes involved [12].*

Severe primary (IL-5) and secondary immunodeficiencies (HIV) are associated with eosinophilia when there is polarization of TH2 by the immunogen (allergen) or drug (antiretroviral); infections such as tuberculosis are the cause of infections and resistance to treatment (**Figure 2**) [11].

## 2.3 Treatment of HES and CEL-NOS

Corticosteroids should be considered a first-line treatment, which are potent anti-eosinophil agents, effective in producing rapid reductions. Maximal dose was 1 mg × kg 2 months, with symptom control and reduction of the eosinophil count to below 1500/mm$^3$ after 1 month of treatment.

Hydroxyurea is an effective first-line agent for HES which may be used in conjunction with corticosteroids or in steroid nonresponders. A typical starting dose is 500–1000 mg daily which can serve as effective palliative to control leukocytosis and eosinophilia but with no proven role in favorably altering the natural history of HES or CEL-NOS (**Figure 2**) [10, 12, 14].

IFN-a has demonstrated hematologic responses and reversion of organ injury in patients with HES and CEL-NOS refractory to therapies including prednisone and/or hydroxyurea. Remissions have been associated with improvement in clinical symptoms and organ disease, including hepatosplenomegaly, cardiac and thromboembolic complications, mucosal ulcers, and skin involvement [5, 10–12].

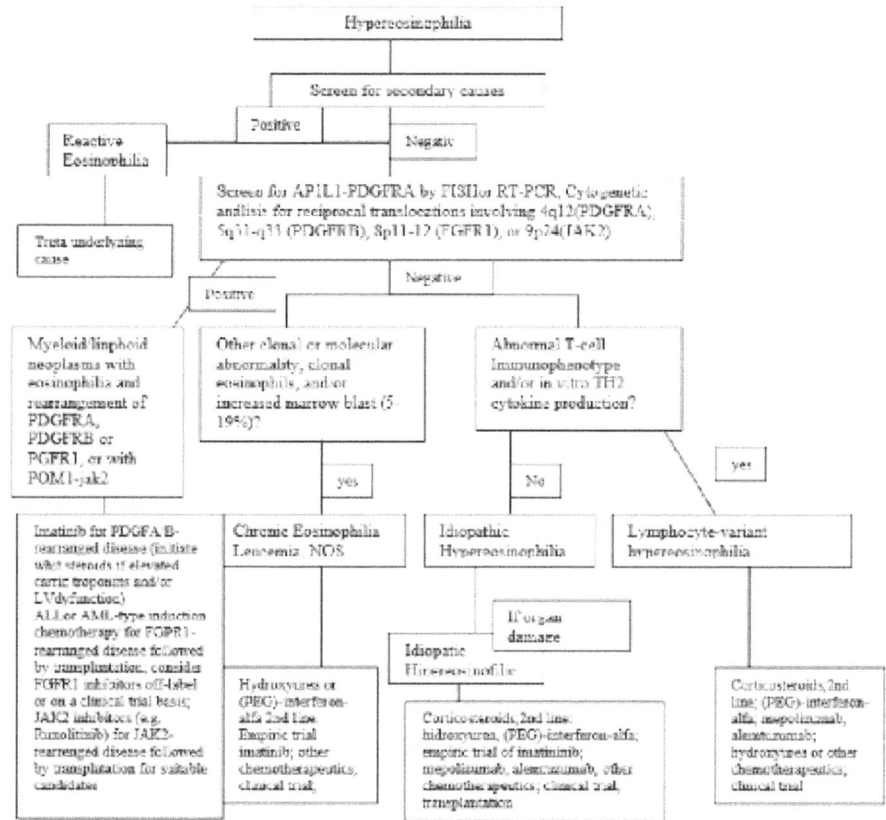

**Figure 3.**
*Diagnostic and treatment algorithm based on revised 2016 WHO classification of eosinophilic disorders. According to the algorithm, the type of eosinophilia can be monitored according to the cases where other drugs other than imatinib should be used, with three pathological options being present: chronic leukemia with eosinophilia, idiopathic hypereosinophilia, and lymphocyte variant, all share the administration of imatinib and corticosteroids (idiopathic hypereosinophilia and lymphocyte variant) [10].*

Mepolizumab anti-IL-5 antibody is a fully monoclonal IgG antibody that inhibits binding of IL-5 chain of the IL-5 receptor expressed on eosinophils [5, 14].

Alemtuzumab is an anti-CD52 monoclonal antibody that has been evaluated in idiopathic HES based on expression of the CD52 antigen on eosinophils. In patients with refractory HES, alemtuzumab was administered intravenously at a dose of 5–30 mg once to thrice weekly.

Bone marrow/peripheral blood stem cell allogeneic transplantation has been attempted in patients with aggressive disease; a disease-free survival ranging from 8 months to 5 years has been reported.

Imatinib is a small-molecule tyrosine kinase inhibitor 100 mg per day; it also shows activity against platelet-derived growth factor receptor (PDGF-R), c-Kit, Abl-related gene (ARG), and their fusion proteins while sparing other kinases (**Figure 3**) [10].

## 3. Hematologic and neoplastic diseases

Mastocytosis: Develops from a neoplastic proliferation of mast cells. It develops from a neoplastic clonal proliferation of mastocytes that accumulate in one or more organ systems and are organize as compact cohesive aggregate groups or multifocal groups of abnormal mastocytes. This disorder is diverse; it can be found as cutaneous lesions that may naturally recede, to highly aggressive neoplasias related with multiple organ failure and short outliving. Mastocytosis subtypes are principally characterized by the clinical manifestations and the spread of the disease. When cutaneous mastocytosis (CM) occurs, mastocyte infiltration is restricted to the skin, whereas systemic mastocytosis (SM) includes at least one extracutaneous organ, with or without skin lesions. Mastocytosis must be distinguished from mastocyte hyperplasia or from the mastocyte activation states, without the morphological or molecular abnormalities that characterize neoplastic proliferation [15]. The WHO classification includes seven types:

a. Cutaneous mastocytosis

b. Indolent systemic mastocytosis (ISM)

c. Systemic mastocytosis with associated clonal, hematologic non-mast cell lineage disease (SM-AHNMD)

d. Aggressive systemic mastocytosis (ASM)

e. Mast cell leukemia (MCL)

f. Mast cell sarcoma (MCS)

g. Extracutaneous mastocytoma

Hypereosinophilic syndrome (HES): It has been described as a condition associated with persistent eosinophilia in the peripheral blood, organ damage, and exclusion of any other underlying disease or condition that may explain eosinophilia or organ damage [4, 16–18]. The diagnostic algorithm must begin with the evaluation of peripheral blood hypereosinophilia (HE), defined as a persistent increase of blood eosinophils, above 1.5 X 109/L blood [4, 16–18]. The term "tissue HE" has also been proposed, and it may be useful in the evaluation and the classification of the disorders related to HES [16, 19]. The establishment of an HES diagnosis must be considered: (a) the existence of an underlying disease or condition and (b) the presence of clinical signs and symptoms or laboratory abnormalities that show organ damage induced by HE (HES) [19]. There are four important groups of underlying disorders in patients with documented HES:

1. Hematopoietic neoplasias

2. Other neoplasias (non-hematopoietic) (paraneoplastic HE)

3. Common allergic, reactive, or immunological conditions

4. Infrequent clinical syndromes that present HE, including rare hereditary disorders [19]

Lymphoid and myeloid leukemias: Many hematologic disorders may present eosinophilia, but only a few present clonal (primary) neoplasias, and just a small number of neoplasms present HE and organ damage. Myeloid neoplasias that present HE include rare acute eosinophilic leukemia types. The most common type of chronic leukemia is chronic eosinophilic leukemia (CEL), which is frequently associated with the FIP1L1-PDGFRA rearrangement in endomyocardial fibrosis/thrombosis and other myeloid neoplasias with rearrangements, such as the 8p11 syndrome [19, 20]. Clonal eosinophilia is frequently observed in advanced cases of systemic mastocytosis [19, 21, 22].

Lymphoid neoplasms may present HE, and in most cases, a T cell lymphoma is diagnosed. Nevertheless, in such patients with 8p11 syndrome and other rare entities, both eosinophils and lymphocytes may be involved in the neoplastic clonal processes [19, 21].

Paraneoplastic conditions associated with hypereosinophilia. Different types of cancers may be preceded or accompanied by eosinophilia. Cancers associated with HE include lung, gastrointestinal tract, pancreas, and thyroid adenocarcinomas, gynecologic tumors, and skin cancer. Although pathogenesis is unclear, there is a widely accepted hypothesis stating that carcinogenic cells or cancer or the cancer microenvironment around fibroblasts produce eosinophilopoietic cytokines [19, 23].

Identification and quantification.

Classic methodology: Clinical manifestations and diagnosis depend on the type of disease and other factors, where different organs may be involved in patients with HES, for example, skin, gastrointestinal tract, heart, and central nervous system.

In order to establish an HES diagnosis, it is recommended to include clinical and laboratory parameters, such as:

a. Physical exam of organs and body systems

b. Laboratory exams: white blood cell count (eosinophils, basophils, neutrophils), hemoglobin, platelet count, B12 vitamin, hepatic enzymes, kidney function tests, and urinalysis

c. Organic functional tests: electrocardiogram, echocardiogram, pulmonary function tests, chest computed tomography and radiography, abdominal ultrasound, and normal endoscopic study [19]

d. Molecular detection of some translocations, such as TCR, BCR/ABL1, JAK2 V617F, KITD816V, PDGFRA/PDGFRB, and FGR1

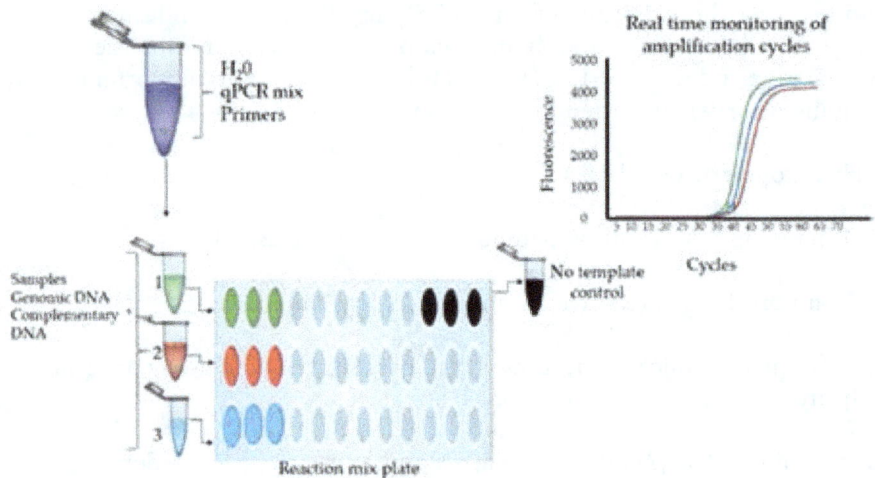

**Figure 4.**
*Flow diagram to perform real-time PCR. In a simplified way, the preparation of the sample with its corresponding primer and the distribution of the samples for its reaction are shown, which can be seen in real time by monitoring the amplification as the cycles in the thermal cycler pass.*

## 3.1 Laboratory diagnosis by molecular parameters

Immunoglobulins rearrangements are detected by real-time polymerase chain reaction with TaqMan molecular probes, such as TCR, BCR/ABL1, JAK2 V617F, KITD816V, PDGFRA/PDGFRB, and FGR1. The most recommended bone marrow exams are cytogenetic assays and fluorescence in situ hybridization (FISH)—other studies which do not include molecular detection are tissue immunohistochemistry and histology (**Figure 4**) [16].

## 4. Allergy and hypersensitivity to drugs (DHRs)

The WHO defines an ADR to any predictable noxious reaction that appears at therapeutic doses, depends on the doses, and is related to pharmacological actions. Other unpredictable reactions: hypersensitivity or allergic (DHRs) associated with immunological mechanisms, susceptibility (atopy), and polymorphism (pharmacogenetic, MHC-HLA) [24–27].

It is considered as a public health problem due to its high morbidity and mortality being 20%; hence, the importance of its clinical diagnosis and laboratory tests is being considered at all stages of life (prenatal, postnatal, childhood, adolescence, adult, and older adult).

### 4.1 Immune response to drugs in DHRs: haptens, pro-haptens, and TCR pi

Medications are usually non-immunogenic haptens of different types:
Pro-haptens. Drugs are generally non-immunogenic haptens of different types: Pro-haptens (non-active reagents) low molecular weight chemicals of less than 1000 D; examples aromatic, heterocyclic, sulfonamides, OH, halogens, resonance, and beta-lactam are processed and presented in the CPA-MHC context and produce a humoral response, IgE, IgG and IgM or cellular.

Active reagents: aromatic, polar, with nitrogen, to induce an immune response CPA-MHC.

Inert TCR pi (pharmacological interaction with immune receptors): Some drugs are able to bind non-covalently to TCR pi receptors pre-developed by a previous immune response to a non-covalently reversible drug and signaling toward a response of hypersensitivity and explain the rapid appearance of symptoms, some cross reactions to the drug, or its metabolites.

Pi concept and HLA restriction in hypersensitivity: In the pi concept, drugs primarily activate TCR, for example, abacavir associated with the HLA-B * 5701 allele in whites, Stevens-Johnson syndrome (SJS) with carbamazepine treatment in Chinese associated in patients with the HLA-B * 1502, and HLA-B * 5801 allele in allopurinol-induced adverse reactions such as SJS and toxic epidermal necrolysis (TEN) [28–31].

## 4.2 Hypersensitivity and diagnosis

Hypersensitivity is an exacerbated immune response, which produces a clinical picture with dermal, systemic disorders, and sometimes sudden death. In 1930 Coombs systematized these reactions according to the period of time in which the symptoms appear, and the dose of challenge has been fundamental to guide the diagnosis, treatment, and monitoring. It has many points in common with autoimmunity, where the antigens are their own; in the case of allergies to medications, the antigens are allergens: drugs or metabolic derivatives. Hypersensitivity reactions require that the individual has been previously sensitized or exposed to at least the antigens in question. The classification of allergic or hypersensitivity reactions into four types (I, II, III, and IV) and subsequently Pichler in 2003 proposed the subdi-vision of type IV into IVa, IVb, IVc, and IVd (**Table 1**) [28, 29].

## 4.3 In vitro tests associated with drug and drug eosinophilia: antibiotics, nonsteroidal anti-inflammatory drugs (NSAIDs) anticonvulsants, and antidiuretics

Modified basophil degranulation (MBD): The test is a basophil activation test (BAT) which consists of incubating the basophils in vitro with the suspected drug to be carried out: epitope-paratope binding, activating the basophils and causing degranulation and release of the aforementioned content (specificity 100%, sensitivity 84.0%) [28, 29].

CD63 flow cytometry: Basophils with specific IgE when incubated with the suspected drug are activated by Fcε I receptors; high affinity and low affinity cause crosslinking and protein kinase signal transduction (MAP, PKC) that stimulate expression of the receptor (CD63) -gp53 (lysosomal-transmembrane protein tetraspanin LAMP-31) on the surface of the basophil while the eosinophilic expresses CD23 [30].

Modified leukocyte migration inhibition factor (MLIF) type IV a, b, and c. Associated with anaphylactic degranulation: It has been reported that leukocytes including basophils (BAT-Chemotaxis) also play a role in directional chemotaxis; therefore, when microhematocrits are incubated in Bloom chambers with medications in two dilutions (1 and 0.1 mg/mL) in an RPMI medium, with negative and positive controls, at 37°C, the first (20 min at 2 hours) and delayed migration can be measured (4, 6, and 18 hours); the % of MLIF can also be calculated against the negative control, as well as the reference values (RV) for MLIF (0–25% inhibition of leukocyte migration) [29].

Eosinophilia in the peripheral blood is a common cause in patients who consume medications, especially in developed countries, who are monitored and can restrict their consumption without changes. However, for the doctor, concern may arise in cases of impending hypersensitivity reaction (HSR). Severe HSRs associated with peripheral blood may include specific reactions of organs (heart, kidney, liver, lungs, joints, central nervous system, and skin) and adverse skin reactions (SCAR) where SJS, TEN, and DRESS are included [32, 33].

| Type | Type of immune response | Clinical symptoms | In vitro diagnostics | In vivo diagnostics |
|------|------------------------|-------------------|---------------------|---------------------|
| I | Measured by IgE eosinophils, mast cells, and basophils (immediate) | Urticaria Angioedema Rhinitis Bronchospasm Anaphylaxis | IgE specific Serum tryptase Cell stimulation test (CAST) BAT(MDB, CD63) | Cutaneous tests (prick, intradermal) Challenge tests Proving tests [Coombs] |
| II | Cytotoxicity dependent on IgG and IGM antibodies (not immediate) and complement | Hemolytic Anemia Thrombocytopenia Neutropenia Autoimmunity | Coombs test Ab vs. platelets Ab vs. neutrophils | Only challenges to the drug can make diagnosis but are high risk [Coombs] |
| III | Deposit of immunocomplexes [IgG and IgM] (not immediate) Complement or FcR | Serum disease Vasculitis, LES-like by medications Glomerulonephritis drug | C3, C4, ANA, ANCA, CCP, antithyroid, etc. Liver and kidney function tests Pathological anatomy | Biopsies with immunofluorescence [Coombs] |
| IVa | TH1 (IFNγ), TNFα, IL12, and macrophages (late) | Contact dermatitis | Lymphocyte transformation test (LT or BT), MLIF, cytotoxic T lymphocyte precursors (CTLp), cytokines (ELISA, PCR) | Patch tests [Pichler] |
| IVb | TH2 (IL-4, IL5, IL13) eosinophils | Maculopapular eruptions (MPE) with eosinophilia (DRESS) | CBC with check eosinophil cellularity, atypical lymphocytes MLIF, BT, LT | Patch tests [Pichler] |
| IVc | CLT, CD4/ CD8 (perforin, granzyme B, Fas L) | Contact dermatitis, maculopapular, and bullous diseases(SJS), TEN | MLIF, liver function tests, CD4/CD8 (death keratinocytes) Activity of IgM vs. herpes virus, Epstein-Barr, and cytomegalovirus (CMV) | Patch tests [Pichler] |
| IVd | T cells, IL8, CXCL8 cells Neutrophils Inflammation | Acute generalized exanthemic pustulosis (AGEP) pharmacodermias associated with neutrophilia | CBC T cells CD4/ CD8 | Patch tests [Pichler] |

*Hypersensitivity reactions require that the individual has been previously sensitized or exposed at least once to the antigens in question. The classification of allergic or hypersensitivity reactions into four types (I, II, III, and IV) and subsequently Pichler in 2003 proposed the subdivision of type IV into IVa, IVb, IVc, and IVd [27–29].*

**Table 1.**
*Hypersensitivity classification according to the Gell and Coombs modified by Sell, Pichler, and ICON.*

The prolongation of eosinophilia can cause tissue damage, although without being clarified specifically, adding to the condition infections as another factor that preserves eosinophilia (parasitic and fungal infestations) or decreases (eosinopenia due to bacterial and viral infections). The diagnosis can be complicated because of the presence of the drug which worsens a preexisting eosinophilia, particularly in atopic patients [33].

DRESS is more common in adult patients than in children, with approximately 50 drugs being described, highlighting anticonvulsants (phenytoin, phenobarbital, and carbamazepine) and antibiotics as the main causes of the syndrome and, to a lesser extent, sulfate derivatives, antidepressants, NSAIDs, and antidiuretics [34]. There is no clear association between variability of the type of drug and the affected organ with the degree of eosinophilia, which can be mild or self-limited and severe when multisystemic complications are generated due to the presence of symptoms that are not appreciated in the mild form [32, 33].

Other proposals that lead to the pathogenesis of DRESS include detoxification defects at the time of the formation of reactive metabolites, slow acetylation, and reactivation of the human herpes virus (HHV-6-7) or EBV [34].

In general, the diagnostic algorithm for eosinophilia linked to SCAR can be visualized as a hypersensitivity response type IVb (SJS and NET) and type IVc (DRESS), which in some way can highlight the pathogenesis proposals previously mentioned not only by DRESS but identify an atopic patient (**Table 1**).

## 5. Conclusions

Eosinophils are leukocytes (white blood cells) found in the peripheral blood, hematopoietic, lymphatic organs, thymus, connective tissue, and digestive tract. They are identified and quantified by manual counting (Neubauer chamber), automated count with autoanalyzer hemocytometers (impedance, colorimetry, and differential in optical microscope), flow cytometry after the advent of monoclonal antibodies, currently the most used to identify surface markers and immunoenzymatic methods (ELISA, RAST, IMMUNOCAP) for cytoplasmic granules.

The classification of eosinophilic diseases "eosinophilic disorders" was revised in 2008 and confirmed in 2016; its study focused on external (extrinsic) and internal (intrinsic) causes (optimized) and optimized and failed diagnosis by precise and timely diagnosis. The algorithms are used and started with the main pillar: The clinical history (clinical criteria, anamnesis, and exploitative maneuvers leading to clinical laboratory algorithms, with initial, basic, and special tests including imaging, tomography, and X-rays to finally improve the prognosis and modify the natural history. The intrinsic and extrinsic disorder algorithm planting is different; this is due to the recognition of molecular altered T cell clones, bone marrow studies, and markers of apoptotic genes, PCM1-JAK2, Fas L, and bcl2.

Some allergies to medications with symptomatology related to specific organ and severe cutaneous against antiepileptics (phenytoin, phenobarbital, carbamazepine) as well as other medications (antibiotics, NSAIDs, antidiuretics) can be related, which rethinks the proposed immunological response algorithm not only in basophil evaluation but also the search for eosinophils in flow cytometry or optical microscopy to assess not only damage but neutralization (eosinophil histaminase).

Corticosteroids are considered the first line of treatment because of their potent anti-eosinophilic effect for disease control, prognosis, and prevention. So the new treatment alternatives could displace steroids with monoclonal antibodies such as the IL-5 inhibitor that show less long-term toxicity.

## Acknowledgements

Thanks to the headquarters and staff of the Department of Allergy and Immunology of the Juarez Hospital of Mexico, Dr. Ruben Humberto Meyer Gomez of the Angeles Hospital, and the laboratory technician Isabel Guerrero Vargas of the LCEIL Laus Deo.

## Appendices and nomenclature

| | |
|---|---|
| AEC | absolute eosinophil count |
| HSR | hypersensitivity reaction |
| SCAR | severe cutaneous adverse reaction |
| SJS | Stevens-Johnson's syndrome |
| TEN | toxic epidermal necrolysis |
| DRESS | drug rash eosinophilia and systemic symptoms |
| CBC | complete blood count |
| DHRs | drug hypersensitivity reaction |

## Author details

Maria-de-Lourdes Irigoyen-Coria[1*], Vilma-Carolina Bekker-Mendez[2], Maria-Isabel Leyva-Carmona[3], Cecilia Rosel-Pech[2], Samuel Moreno-Olivares[4] and David Solis-Hernandez[5]

1 Lindavista Integral Specialized Clinics Laboratory (LCEIL), Mexican Social Security Institute (IMSS), Mexico City, Mexico

2 Biomedical Research Unit Hospital of CMN Infectology "La Raza" IMSS, Mexico City, Mexico

3 Institute of Social Security and Services of State Workers (ISSSTE), Mexico City, Mexico

4 Mexican Social Security Institute (IMSS), Mexico City, Mexico

5 National Autonomous University of Mexico (UNAM) and Lindavista Integral Specialized Clinics Laboratory (LCEIL), Mexico City, Mexico

*Address all correspondence to: luluirigoyen@yahoo.es

# References

[1] Davoine F, Lacy P. Eosinophil cytokines and growth factors: Emerging roles in immunity. Frontiers in Immunology. 2014;**10**:570. DOI: 10.3389/fimmu.2014. 00570

[2] Lorente F, Pellegrini J, de Arriba S. Immune Function of the Eosinophil in Health and Disease XXXIX Congress of the Spanish Society of Clinical Immunology and Pediatric Allergology. Spain: Spanish Pediatric Association (AEP); 2015

[3] Buckland K, Matin MC Traductor. Eosinophils [Internet]. Available from: http://inmunologia.eu/celulas-inmunologia-en-un-mordisco/eosinofilos [Accessed on: 18-06-2019]

[4] Dagmar S, Hans-Uwe S. Eosinophilic disorders. The Journal of Allergy and Clinical Immunology. 2007;**119**(6):1291-1300. DOI: 10.1016/j.jaci.2007.02.010

[5] Bailon F, Huerta L, Gutierrez H. Differential diagnosis of peripheral eosinophilia and new treatment options. Pediatric Allergy, Asthma and Immunology. 2012;**21**(2):63-71. Available from: https://www.medigraphic.com/cgi-bin/new/resumen.cgi?IDARTICULO=37666

[6] Muniz VS, Weller PF, Neves JS. Eosinophil crystalloid granules: Structure, function, and beyond. Journal of Leukocyte Biology. 2012;**92**:281-288. DOI: 10.1189/jlb.0212067

[7] Rothenberg ME, Hogaan SP. The eosinophil. Annual Review of Immunology. 2006;**24**:147-174. DOI: 10.1146/annurev.immunol.24.021605.090720

[8] Mora N, Rosales C. Fc receptor functions defense mechanisms and immune regulation. Revista de Investigación Clínica. 2009;**61**(4):313-326. Available from: https://www.medigraphic.com/pdfs/revinvcli/nn-2009/nn094i.pdf

[9] Kita H. Eosinophils: Multifaceted biological properties and roles health and disease. Immunological Reviews. 2011;**242**:161-177. DOI: 10.1111/j.1600-065X.2011.01026.x

[10] Gotlib J. World Health Organization defined eosinophilic disorders: 2017 update on diagnosis, risk stratification, and management. American Journal of Hematology. 2017;**92**:1242-1259

[11] Simon D et al. Eosinophilic disorders. The Journal of Allergy and Clinical Immunology. 2007;**119**:1291-1300

[12] Grzegorz H et al. Diagnostic and therapeutic management in patients with hypereosinophilic syndromes. Polskie Archiwum Medycyny Wewnętrznej. 2011;**121**:1-2

[13] Fichman L. Síndrome Hipereosinofílico. Hema. 2007;**11**(3):220-242

[14] Busse WW, Ring J, Huss-Marp J, Kahn JE. A review of treatment with mepolizumab, an anti–IL-5 mAb, in hypereosinophilic syndromes and asthma. The Journal of Allergy and Clinical Immunology. 2010;**125**(4):803-813

[15] Vardiman J, Bennett J, Bain B, Brunning RTJ. WHO Classification of Tumours of Haematopoietic and Lymphoid Tissues. In: Swerdlow SH, Campo E, Harris NL, Jaffe ES, Pileri SA, Stein H, Thiele J, Vardiman JW, editors. 2008. pp. 80-81

[16] Valent P, Klion AD, Horny HP, Roufosse F, Gotlib J, Weller PF, et al. Contemporary consensus proposal on criteria and classification

of eosinophilic disorders and related syndromes. The Journal of Allergy and Clinical Immunology. 2012;**130**(3):607-612

[17] Wilkins HJ, Crane MM, Copeland K, Williams WV. Hypereosinophilic syndrome: An update. American Journal of Hematology. 2005;**80**(2):148-157

[18] Leiferman KM, Butterfield JH, Valent P, Vandenberghe P, Roufosse F, Cerny-Reiterer S, et al. Pathogenesis and classification of eosinophil disorders: A review of recent developments in the field. Expert Review of Hematology. 2012;**5**(2):157-176. Available from: http://www.ncbi.nlm.nih.gov/pubmed/22475285%0Ahttp://www.pubmedcentral.nih.gov/articlerender.fcgi?artid=PMC3625626

[19] Valent P, Klion AD, Rosenwasser LJ, Arock M, Bochner BS, Butter JH, et al. World Allergy Organization Journal. 2012;**5**:174-181

[20] Gotlib J, Cools J. Five years since the discovery of FIP1L1-PDGFRA: What we have learned about the fusion and other molecularly defined eosinophilias. Leukemia. 2008;**22**(11):1999-2010

[21] Böhm A, Födinger M, Wimazal F, Haas OA, Mayerhofer M, Sperr WR, et al. Eosinophilia in systemic mastocytosis: Clinical and molecular correlates and prognostic significance. The Journal of Allergy and Clinical Immunology. 2007;**120**(1):192-199

[22] Ornitz DM, Itoh N. The fibroblast growth factor signaling pathway. Wiley Interdisciplinary Reviews: Developmental Biology. 2015;**4**(3):215-266. DOI: 10.1002/wdev.176

[23] Lowe D, Jorizzo J, Hutt MSR. Tumour-associated eosinophilia: A review. Journal of Clinical Pathology. 1981;**34**:1343-1348

[24] Lares-Asseff I, Trujillo-Jimenez F. Pharmacogenetics and its importance in the clinic. Gaceta Médica de México. 2001;**137**(3):227-236

[25] Gibaldi M. Pharmacogenetics: Part I. The Annals of Phannacotherapy. 1992;**26**:121-126. DOI: 10.1177/106002809202600123

[26] Giner-Muñoz. MT hypersensitivity to medications. Pediatria Integral. 2009;**13**:819-834

[27] Demoly P, Adkinson NF, Brockow K, Castells M, Chiriac AM, et al. International consensus on drug allergy. Allergy. 2014;**69**(4):420-437

[28] Giner-Munoz MT. Allergy to medicines. Basic concepts and attitude to be followed by the pediatrician. Protoc Diagn Ter Pediatr. 2013;**1**:1-24. https://www.aeped.es/sites/default/files/documentos/1-alergia_farmacos_0. pdf

[29] Irigoyen-Coria ML, Rojo- Gutierrez MI, Meyer-Gomez RH, Leyva-Carmona I, Zendejas- Buitron VM, et al. Modified tests basophil degranulation and leukocyte migration inhibition factor in drug allergy. Study 2009-2014. Revista Alergia México. 2016;**63**(4):342-350

[30] McGowan EC, Saini S. Update on the performance and application of basophil activations test. Current Allergy and Asthma Reports. 2013;**13**(1):101-109

[31] Mallal S, Phillips E, Carosi G, Molina JM, Workman C, et al.; PREDICT-1 Study TeamHLA-B*5701 screening for hypersensitivity to abacavir. The New England Journal of Medicine. 2008;**358**(6):568-579

[32] Blumenthal K, Youngster I, Rabideau DJ, Parker RA, Manning KS, et al. Peripheral blood eosinophilia and hypersensitivity reactions among

patients receiving outpatient parenteral antibiotics. The Journal of Allergy and Clinical Immunology. 2015;**136**(5):1288- 1294. DOI: 10.1016/j.jaci.2015.04.005

[33] Maidment I, Williams C. Drug-induced eosinophilia. The Pharmaceutical Journal. 2000;**264**(7078):71-76. Available from https://www.pharmaceutical-journal.com/learning/learning-article/drug-induced-eosinophilia/20000049.article?firstPass=false

[34] Karakayali B, Yazar AS, Cakir D, Cetemen A, Kariminikoo M, et al. Drug reaction with eosinophilia and systemic symptoms (DRESS) syndrome associated with cefotaxime and clindamycin use in a 6 years-old boy: A case report. The Pan African Medical Journal. 2017;**28**:218. DOI: 10.11604/pamj.2017.28.218.108.28

# 13

# The Immune System of Mesothelioma Patients: A Window of Opportunity for Novel Immunotherapies

*Fabio Nicolini and Massimiliano Mazza*

## Abstract

The interplay between the immune system and the pleural mesothelium is crucial both for the development of malignant pleural mesothelioma (MPM) and for the response of MPM patients to therapy. MPM is heavily infiltrated by several immune cell types which affect the progression of the disease. The presence of organized tertiary lymphoid structures (TLSs) witness the attempt to fight the disease *in situ* by adaptive immunity which is often suppressed by tumor expressed factors. In rare patients physiological, pharmacological or vaccine-induced immune response is efficient, rendering their plasma a valuable resource of anti-tumor immune cells and molecules. Of particular interest are human antibodies targeting antigens at the tumor cell surface. Here we review current knowledge regarding MPM immune infiltration, MPM immunotherapy and the harnessing of this response to identify novel biologics as biomarkers and therapeutics through innovative screening strategies.

**Keywords:** Malignant pleural mesothelioma (MPM), Immunotherapy, Fully human antibody, Tertiary lymphoid structure (TLS), BCR repertoire

## 1. Introduction

Malignant pleural mesothelioma (MPM) is an aggressive neoplasm principally due to asbestos exposure with a poor prognosis and a median overall survival (OS) of only 14 months [1]. Heavy asbestos utilization during earlier decades in Europe is the cause of actual disease incidence [2] and, despite many countries have banned asbestos use in recent years, a peak of MPM incidence is expected for 2020s due to a long latency and delayed disease onset [1, 3–5]. On the contrary, other countries that still make use asbestos are very likely to observe a substantial increase of asbestos-related disease and MPM in the future. BRCA1 associated protein-1 (*BAP1*) protein is an important player in DNA repair mechanisms, cell cycle control, carcinogenesis and apoptosis and almost 60% of MPM patients have BAP1 mutation [6–13]. BAP1 mutational status determines the insurgence of MPM [9, 10, 12–15], and influences the response to chemotherapy [16] and patient' s clinical outcome [17]. When other gene alterations are coupled to BAP1 mutation, synthetic lethality approaches could be evaluated as therapeutic options [18, 19]. Other frequent mutations are in the genes NF2, LATS2, TP53, SETD2 and TERT promoter as recently reported and are associated with different histotypes of MPM with epithelioid, biphasic and sarcomatoid features [20]. MPM is characterized by a lack of early and specific symptom-atology and few reliable biomarkers and screening tools are available causing a late prognosis. As we recently reviewed [21], current therapies in clinical practice consist of surgery, radiotherapy and chemotherapy and innovative therapeutic approaches are being explored. From this survey emerged that new therapeutic modalities and prognostic biomarkers are urgently needed in order to grant a fair chance of survival to all MPM patients. Here we describe the interplay of the immune system and MPM at the tumor tissue level and envision strategies to take advantage of it and derive novel fully human MPM-targeting antibodies to be used as biomarkers and for the design of novel immunotherapies.

## 2. Inflammatory response and carcinogenesis in MPM

MPM's development is intertwined with the inflammatory response provoked by asbestos exposure. Asbestos fibers and fluid enter the pleural space where they reach the outer pulmonary parenchyma inducing an inflammatory response [22]. Later steps see macrophage infiltration guided by the presence of the chemokine CCL2 generated by mesothelial cells in response to asbestos fibers contact. Reactive oxygen species (ROS) and nitrogen species are produced by macrophages that, together with already present nitrogen and oxygen species generated from iron particles associated with the fibers, create reactive and dangerous free radicals responsible for mutagenic events and genomic instability [23–25].

Normally, cells which suffer genotoxic DNA damage undergo PARP-dependent apoptosis. Despite that, an *in vitro* study [26] demonstrated that damaged human mesothelial cells could be rescued and skip apoptosis by TNF-alfa produced by macrophages and by other intracellular pathways activated in mesothelial cells, such as NFkB [26–28]. Conversely, TNF-alfa receptor knock-out mice are protected from fibroproliferative lesions when exposed to asbestos fibers [29]. In summary, among innate immune system players, macrophages contribute to genomic altera-tions as well as survival of mesothelial cells in a context of inflammatory response to asbestos fibers.

## 3. Immune cell infiltrate in MPM

### 3.1 Tumor-Associated Macrophages

Tumor-Associated Macrophages (TAMs) are the most abundant cells infiltrating the pleural effusions [30–33] and are associated with poor prognosis [32, 34, 35]. *In vitro* and *in vivo* experiments support TAMs as potential targets for MPM treatment. Chemokines released by mesothelioma cells such as CCL4, CCL5, CXCL12 and, in particular, CCL2, are chemoattractants for monocytes [36–38]. CCL2 concentration is particularly high in malignant pleural effusions with respect to benign lesions or lung adenocarcinoma pleural effusions [39, 40] and affects CCR2-expressing monocyte trafficking in MPM [41]. When recruited to MPM lesions, monocytes and macrophages switch to immunosuppressive cells under the influence of growth factors such as M-CSF, IL-34, MCSF [41, 42] and cytokines such as IL-10 and TGF-β released by MPM cells. Those cytokines act both on monocyte and macro-phage development and activation but also exert autocrine feedback loop functions on MPM cells [42, 43]. Also, the macrophage checkpoint marker and " do not eat me" signal CD47 is found to be highly expressed in the majority of patients with epithelioid mesothelioma [44]. In mesothelioma, TAMs show an immunosuppressive phenotype, characterized by CD14$^{mid}$CD16$^{hi}$ expression, reduced phagocytic activity and increased IL-10 production [45]. In addition, in vitro co-culture of TAMs with MPM cells boosts tumor proliferation and concomitantly reduces sensitivity to chemotherapy treatment [41]. Pro-tumoral activity of TAMs is also evident in mesothelioma mouse models where the removal of macrophages reduces the number of tumor nodules, metastases and tissue invasiveness [46].

## 3.2 Myeloid-Derived Suppressor Cells

Granulocytes and neutrophils are also present in MPM microenvironment and recruited by CXCR2 or CXCL5 and CXCL1 chemokines, respectively [36, 47]. Also, polarization and phenotype of granulocytes are affected by growth factors from the mesothelioma secretome which increases their expression of CD11b, CD15 and CD66b markers. These cells function as Myeloid-Derived Suppressor Cells (MDSC) and negatively affect T-cell proliferation via the production and release of ROS [48]. Also, the presence of consistent neutrophilic infiltrate as well as high numbers of neutrophils in the peripheral blood is associated with poor prognosis in epithelioid mesothelioma [49, 50]. However, MDSC targeting in MPM is still debated and controversial and requires further investigations.

## 3.3 T-lymphocytes

CD4$^+$ and CD8$^+$ T-lymphocytes are present in MPM microenvironment but in lower numbers compared to macrophages [32, 51–53]. T-regulatory cells (Tregs) are also present in MPM tissue but are less abundant compared to other solid tumors [54]. Principal chemokines present in mesothelioma secretome involved in T-cell trafficking are CXCL12, CXCL10 and CCL5. CXCR3, the receptor of CXCL10 chemokine, is upregulated in mouse models of MPM [47]. CCL5 concentration is high in MPM patients' peripheral blood with respect to asbestos workers and healthy individuals [55] while its receptor CCR5 is expressed on T-cell infiltrating pleural effusions [56]. As discussed in the following chapters, T-cells activation and programming is determined by the presence of neo antigenic stimuli [57, 58] and immune checkpoint expression [59, 60] in specialized immune structures organized *in situ*.

## 4. Tertiary lymphoid structures in solid tumors and MPM: where the anti-tumor response begins

Secondary lymphoid organs (SLOs) are lymphoid regions wherein dendritic cells (DCs) present antigens to T-cells in a major histocompatibility complex (MHC)-dependent way acting an efficient adaptive response against cancer, requiring the migration of DCs from the tumor site to the SLOs [61]. Consequently, B-cells are also activated in the SLOs by CD4+ T-cells, begin to proliferate and form a secondary follicle that will be converted to a germinal center (GC). This process induces T and B-lymphocyte proliferation and differentiation into effector T-cells and memory B-cells (MBCs), respectively, that migrate into the tumor contributing to cancer cells elimination, unless unfavorable/antagonizing events or exhaustive signals are in place. However, studies on the role of the immune system in tumors revealed that anti-tumor mechanisms can take place also at the tumor site within organized lymphoid aggregates similar to SLOs [62] called tertiary lymphoid structures (TLSs) [63].

TLSs are also present in the stroma, at the invasive margin and/or in the core of different tumor types [63, 64]. TLSs are composed of a T-cell-rich zone together with mature DCs but also by B-cell rich-GC surrounded by plasma cells (PCs). Inside TLSs tumor antigens are presented to T-cells by DCs. and both T- and B- cells are activated, begin to proliferate and to differentiate to effector memory T helper (TH) cells, effector memory cytotoxic T-cells, MBCs or antibody-producing PCs [53, 65–69]. High numbers of CD8+ and CD4+ T-cells in tumors determine TLS density [70] and evi-dence indicates a positive correlation of TLS density on OS and disease-free survival in lung cancer [66, 70–72], colorectal cancer [73, 74], pancreatic cancer [75, 76], oral squamous cell carcinoma [77] and invasive breast cancer [65, 78–80].

Importantly, its prognostic value is independent of tumor–node–metastasis (TNM) staging in most malignancies suggesting TLS can induce a systemic long-lasting anti-tumor response. High endothelial venules (HEVs) similar to those that allow entry of lymphocytes into SLOs could be detected near TLSs [65]. In this context HEVs allow lymphocytes to enter into tumors. Therefore, therapeutic approaches that enhance HEV formation would be beneficial to improve anti-tumor immune responses. Tregs negatively regulate HEV formation and their absence in cancer murine models promotes T-cell activation and tumor infiltra-tion, favoring the eradication of the lesions [81, 82]. Also other immunosup-pressive cell types, such as MDSCs, regulatory B-cell (Bregs) and cytokines, like TGFβ and IL-10, play a part in the development of an immunosuppressive tumor microenvironment (TME).

Tumor-resident Tregs co-express high levels of CTLA-4, OX-40 and GITR compared to effector T-cells and In murine models of MPM, the combination of anti-OX-40 and anti-CTLA-4 antibodies has synergistic effect on CTLA-4$^+$, OX-40$^+$ tumor resident T-regs and contributing to a clear tumor regression when compared to single-antibody treatment [83]. Coherently with this point, combined anti-angiogenic and anti-PD-L1 therapies favor HEV and TLS formation in murine models of breast cancer and neuroendocrine pancreatic tumors [84] suggesting that a powerful anti-tumor systemic response by ICIs is sustained, if not triggered, by the presence of TLSs *in situ*. TLS heterogeneity among human cancers has been analyzed via a pan-cancer gene expression analysis of TME cellular composition on The Cancer Genome Atlas (TCGA) data and MPM, as well as lung adenocarcinoma and lung squamous cell carcinoma, display high expression of a 12-chemokine gene signature associated with TLS presence [85] suggesting TLSs are frequent, but also heterogeneous [86].

Seventy percent of MPM cases contain lymphoid aggregates and about 30% of them contain GCs [31]. These aggregates are functionally similar to TLSs, in which T- and B- lymphocytes are apart in two adjacent regions surrounded by HEV, as already shown for ovarian and prostate cancer [87, 88]. Intratumoral CD8 + T-lymphocytes in high numbers are an independent good prognostic marker for MPM patients [68]. Additionally, structural inter- or intra-chromosomal rearrange-ments and single nucleotide variants have been recently reported from mate-pair and RNA sequencing-based analyses on mesothelioma specimens predicting the expression of potentially-targetable neoantigens [58]. Moreover, some of these neo-antigens bind patient-specific MHC and specific tumor-infiltrating T-cell clones are expanded as observed through TCR repertoire analysis [58]. Indeed, TCR diversity and mutation/neoantigen load are inversely correlated, but both active and suppres-sive TME immune components, such as Treg and CD8 + T-cells, were present and equally balanced suggesting a scenario where activated anti-tumor CD8+ T-cells are counteracted by pro-tumoral immune suppressive molecules and Treg cells [57] or activated CD8+ T and CD4+ T-helper cells displaying phenotypic markers of exhaustion like PD-1, TIM-3 and LAG3 [59].

## 5. The importance of B-cell infiltration in solid tumors and MPM

B-cell follicles in TLS from non-small cell lung cancer and ovarian cancers contain bona fide Ki67+ GC B-cells expressing the activation-induced deaminase (AID) gene, that codes a critical enzyme in somatic hypermutation and class switch recombination processes typical of immunoreceptor genes, as well as, of BCL-6, the transcription factor involved in the late stage of B-cell maturation [66, 89]. Additionally, the presence of CD38+ CD138+ PCs around the follicle is highly sugges-tive of antibody production *in situ* [90]. Indeed, micro-dissected follicles subjected to BCR repertoire analysis revealed clonal amplification compared to peripheral B-cells, supporting the idea that locally presented antigens can elicit specific B-cell responses in several malignancies [87, 89, 91–94].

Additionally, PCs isolated from dense aggregates in tumor stroma [90], produce anti-tumor antibodies of the immunoglobulin G (IgG) isotype *in vivo* whose mech-anism of action has not been yet determined. One possibility is that anti-tumor IgGs produced locally increase antigen presentation by DCs and/or directly promote the activity of specific subsets of CD4+ T-cells endowed with Fcγ receptors (FcγRs) [95]. The presence of IgG deposits in TLS, the spatial organization of TLSs that may favor DC priming by locally produced IgGs and the observation that tumor-derived immune complexes increase the expression of the co-stimulatory molecule CD86 on DCs *in vivo* [87] suggest that these mechanisms take place. In favor of the latter are the results of a meta-analysis in a large set of human cancers showing that the prognostic effect of T-cells is generally stronger when tumor-infiltrating B-cells or PCs are present, supporting the hypothesis that a coordination between cellular and humoral adaptive immune responses is crucial for effective anti-tumor adaptive responses [96].

The role of B-cells and the association of B-cell rich TLSs with survival and anti-PD-1 immunotherapy response in sarcoma and melanoma have been recently established [97, 98]. Interestingly B-cells are the strongest prognostic factor even in the context of low CD8+ T-cells [97] in sarcoma and class-switched MBCs are specifically enriched in melanoma ICI-treated responders [99]. In murine models of MPM treated with immunotherapy, the presence of B-cells is essential for good prognosis, indicating that antibodies are generated and contribute significantly and essentially to the therapeutic effect [100]. Consistently, B-lymphocyte infiltration in MPM tissue positively correlates with prognosis [38] although variable in its extent [101]. Moreover clinical [52] and preclinical data on B-lymphocytes contribution to MPM prognosis suggest that they elicit an adaptive cytotoxic immune response rather than acting directly as antigen presenting cells (APCs) [100, 102]. In this respect MPM and other solid tumors share many similarities and provide a solid opportunity to develop novel immunotherapies via the identification of MPM targeting molecules in patients.

## 6. Immunotherapy in MPM

Immune checkpoint (IC) proteins, such as cytotoxic T-lymphocyte-associated antigen 4 (CTLA-4), programmed death 1 (PD-1) and PD-L1, are regulators of the immune system that preserve homeostasis and hinder autoimmunity in physi-ological conditions [103]. ICs overexpression in MPM keeps anti-tumor immune response in check contributing to the creation of a local immunosuppressive TME [31, 104]. IC inhibitors (ICIs), i.e. antibodies targeting ICs, are used as immuno-modulatory agents to interfere with the CTLA-4/B7.1/2 or PD-1/PD-L1 axes thereby helping to overcome tumor-immune escape [95, 105, 106].

Recently, PD-L1 expression in MPM has been assessed on tissue microarrays using two different FDA-approved antibodies and 22–27% of cases were positive for PD-L1 (1% cut off) [107]. PD-L1 is expressed in a high proportion of biphasic and sarcomatoid MPM cases and its positivity >1% is associated with a significant 10-months reduction in median OS compared to PD-L1 negative tumors [108, 109]. Similarly, high PD-L1 expression (>50%) in epithelioid MPM patients correlates with shorter PFS (6.7 vs. 9.9 months) [108]. Despite its prognostic value [59, 60, 110], PD-L1 expression is not a valid predictive marker of response to anti-PD-L1 therapies for several tumor types [111, 112], including MPM [113]. Anti-PD-1/PD-L1 therapies were tested in different trials in MPM patients [114–121]. Combination of pembrolizumab with PPC in first-line treatment compared to pembrolizumab or PPC alone, is currently being evaluated in the phase III trial NCT0278417, while nivolumab is being investigated in the randomized phase III trial CONFIRM (NCT03063450) in comparison with placebo [119]. Durvalumab activity, a PD-L1 inhibitor, in combination with first-line CCP was tested in the DREAM study (ANZ clinical trial registry number: ACTRN12616001170415). This combination resulted in an ORR of 61% using mRECIST and 53% using iRECIST criteria and in a 6 months PFS of 71% (mRECIST). On the basis of these observations a randomized phase 3 trial will be started [122].

ICs expression is controlled at different stages of T-lymphocyte activation and variable in tumor cells. For these reasons, a combination strategy employing two different ICIs in addition to chemotherapy has been proposed to achieve a synergistic effect by overcoming immune-resistance observed in some MPM patients. Encouraging results observed for different ICIs in combination [113, 123, 124] prompted the investigation of the nivolumab plus ipilimumab combination in comparison to standard PPC alone as first-line option in the phase III clinical trial Checkmate-743 (NCT02899299). Checkmate-743 has clearly demonstrated the benefit of nivolumab in combination with ipilimumab in first line mesothelioma treatment and based on those results obtained approval from FDA from October 2020. On 22 April 2021, the Committee for Medicinal Products for Human Use (CHMP) adopted a positive opinion recommending a change to the terms of the marketing authorization for the medicinal product Opdivo (nivolumab) in combination with ipilimumab for the first line treatment of adult patients with unresectable malignant pleural mesothelioma in Europe as well.

At present, efficacy and safety of adoptive T-cell therapies, in particular chimeric antigen receptor-transduced T-cells (CAR-T), in MPM and other solid tumors are under investigation [125, 126]. CAR-T-cells directed against mesothelin (MSLN), a glycoprotein expressed on MPM and other solid tumor cells, with a limited presence on normal tissues [127], represent a promising therapeutic option [128, 129]. Recently, Adusumilli and colleagues reported the outcome of a phase I clinical trial, NCT02414269, [130, 131] on MPM patients with pleural metastases from lung or breast cancer treated with anti-MSLN CAR-T-cells. Of note, the inclusion of anti-PD-1 therapy was crucial to elicit clinical efficacy and avoid T-cell exhaustion since no patient had an objective response before pembrolizumab addition showing the importance of conditioning the immune suppressive features of the TME also in this therapeutic setting.

Pembrolizumab plus anti-MSLN CAR-T-cell combination showed the best clini-cal outcome with an ORR of 63% (10/16) and a DCR of 75% (12/16). No evidence of on-target, off-tumor or therapy related toxicities higher than grade 1 was observed. Although applied to a limited number of patients so far, CAR-T therapies against MPM have shown really impressive results highlighting the different efficacy for advanced cell therapies compared to small molecule drugs or antibodies. Recently, a comprehensive review about immunotherapy in MPM has been published [132]. However, the limited availability of therapeutic targetable antigens hinders the efficacy of CAR based strategies for MPM patients. More targets are needed for MPM treatment in the future.

## 7. Making a hot tumor microenvironment

ICIs effectiveness in MPM treated patients highlight the presence of potentially active immune cells *in situ that* if properly unleashed can elicit antitumor responses. However, to achieve this goal, TME must be modified in order to abolish/interfere with specific immune suppressive cues. Interestingly, Barsky and colleagues recently reported a case of a man with MPM treated with a combination of palliative radiation and immune-gene therapy (GM-CSF) [133]. The outcome of this treatment combination was outstanding, resulting in a so-called "abscopal effect".

The abscopal effect is observed when a localized radiation induces an antitumor response at distant sites. RT can trigger an immunogenic cell death (ICD) [134, 135] and can stimulate antigen-specific, adaptive immunity [136]. ICD sets the stage for anti-tumor immune responses which include the release of tumor antigens by irradiated tumor cells, the cross-presentation of tumor-derived antigens to T-cells by antigen-presenting cells (APCs), and the migration of effector T-cells from the lymph nodes to distant tumor sites, suggesting that irradiated tumors can act as an *in situ* vaccine if appropriate conditions are in place [137–139]. The overall incidence of the abscopal effect of RT alone is low with 46 clinical cases reported from 1969 [139]. Those poor numbers witness the insufficiency of RT alone to overcome the immune resistance of malignant tumors. Immunotherapy can lower host immune tolerance towards tumors, therefore the combination of RT and immunotherapy can amplify the anti-tumor immune response, a hypothesis currently under investigation in the trial NCT02959463 where adjuvant pembrolizumab after RT in lung-intact MPM patients is tested. In a murine model of MPM, the abscopal effect can be induced by local RT and enhanced by immune suppressive CTLA-4 blockade as infiltrated T-cells, both in primary and secondary tumor sites, are predominantly cytotoxic CD8+ T-cells while Tregs are reduced [140]. Those observations corroborate the idea that a systemic tumor response can be unleashed by a local treatment thereby modifying the features of the TME.

## 8. The quest for specificity in malignant mesothelioma: how can we fill this gap?

Adoptive cell therapies in combination with ICIs are showing promising results for MPM patients. Their specificity or preference of targeting is granted almost exclusively by the use of antibodies or their derived fragments that are directed to tumor specific/associated antigens. First attempts of therapy using murine monoclonal antibodies (mAbs) in cancer patients failed due to neutralizing antibodies generation and to mismatch with components of the human immune system. These results highlighted the importance of using human or human compatible/tolerable biomolecules and prompted the design of novel screening platforms to find them. Antigen unbiased screening methods (**Figure 1**) can be used to this end to test *a priori* the targeting ability of antibodies to cells postponing the identification of antigens to lead candidates only.

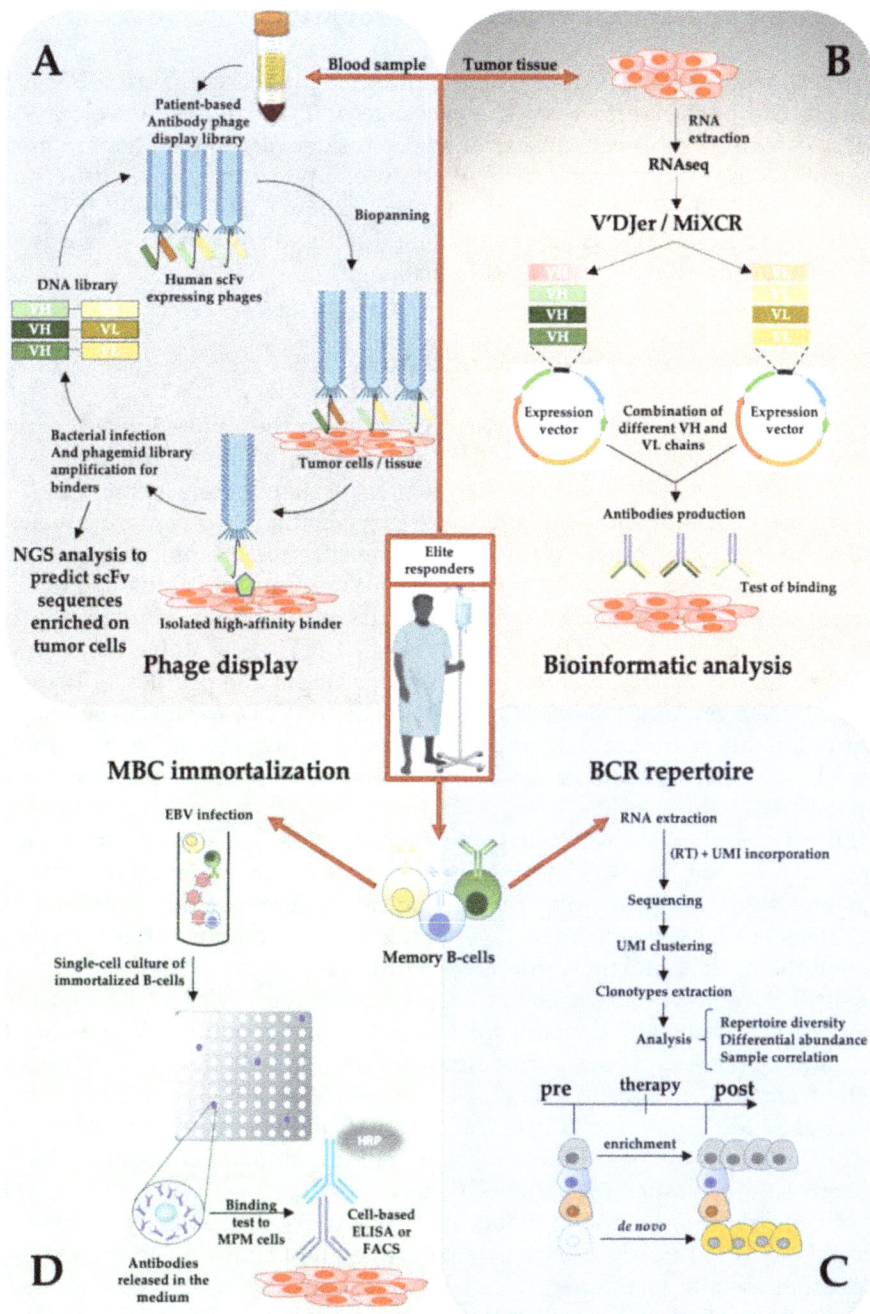

**Figure 1.**

*Schematic representation of 4 antigen-unbiased screening strategies to obtain fully human tumor targeting antibodies. Panel **A**: Patient derived scFv phage display libraries can be generated from MPM patient peripheral blood B cells. Those libraries are used to screen for novel specificities. Phage displayed scFvs undergo selection through consecutive rounds of panning on tumor cells to enrich for specific binders. NGS analysis allows the prediction of scFv sequences enriched on tumor cells. Panel **B**: de novo formed sequences, like those codifying the BCRs of infiltrated immune cells in tumor tissue can be retrieved using specific bioinformatic tools. Combinations of different heavy (VH) and light (VL) variable chains are used to generate candidate antibodies to be screened on cell or tumor tissues. Panel **C**: Analysis of BCR repertoire could be performed from memory B-cells from MPM patients. Enriched or de novo formed sequences could be monitored before and after a specific treatment in order to identify specific clones. Panel **D**: Memory B-cells from MPM patients can be immortalized through EBV infection and the immunoglobulins released in the medium of clonal cell cultures are tested on tumor cells by FACS or ELISA assays.*

## 9. From today's patients the future cures for MPM

As explained above, patients develop an immune response against MPM that, if unleashed, can be very effective. The presence of TLSs and the development of oligoclonal families of B-cells inside or at the border of MPM tissue are positive prognostic features and constitute a window of opportunity to capture human therapeutic antibodies. Now the next question is: how can we exploit this powerful reservoir of biologics to isolate or design targeting drugs? In other words: what technologies are available to take up this challenge?

## 10. BCR repertoire from sequencing data

Bulk RNA-Seq data from tumor tissue contain a hitherto overlooked picture of tumor and its ecosystem. Typically, data are analyzed to assess the expression of known transcripts, while *de novo* formed sequences, like those generated by T- and B-cells in the assembly and generation of their specific receptors, are usually disregarded since they fall off from the comparison with the reference transcriptome. However, these sequences can be retrieved from raw data and employed to extract the sequence of TCRs and BCRs from tumor tissue infiltrated immune cells using specific bioinformatic tools. One of them is MiXCR [141], a universal tool which takes raw sequencing data, including RNA-seq, as input and profiles TCR and BCR repertoires. As a reference, it uses a built-in library of V, D, J and C gene sequences from the human or mouse genome. MixCR output provides a list of clonotypes derived by assembling identical and homologous reads, corrected for sequencing errors.

V'DJer is another software that can process RNA-seq data for this purpose [142]. It can be run on BCR light and heavy chain data and employs unmapped paired end short reads aligning them against a reference transcriptome. Then, V'DJer detects VDJ rearrangements, generates contigs and quantifies the ones that represent the most abundant portions of the BCR repertoire. When the expression levels of BCR are low, there is an option to increase sensitivity of the algorithm at the cost of increasing the demand for computational resources. V'DJer has been used, for example, to retrieve antibodies from RNA sequencing data of melanoma patients from TCGA repository [142, 143]. At present, TCGA contains expression analyses of 87 MPM patients (TCGA-MESO) that could be used for this purpose. In addi-tion, RNA can be obtained from FFPE samples containing TLSs in prospective and retrospective patients' cohorts.

It is possible to infer the sequence of resident B-cell clones by applying bio-informatic tools to RNA-Se q o r b y sequencin g amplicon s fo r immunoglobuli n chains using specific sets of degenerate universal primers from whole tissue DNA or RNA/cDNA. The latter approach is implemented by the immunoSEQ platform (Adaptive Biotechnologies, Seattle, WA). In contrast to profiling using bulk RNA-Seq data, it is more precise since the experimental design is optimized to identify the BCR repertoire through the ImmunoSeq Analyzer software which is specific for this purpose. Its starting material can be both genomic DNA (gDNA) and cDNA: in order to assess clonal expansion of B-cells in tissues, gDNA is the best solution since each cell contains the same copy number, while mRNA transcripts can be very different among cells, depending on cellular activation and even the retrotranscription procedure can add other confounding factors. However, cDNA is a better choice if the goal is to find the most abundantly produced antibodies in situ, since there is a difference in the mRNA expression between activated and naive B-cells. Finally, independently of the method employed for their derivation, identified immunoglobulin heavy and light chain sequences can be assembled to produce candidate antibodies and test them for MPM target cells binding.

## 11. Memory B-cell receptor repertoire in MPM patients

A second powerful approach to obtain human antibodies targeting MPM cancer cells exploits directly the immune system of patients. Individuals exposed to viral agents, parasites and tumors develop an adaptive response against non-self and neoantigens. Anti-cancer treatments such as vaccines and ICIs elicit impressive clinical responses (reviewed in [95]) and an immunological memory in subgroups of cancer patients ("elite responders") has been reported. MPM is not characterized by high mutational burden [15] an important determinant of the response to checkpoint blockade.

The efficacy of the anti-PD-1 pembrolizumab was shown by Alley and colleagues in KEYNOTE-028 [116]. In addition, ipilimumab in combination with anti-TGFβ and anti-CD25 antibodies of syngeneic MPM in BALB/c animals resulted in: i) disease eradication in treated mice; ii) elevated levels of tumor-specific IgG antibodies in healed animals; iii) failure to regrow tumors in cured mice when re-challenged with the same tumor; iv) importantly, no response in the absence of B-cells, suggesting that antibodies generated upon treatment contribute significantly to the curative effect [100]. Besides that, CD20+ B-cells infiltration in MPM tumor tissue is a positive prognostic factor as previously discussed [38].

Therefore, the immune system of elite responders can be mined to isolate MBCs producing targeting antibodies. MBCs derive mostly from affinity matured and somatically hypermutated B-cells arising in the germinal centers [144] and constitute a reservoir of high-affinity antibody producers. These features make the MBC pool very attractive so biotech and pharma companies invest in the design of screening platforms to exploit it. For example, Oncoresponse, a company that developed a proprietary, clinically validated human-antibody discovery platform in partnership with MD Anderson Cancer Center follows this paradigm and identifies therapeutically relevant antibodies from patients showing elite response against cancer after immunotherapy. MBCs are easily accessible from the peripheral blood of donors and are suitable for viral immortalization to generate lymphoblastoid cultures for high throughput screens. MBC immortalization is usually performed by infection of peripheral MBCs by Epstein Barr Virus (EBV) [145] or by BCL-6/BCL-XL expressing vectors [146]. Those procedures generate cells that express BCR on the membrane and release their antibody into culture medium at the same time. BCR presence is exploited to isolate cells binding to labeled soluble antigens by cell sorting [146] so that subsequently immunoglobulin sequences from isolated cells can be cloned into expression vectors for large-scale antibody production. Companies like Humabs and AIMM therapeutics exploit those strategies to raise antibodies against specific targets. However, the same technology can be used to isolate targeting antibodies in an antigen unbiased manner as shown for melanoma via cell-based screenings of EBV immortalized B-cells [147]. In addition, human plasmablasts and MBCs can be cultured for a limited time using specific cytokines [147–152].

Importantly, these approaches to retrieve targeting antibodies do not rely on a prior knowledge of the target. Target identification in this case is postponed, initially drawing on the demonstration of efficacy and specificity towards MPM cancer cells. MBCs receptor repertoire can be obtained also from peripheral blood or draining lymph node purified MBCs by RNA-Seq mining for *de novo* formed or highly enriched variants after treatment in elite responders [142]. Advantages and

| Approach | Antigen display | Advantages | Disadvantages |
|---|---|---|---|
| **Phage-display technology with patient derived scFv antibody libraries** | Antigen on cell surface | • Cheap instrumentation<br>• Used with any cell type<br>• Established technology<br>• Fastest strategy to lead candidates<br>• NGS driven selection of candidates | • Affinity maturation step is often needed<br>• Reformatting in IgG format, if needed<br>• Binding to normal human tissues to establish specificity *a posteriori* |
| **BCR repertoire from the peripheral blood of elite responders pre and post therapy** | Antigen on cell surface | • Availability of blood samples from elite responders<br>• Antibodies are derived from affinity matured human immunoglobulins | • Possible downsampling<br>• Cloning and production of candidate antibodies is required<br>• VH and VL pairs are not known (unless single cell sequencing is used)<br>• Requires a test of binding specificity to normal human tissues *a posteriori* |
| **Bioinformatic analysis of BCR repertoire in tumor tissue** | Antigen on cell surface | • Availability of large number of FFPE samples<br>• Applicable to retrospective case series<br>• Applicable to any RNA-Seq dataset | • Requires cloning and production of the antibodies<br>• Possible downsampling due to low quality or limited sample material<br>• VH and VL pairs cannot be known<br>• Requires a test of binding specificity to normal human tissues *a posteriori* |
| **MBC immortalization** | Antigen on cell surface | • Easy availability of elite responder samples (blood/PBMCs)<br>• Established protocols<br>• Isolation of *in vivo* high-affinity matured and human compatible immunoglobulins<br>• Basic technical expertise on viral manipulation | • Requires a BSL2 area<br>• Identification of the antigens can be technically challenging<br>• Requires a test of binding specificity to normal human tissues *a posteriori* |

**Table 1.**
*Advantages and drawbacks of antigen-unbiased screens to obtain fully human antibodies.*

drawbacks of the different screening strategies for fully human antibody selection are summarized in **Table 1**.

## 12. Phage display screening using patient-derived scFv antibody libraries

A useful strategy to select human antibody fragments (Fabs and scFvs) against specific antigens or cells is phage display (reviewed in [153]). The importance of phage display has been restated in 2018 by the award of Nobel Prize in Chemistry to George P. Smith and Sir Gregory P. Winter"for the phage display of peptides and antibodies". Phage display has allowed the production of clinically relevant antibod-ies (reviewed in [154]). The presence of BCRs in TME, SLOs and in the peripheral blood of MPM and other tumor patients allows for the generation of patient derived scFv phage display libraries [155] that can be used to screen for novel specificities. Phage displayed scFvs undergo selection through consecutive rounds of panning on tumor cells to enrich for specific binders (**Figure 1**). Identified antibodies can be reformatted to fully human antibodies or used as fragments or building blocks for CAR constructs.

Importantly those antibodies will derive from the permutation of original VH and VL sequences of the B-cell repertoire during library preparation while for EBV immortalized cells VH and VL pairs will be the original ones as in the patient. Classically single bacterial clones were selected and grown to produce antibodies or phages displaying specific antibodies in order to test individually their targeting of a cell of interest. Nowadays, next generation sequencing provides an efficient, quantitative and quick analytical tool to assess the evolution of complexity of phage antibody-display libraries during consecutive biopanning enrichment stages. Phage clonal evolution during screening can be studied and used to identify putative candidate antibodies and promote their cloning and production for further testing their binding to cells [156].

An unbiased phage display approach has been used to identify tumor-targeting scFvs for both sarcomatoid and epithelioid MPM. In this study, 95 mesothelioma-targeting scFvs were identified and 21 candidates were characterized for binding by FACS and IHC and for their *in vitro* internalization capacity by MPM cells with the goal to deliver conjugated anti-tumor drugs directly inside tumor cells [157]. Further analyses identified MCAM/CD146 as one of the antigens. CD146 had been previously described as a marker in advanced melanoma [158] and other tumors [159, 160], it is expressed in all MPM histotypes and by a limited spectrum of normal human adult tissues [161]. The clinical utility of MCAM/CD146 detection in pleural effusion fluid and peripheral blood samples as a diagnostic and prognostic marker for MPM [162] is under evaluation. The generation of a phage antibody-display library from the entire antibody genes repertoire of a cancer patient has been also attempted. Rare cancer targeting antibodies have been identified by this strategy [163]. However, the immunodominance phenomenon typical of certain cancers [153, 164, 165] has hindered a wider use of this strategy in early attempts.

## 13. Conclusions

Despite amazing efforts made by the scientific community and the therapeutic options developed over the last decades, the discovery of a curative treatment for MPM is still elusive and constitutes an unmet clinical need. To-date, the most promising therapeutic approaches comprise immunotherapies and CAR-based therapies that have shown impressive although preliminary clinical results. The field needs to bet on and implement these novel approaches towards novel targets and antigens to cope with tumor heterogeneity and to provide effective treatments to be used in combination. The most innovative screening technologies for the generation of fully human antibodies are in place and combine elements from fields of science that started far apart and came together to serve the purpose. These include protein engineering, next-generation sequencing (NGS), virology and cell biology providing an opportunity to find novel and unknown therapeutic targets for MPM and cancer in general. Based on these premises, we believe that a future breakthrough in MPM management will come from the design of novel

ATMPs engineered to target antigens that are still unknown but that can be identified via unbiased screening strategies.

## Acknowledgements

We thank Alicja M. Gruszka for her help in proofreading and editing this
manuscript.

## Author details

Fabio Nicolini* and Massimiliano Mazza*
Immunotherapy, Cell Therapy and Biobank (ITCB), IRCCS Istituto Romagnolo per
lo Studio dei Tumori (IRST) "Dino Amadori", Meldola, Italy

*Address all correspondence to: fabio.nicolini@irst.emr.it  and
massimiliano.mazza@irst.emr.it

# References

[1] Carbone M, Adusumilli PS, Alexander HR Jr, Baas P, Bardelli F, Bononi A, et al. Mesothelioma: Scientific clues for prevention, diagnosis, and therapy. CA A Cancer J Clin. 2019 Jul 30;69(5):402-29.

[2] Kameda T, Takahashi K, Kim R, Jiang Y, Movahed M, Park E-K, et al. Asbestos: use, bans and disease burden in Europe. Bull World Health Organ. 2014 Nov 1;92(11):790-7.

[3] Peto J, Decarli A, La Vecchia C, Levi F, Negri E. The European mesothelioma epidemic. Br J Cancer. 1999 Feb;79(3-4):666-72.

[4] Henley SJ, Larson TC, Wu M, Antao VCS, Lewis M, Pinheiro GA, et al. Mesothelioma incidence in 50 states and the District of Columbia, United States, 2003-2008. Int J Occup Environ Health. 2013 Jan;19(1):1-10.

[5] Beckett P, Edwards J, Fennell D, Hubbard R, Woolhouse I, Peake MD. Demographics, management and survival of patients with malignant pleural mesothelioma in the National Lung Cancer Audit in England and Wales. Lung Cancer 2015 Jun;88(3):344-8.

[6] Cheung M, Testa JR. BAP1, a tumor suppressor gene driving malignant mesothelioma. Transl Lung Cancer Res. 2017 Jun;6(3):270-8.

[7] Yu H, Pak H, Hammond-Martel I, Ghram M, Rodrigue A, Daou S, et al. Tumor suppressor and deubiquitinase BAP1 promotes DNA double-strand break repair. Proc Natl Acad Sci USA. 2014 Jan 7;111(1):285-90.

[8] Carbone M, Yang H, Pass HI, Krausz T, Testa JR, Gaudino G. BAP1 and cancer. Nature Publishing Group. 2013 Mar;13(3):153-9.

[9] Affar EB, Carbone M. BAP1 regulates different mechanisms of cell death. Cell Death Dis. Nature Publishing Group; 2018 Nov 19;9(12):1151-3.

[10] Zhang Y, Shi J, Liu X, Feng L, Gong Z, Koppula P, et al. BAP1 links metabolic regulation of ferroptosis to tumour suppression. Nat Cell Biol. Nature Publishing Group; 2018 Oct;20(10):1181-92.

[11] Dey A, Seshasayee D, Noubade R, French DM, Liu J, Chaurushiya MS, et al. Loss of the tumor suppressor BAP1 causes myeloid transformation. Science. 2012 Sep 21;337(6101):1541-6.

[12] Bononi A, Giorgi C, Patergnani S, Larson D, Verbruggen K, Tanji M, et al. BAP1 regulates IP3R3-mediated $Ca^{2+}$ flux to mitochondria suppressing cell transformation. Nature Publishing Group; 2017 Jun 22;546(7659):549-53.

[13] Bononi A, Yang H, Giorgi C, Patergnani S, Pellegrini L, Su M, et al. Germline BAP1 mutations induce a Warburg effect. Cell Death Differ. 2017 Oct;24(10):1694-704.

[14] Betti M, Casalone E, Ferrante D, Aspesi A, Morleo G, Biasi A, et al. Germline mutations in DNA repair genes predispose asbestos-exposed patients to malignant pleural mesothelioma. Cancer Letters. 2017 Oct 1;405:38-45.

[15] Bueno R, Stawiski EW, Goldstein LD, Durinck S, De Rienzo A, Modrusan Z, et al. Comprehensive genomic analysis of malignant pleural mesothelioma identifies recurrent mutations, gene fusions and splicing alterations. Nat Genet. Nature Publishing Group; 2016 Apr; 48(4):407-16. [16] Hassan R, Morrow B, Thomas A, Walsh T, Lee MK, Gulsuner S, et al.

Inherited predisposition to malignant mesothelioma and overall survival following platinum chemotherapy. Proc Natl Acad Sci USA. National Academy of Sciences; 2019 Apr 30;116(18): 9008-13.

[17] Farzin M, Toon CW, Clarkson A, Sioson L, Watson N, Andrici J, et al. Loss of expression of BAP1 predicts longer survival in mesothelioma. Pathology. 2015 Jun;47(4):302-7.

[18] Srinivasan G, Sidhu GS, Williamson EA, Jaiswal AS, Najmunnisa N, Wilcoxen K, et al. Synthetic lethality in malignant pleural mesothelioma with PARP1 inhibition. Cancer Chemother Pharmacol. Springer Berlin Heidelberg; 2017 Oct;80(4): 861-7.

[19] Zauderer MG, Szlosarek P, Le Moulec S, Popat S, Taylor P, Planchard D, et al. Phase 2, multicenter study of the EZH2 inhibitor tazemetostat as monotherapy in adults with relapsed or refractory (R/R) malignant mesothelioma (MM) with BAP1 inactivation. JCO. 2018; 36 (15_ suppl) :8515-5.

[20] Quetel L, Meiller C, Assié J-B, Blum Y, Imbeaud S, Montagne F, et al. Genetic alterations of malignant pleural mesothelioma: association with tumor heterogeneity and overall survival. Mol Oncol. John Wiley & Sons, Ltd; 2020 Jun;14(6):1207-23.

[21] Nicolini F, Bocchini M, Bronte G, Delmonte A, Guidoboni M, Crinò L, et al. Malignant Pleural Mesothelioma: State-of-the-Art on Current Therapies and Promises for the Future. Front Oncol. 2019;9:1519.

[22] Donaldson K, Murphy FA, Duffin R, Poland CA. Asbestos, carbon nanotubes and the pleural mesothelium: a review of the hyp-othesis regarding the role of long fibre retention in the parietal pleura, inflammation and

mesothelioma. Part Fibre Toxicol. BioMed Central; 2010 Mar 22;7(1):5-17.

[23] Park SH, Aust AE. Participation of iron and nitric oxide in the mutagenicity of asbestos in hgprt-, gpt+ Chinese hamster V79 cells. Cancer Res. Cancer Res; 1998 Mar 15;58(6):1144-8.

[24] Kamp DW, Israbian VA, Preusen SE, Zhang CX, Weitzman SA. Asbestos causes DNA strand breaks in cultured pulmonary epithelial cells: role of iron-catalyzed free radicals. Am J Physiol. American Physiological Society Bethesda, MD; 1995 Mar;268 (3 Pt 1):L471-80.

[25] Hei TK, Piao CQ, He ZY, Vannais D, Waldren CA. Chrysotile fiber is a strong mutagen in mammalian cells. Cancer Res. Cancer Res; 1992 Nov 15;52(22):6305-9.

[26] Yang H, Bocchetta M, Kroczynska B, Elmishad AG, Chen Y, Liu Z, et al. TNF-alpha inhibits asbestos-induced cytotoxicity via a NF-kappaB-dependent pathway, a possible mechanism for asbestos-induced oncogenesis. Proc Natl Acad Sci USA. National Academy of Sciences; 2006 Jul 5;103(27):10397-402.

[27] Yang H, Rivera Z, Jube S, Nasu M, Bertino P, Goparaju C, et al. Programmed necrosis induced by asbestos in human mesothelial cells causes high-mobility group box 1 protein release and resultant inflammation. Proc Natl Acad Sci USA. National Academy of Sciences; 2010 Jul 13;107(28):12611-6.

[28] Padmore T, Stark C, Turkevich LA, Champion JA. Quantitative analysis of the role of fiber length on phagocytosis and inflammatory response by alveolar macrophages. Biochim Biophys Acta Gen Subj. 2017 Feb;1861(2):58-67.

[29] Liu JY, Brass DM, Hoyle GW, Brody AR. TNF-alpha receptor

knockout mice are protected from the fibroproliferative effects of inhaled asbestos fibers. Am J Pathol. 1998 Dec;153(6):1839-47.

[30] Lievense LA, Cornelissen R, Bezemer K, Kaijen-Lambers MEH, Hegmans JPJJ, Aerts JGJV. Pleural Effusion of Patients with Malignant Mesothelioma Induces Macrophage-Mediated T Cell Suppression. J Thorac Oncol. 2016 Oct;11(10):1755-64.

[31] Marcq E, Siozopoulou V, De Waele J, van Audenaerde J, Zwaenepoel K, Santermans E, et al. Prognostic and predictive aspects of the tumor immune microenvironment and immune checkpoints in malignant pleural mesothelioma. Oncoimmunology. Taylor & Francis; 2017 Jan 20;6(1):1-10.

[32] Burt BM, Rodig SJ, Tilleman TR, Elbardissi AW, Bueno R, Sugarbaker DJ. Circulating and tumor-infiltrating myeloid cells predict survival in human pleural mesothelioma. Cancer. John Wiley & Sons, Ltd; 2011 Nov 15;117(22): 5234-44.

[33] Awad MM, Jones RE, Liu H, Lizotte PH, Ivanova EV, Kulkarni M, et al. Cytotoxic T Cells in PD-L1-Positive Malignant Pleural Mesotheliomas Are Counterbalanced by Distinct Immunosuppressive Factors. Cancer Immunology Research. American Association for Cancer Research; 2016 Dec;4(12):1038-48.

[34] Cornelissen R, Hegmans JPJJ, Maat APWM, Kaijen-Lambers MEH, Bezemer K, Hendriks RW, et al. Extended Tumor Control after Dendritic Cell Vaccination with Low-Dose Cyclophosphamide as Adjuvant Treatment in Patients with Malignant Pleural Mesothelioma. Am J Respir Crit Care Med. 2016 May; 193 (9): 1023-31.

[35] Tanrikulu AC, Abakay A, Komek H, Abakay O. Prognostic value of the lymphocyte-to-monocyte ratio and other inflammatory markers in malignant pleural mesothelioma. Environ Health Prev Med. BioMed Central; 2016 Sep;21(5):304-11.

[36] Hegmans JPJJ, Hemmes A, Hammad H, Boon L, Hoogsteden HC, Lambrecht BN. Mesothelioma environment comprises cytokines and T-regulatory cells that suppress immune responses. Eur Respir J. European Respiratory Society; 2006 Jun;27(6): 1086 -95.

[37] Li T, Li H, Wang Y, Harvard C, Tan J-L, Au A, et al. The expression of CXCR4, CXCL12 and CXCR7 in malignant pleural mesothelioma. J Pathol. John Wiley & Sons, Ltd; 2011 Mar ;223(4):519-30.

[38] Ujiie H, Kadota K, Nitadori J-I, Aerts JG, Woo KM, Sima CS, et al. The tumoral and stromal immune microenvironment in malignant pleural mesothelioma: A comprehensive anal-ysis reveals prognostic immune markers. Oncoimmunology. Taylor & Francis; 2015 Jun;4(6):e1009285.

[39] Blanquart C, Gueugnon F, Nguyen J-M, Roulois D, Cellerin L, Sagan C, et al. CCL2, galectin-3, and SMRP combination improves the diagnosis of mesothelioma in pleural effusions. J Thorac Oncol. 2012 May;7(5):883-9.

[40] Gueugnon F, Leclercq S, Blanquart C, Sagan C, Cellerin L, Padieu M, et al. Identification of novel markers for the diagnosis of malignant pleural mesothelioma. Am J Pathol. 2011 Mar;178(3):1033-42.

[41] Chéné A-L, d'Almeida S, Blondy T, Tabiasco J, Deshayes S, Fonteneau J-F, et al. Pleural Effusions from Patients with Mesothelioma Induce Recruitment of Monocytes and Their Differentiation into M2 Macrophages. J Thorac Oncol. 2016 Oct;11(10):1765-73.

[42] Cioce M, Canino C, Goparaju C, Yang H, Carbone M, Pass HI. Autocrine

CSF-1R signaling drives mesothel-ioma chemoresistance via AKT activ-ation. Cell Death Dis. Nature Pub-lishing Group; 2014 Apr 10;5 (4):e 1167-7.

[43] Fujii M, Toyoda T, Nakanishi H, Yatabe Y, Sato A, Matsudaira Y, et al. TGF-β synergizes with defects in the Hippo pathway to stimulate human malignant mesothelioma growth. J Exp Med. 2012 Mar 12;209(3):479-94.

[44] Schürch CM, Forster S, Brühl F, Yang SH, Felley Bosco E, Hewer E. The "don't eat me" signal CD47 is a novel diagnostic biomarker and potential therapeutic target for diffuse malig-nant mesothelioma. Oncoimmunolo-gy. Taylor & Francis; 2017;7(1): e13732 35.

[45] Izzi V, Chiurchiù V, D'Aquilio F, Palumbo C, Tresoldi I, Modesti A, et al. Differential effects of malignant mesothelioma cells on THP-1 mono-cytes and macrophages. Int J Oncol. Int J Oncol; 2009 Feb;34(2):543-50.

[46] Miselis NR, Wu ZJ, Van Rooijen N, Kane AB. Targeting tumor-associated macrophages in an orthotopic murine model of diffuse malignant mesoth-elioma. Molecular Cancer Therapeu-tics. American Association for Can-cer Research; 2008 Apr;7(4): 788-99.

[47] Rehrauer H, Wu L, Blum W, Pecze L, Henzi T, Serre-Beinier V, et al. How asbestos drives the tissue towards tumors: YAP activation, macrophage and mesothelial precur-sor recruitment, RNA editing, and somatic mutations. Oncogene. Nature Publishing Group; 2018 May;37(20): 2645-59.

[48] Khanna S, Graef S, Mussai F, Thomas A, Wali N, Yenidunya BG, et al. Tumor-Derived GM-CSF Promotes Granulocyte Immunosuppression in Mesothelioma Patients. Clin Cancer Res. American Association for Cancer Research; 2018 Jun 15;24(12):2859-72.

[49] Kao SCH, Pavlakis N, Harvie R, Vardy JL, Boyer MJ, van Zandwijk N, et al. High blood neutrophil-to-lympho-cyte ratio is an indicator of poor prognosis in malignant mesothelioma patients undergoing systemic therapy. Clin Cancer Res. American Association for Cancer Research; 2010 Dec 1;16 (23): 5805-13.

[50] Chee SJ, Lopez M, Mellows T, Gankande S, Moutasim KA, Harris S, et al. Evaluating the effect of immune cells on the outcome of patients with mesothelioma. Br J Cancer. Nature Publishing Group; 2017 Oct 24;117(9): 1341-8.

[51] Marcq E, Siozopoulou V, De Waele J, van Audenaerde J, Zwaenepoel K, Santermans E, et al. Prognostic and predictive aspects of the tumor immune microenvironment and immune che-ckpoints in malignant pleural meso-thelioma. Oncoimmunology. Tay-lor & Francis; 2017 Jan 20;6(1):1-10.

[52] Chee SJ, Lopez M, Mellows T, Gankande S, Moutasim KA, Harris S, et al. Evaluating the effect of immune cells on the outcome of patients with mesothelioma. Nature Publishing Group; 2017 Aug 17;117(9):1341-8.

[53] Anraku M, Cunningham KS, Yun Z, Tsao M-S, Zhang L, Keshavjee S, et al. Impact of tumor-infiltrating T cells on survival in patients with malignant pleural mesothelioma. J Thorac Car-diovasc Surg. 2008 Apr; 135(4): 823-9.

[54] DeLong P, Carroll RG, Henry AC, Tanaka T, Ahmad S, Leibowitz MS, et al. Regulatory T cells and cytokines in malignant pleural effusions secondary to mesothelioma and carcinoma. Cancer Biol Ther. Taylor & Francis; 2005 Mar;4(3):342-6.

[55] Comar M, Zanotta N, Bonotti A, Tognon M, Negro C, Cristaudo A, et al. Increased levels of C-C chemokine RANTES in asbestos exposed workers and in malignant mesothelioma patients

from an hyperendemic area. PLOS ONE. Public Library of Science; 2014;9(8): e104848.

[56] Davidson B, Dong HP, Holth A, Berner A, Risberg B. Chemokine receptors are infrequently expressed in malignant and benign mesothelial cells. Am J Clin Pathol. 2007 May;127(5): 752-9.

[57] Kiyotani K, Park J-H, Inoue H, Husain A, Olugbile S, Zewde M, et al. Integrated analysis of somatic mutations and immune microenvironment in malignant pleural mesothelioma. Oncoimmunology. Taylor & Francis; 2017;6(2):e1278330.

[58] Mansfield AS, Peikert T, Smadbeck JB, Udell JBM, Garcia-Rivera E, Elsbernd L, et al. Neoantigenic Potential of Complex Chromosomal Rearrangements in Mesothelioma. J Thorac Oncol. 2019 Feb;14(2): 276-87.

[59] Marcq E, Waele JD, Audenaerde JV, Lion E, Santermans E, Hens N, et al. Abundant expression of TIM-3, LAG-3, PD-1 and PD-L1 as immunotherapy checkpoint targets in effusions of mesothelioma patients. Oncotarget. 2017 Oct 27;8(52):89722-35.

[60] Cedrés S, Ponce-Aix S, Zugazagoitia J, Sansano I, Enguita A, Navarro-Mendivil A, et al. Analysis of expression of programmed cell death 1 ligand 1 (PD-L1) in malig-nant pleural mesothelioma (MPM). Gangopadhyay N, editor. PLOS ONE. 2015;10(3):e0121071.

[61] Mellman I, Coukos G, Dranoff G. Cancer immunotherapy comes of age. Nature. 2011;480(7378):480-9.

[62] Drayton DL, Liao S, Mounzer RH, Ruddle NH. Lymphoid organ devel-opment: from ontogeny to neogenesis. NatImmunol.2006;7(4):34 4- 53.

[63] Dieu-Nosjean M-C, Giraldo NA, Kaplon H, Germain C, Fridman WH, Sautès-Fridman C. Tertiary lymphoid structures, drivers of the anti-tumor responses in human cancers. Immunol Rev. John Wiley & Sons, Ltd (10.1111); 2016 May;271(1):260-75.

[64] Sautès-Fridman C, Lawand M, Giraldo NA, Kaplon H, Germain C, Fridman WH, et al. Tertiary Lymphoid Structures in Cancers: Prognostic Value, Regulation, and Manipulation for Therapeutic Intervention. Front Immunol. 2016 Oct 3;7(27):4410-1.

[65] Martinet L, Garrido I, Filleron T, Le Guellec S, Bellard E, Fournie JJ, et al. Human Solid Tumors Contain High Endothelial Venules: Association with T- and B-Lymphocyte Infiltration and Favorable Prognosis in Breast Cancer. Cancer Res. 2011 Aug 30;71(17):5678-87.

[66] Germain C, Gnjatic S, Tamzalit F, Knockaert S, Remark R, Goc J, et al. Presence of B Cells in Tertiary Lymphoid Structures Is Associated with a Protective Immunity in Patients with Lung Cancer. Am J Respir Crit Care Med. 2014 Apr;189(7):832-44.

[67] Ettinger DS, Wood DE, Akerley W, Bazhenova LA, Borghaei H, Camidge DR, et al. NCCN Guidelines Insights: Malignant Pleural Meso-thelioma, Version 3.2016. Vol. 14, Journal of the National Comprehensive Cancer Net - work: JNCCN. 2016. pp. 825-36.

[68] Yamada N, Oizumi S, Kikuchi E, Shinagawa N, Konishi-Sakakibara J, Ishimine A, et al. CD8+ tumor-infiltrating lymphocytes predict favorable prognosis in malignant pleural mesothelioma after resection. Cancer Immunol Immunother. 2010 Oct; 59 (10): 1543-9.

[69] Suzuki K, Kadota K, Sima CS, Sadelain M, Rusch VW, Travis WD, et al. Chronic inflammation in tumor

stroma is an independent predictor of prolonged survival in epithelioid malignant pleural mesothelioma patients. Cancer Immunol Immunother. 3rd ed. 2011 Dec;60(12):1721-8.

[70] Goc J, Germain C, Vo-Bourgais TKD, Lupo A, Klein C, Knockaert S, et al. Dendritic Cells in TumorAssociated Tertiary Lymphoid Structures Signal a Th1 Cytotoxic Immune Contexture and License the Positive Prognostic Value of Infilt-rating CD8+ T Cells. Cancer Res. 2014 Feb 2; 74(3):705-15.

[71] Dieu-Nosjean M-C, Antoine M, Danel C, Heudes D, Wislez M, Poulot V, et al. Long-Term Survival for Patients With Non–Small-Cell Lung Cancer With Intratumoral Lymphoid Structures. JCO. 2008 Sep 20;26(27): 4410-7.

[72] Silina K, Soltermann A, Attar FM, Casanova R, Uckeley ZM, Thut H, et al. Germinal Centers Determine the Prognostic Relevance of Tertiary Lymphoid Structures and Are Impaired by Corticosteroids in Lung Squamous Cell Carcinoma. Cancer Res. American Association for Cancer Research; 2018 Mar 1;78(5):1308-20.

[73] Di Caro G, Bergomas F, Grizzi F, Doni A, Bianchi P, Malesci A, et al. Occurrence of Tertiary Lymphoid Tissue Is Associated with T-Cell Infiltration and Predicts Better Prognosis in Early-Stage Colorectal Cancers. Clin Cancer Res. 2014 Apr 15;20(8):2147-58.

[74] Posch F, Silina K, Leibl S, Mündlein A, Moch H, Siebenhüner A, et al. Maturation of tertiary lymphoid structures and recurrence of stage II and III colorectal cancer. Oncoimmunology. Taylor & Francis; 2017 Dec 20;7(2):1-13.
[75] Hiraoka N, Ino Y, Yamazaki-Itoh R, Kanai Y, Kosuge T, Shimada K. Intratumoral tertiary lymphoid organ is a favourable prognosticator in patients with pancreatic cancer. Br J Cancer. Nature Publishing Group; 2015 May 5;112(11):1782-90.

[76] Castino GF, Cortese N, Capretti G, Serio S, Di Caro G, Mineri R, et al. Spatial distribution of B cells predicts prognosis in human pancreatic adenocarcinoma. Oncoimmunology. Taylor & Francis; 2016 Apr 5;5(4):1-14.

[77] Wirsing AM, Ervik IK, Seppola M, Uhlin-Hansen L, Steigen SE, Hadler-Olsen E. Presence of high-endothelial venules correlates with a favorable immune microenvironment in oral squamous cell carcinoma. Modern Pathology. Springer US; 2018 Jun 7;:1-13.

[78] Gu-Trantien C, Loi S, Garaud S, Equeter C, Libin M, de Wind A, et al. CD4+ follicular helper T cell infiltration predicts breast cancer survival. Journal of Clinical Investigation. 2013 Jun 17;123(7):2873-92.

[79] Lee HJ, Kim JY, Park IA, Song IH, Yu JH, Ahn J-H, et al. Prognostic Significance of Tumor-Infiltrating Lymphocytes and the Tertiary Lymphoid Structures in HER2-Positive Breast Cancer Treated With Adjuvant Trastuzumab. Am J Clin Pathol. 2015 Aug 1;144(2):278-88.

[80] Savas P, Salgado R, Denkert C, Sotiriou C, Darcy PK, Smyth MJ, et al. Clinical relevance of host immunity in breast cancer: from TILs to the clinic. Nat Rev Clin Oncol. Nature Publishing Group; 2016 Apr;13(4):228-41.

[81] Colbeck EJ, Jones E, Hindley JP, Smart K, Schulz R, Browne M, et al. Treg Depletion Licenses T Cell-Driven HEV Neogenesis and Promotes Tumor Destruction. Cancer Immunology Research. 2017 Nov;5(11):1005-15.

[82] Joshi NS, Akama-Garren EH, Lu Y, Lee D-Y, Chang GP, Li A, et al. Regulatory T Cells in Tumor-Associated Tertiary Lymphoid Structures Suppress

Anti-tumor T Cell Responses. Immunity. 2015 Sep 15;43(3):579-90.

[83] Fear VS, Tilsed C, Chee J, Forbes CA, Casey T, Solin JN, et al. Combination immune checkpoint blockade as an effective therapy for mesothelioma.Oncoimmunology. Taylor & Francis; 2018 Sep 12; 7(10): 1-14.

[84] Allen E, Jabouille A, Rivera LB, Lodewijckx I, Missiaen R, Steri V, et al. Combined antiangiogenic and anti-PD-L1 therapy stimulates tumor immunity through HEV formation. Sci Transl Med. 2017 Apr 12;9(385): eaak9679.

[85] Coppola D, Nebozhyn M, Khalil F, Dai H, Yeatman T, Loboda A, et al. Unique ectopic lymph node-like structures present in human primary colorectal carcinoma are identified by immune gene array profiling. Am J Pathol. 2011 Jul;179(1):37-45.

[86] Sautès-Fridman C, Petitprez F, Calderaro J, Fridman WH. Tertiary lymphoid structures in the era of cancer immunotherapy. Nature Publishing Group. Nature Publishing Group; 2019 Jun;19(6):307-25.

[87] Montfort A, Pearce O, Maniati E, Vincent BG, Bixby L, Böhm S, et al. A Strong B-cell Response Is Part of the Immune Landscape in Human High-Grade Serous Ovarian Metastases. Clin Cancer Res. 2017 Jan 2;23(1): 250-62.

[88] García-Hernández M de LL, Uribe-Uribe NO, Espinosa-González R, Kast WM, Khader SA, Rangel-Moreno J. A Unique Cellular and Molecular Microenvironment Is Present in Tertiary Lymphoid Organs of Patients with Spontaneous Pro-state Cancer Regression. Front Immunol. 2017 May 17;8:87-21.

[89] Nielsen JS, Sahota RA, Milne K, Kost SE, Nesslinger NJ, Watson PH, et al. CD20+ Tumor-Infiltrating Lymphocytes Have an Atypical CD27- Memory Phenotype and Together with CD8+ T Cells Promote Favorable Pro-gnosis in Ovarian Cancer. Clin Cancer Res. 2012 Jun 14;18(12):3281-92.

[90] Kroeger DR, Milne K, Nelson BH. Tumor-Infiltrating Plasma Cells Are Associated with Tertiary Lymphoid Structures, Cytolytic T-Cell Responses, and Superior Prognosis in Ovarian Cancer. Clin Cancer Res. 2016 Jun 14;22(12):3005-15.

[91] Coronella JA, Spier C, Welch M, Trevor KT, Stopeck AT, Villar H, et al. Antigen-Driven Oligoclonal Expansion of Tumor-Infiltrating B Cells in Infiltrating Ductal Carcinoma of the Breast. JI. 2002 Aug 15;169(4):1829-36.

[92] Schlößer HA, Thelen M, Lechner A, Wennhold K, Garcia-Marquez MA, Rothschild SI, et al. B cells in esophago-gastric adenocarcinoma are highly differentiated, organize in tertiary lymphoid structures and produce tumor-specific antibodies. Oncoimmunology. Taylor & Francis; 2018 Oct 29;8(1):e1512458.

[93] Nzula S, Going JJ, Stott DI. Antigen-driven clonal proliferation, somatic hypermutation, and selection of B lymphocytes infiltrating human ductal breast carcinomas. Cancer Res. 2003 Jun 15;63(12):3275-80.

[94] Cipponi A, Mercier M, Seremet T, Baurain J-F, Théate I, van den Oord J, et al. Neogenesis of Lymphoid Structures and Antibody Responses Occur in Human Melanoma Metastases. Cancer Res. 2012 Aug 14;72(16):3997-4007.

[95] Darvin P, Toor SM, Sasidharan Nair V, Elkord E. Immune checkpoint inhibitors: recent progress and potential biomarkers. Exp Mol Med. Nature

Publishing Group; 2018 Dec 13;50 (12):165-11.

[96] Wouters MCA, Nelson BH. Prognostic Significance of Tumor-Infiltrating B Cells and Plasma Cells in Human Cancer. Clin Cancer Res. 2018 Dec 15;24(24):6125-35.

[97] Petitprez F, de Reyniès A, Keung EZ, Chen TW-W, Sun C-M, Calderaro J, et al. B cells are associated with survival and immunotherapy response in sarcoma. Nature. Nature Publishing Group; 2020 Jan; 577(7791): 556-60.

[98] Cabrita R, Lauss M, Sanna A, Donia M, Skaarup Larsen M, Mitra S, et al. Tertiary lymphoid structures improve immunotherapy and survival in melanoma. Nature. Nature Publishing Group; 2020 Jan;577(7791):561-5.

[99] Helmink BA, Reddy SM, Gao J, Zhang S, Basar R, Thakur R, et al. B cells and tertiary lymphoid structures promote immunotherapy response. Nature. Nature Publishing Group; 2020 Jan;577(7791):549-55.

[100] Krishnan S, Bakker E, Lee C, Kissick HT, Ireland DJ, Beilharz MW. Successful combined intratumoral immunotherapy of established murine mesotheliomas requires B-cell involvement. J Interferon Cytokine Res. Mary Ann Liebert, Inc. 140 Huguenot Street, 3rd Floor New Rochelle, NY 10801 USA; 2015 Feb;35(2):100-7.

[101] Minnema-Luiting J, Vroman H, Aerts J, Cornelissen R. Heterogeneity in Immune Cell Content in Malignant Pleural Mesothelioma. Int J Mol Sci. Multidisciplinary Digital Publishing Institute; 2018 Apr;19(4):1041-12.

[102] Jackaman C, Cornwall S, Graham PT, Nelson DJ. CD40-activated B cells contribute to mesothelioma tumor regression. Immunol Cell Biol. 2011 Feb;89(2):255-67.

[103] Buchbinder EI, Desai A. CTLA-4 and PD-1 Pathways: Similarities, Differences, and Implications of Their Inhibition. Am J Clin Oncol. 2016 Feb;39(1):98-106.

[104] Pasello G, Zago G, Lunardi F, Urso L, Kern I, Vlacic G, et al. Malignant pleural mesothelioma immune microenvironment and checkpoint expression: correlation with clinical-pathological features and intratumor heterogeneity over time. Ann Oncol. 2018 May 1;29(5):1258-65.

[105] Nowak AK, Forde PM. Immunotherapy trials in mesothelioma-promising results, but don't stop here. Nat Rev ClinOncol. 2019 Dec; 16(12): 726-8.

[106] Wei SC, Duffy CR, Allison JP. Fundamental Mechanisms of Immune Checkpoint Blockade Therapy. Cancer Discov. American Association for Cancer Research; 2018 Sep;8(9): 1069-86.

[107] Chapel DB, Stewart R, Furtado LV, Husain AN, Krausz T, Deftereos G. Tumor PD-L1 expression in malignant pleural and peritoneal mesothelioma by Dako PD-L1 22C3 pharmDx and Dako PD-L1 28-8 pharmDx assays. Human Pathology. 2019 May;87:11-7.

[108]B rosseau S, Danel C, Scher-pereel A, Mazieres J, Lantuejoul S, Margery J, et al. Shorter Survival in Malignant Pleural Mesothelioma Patients With High PD-L1 Expression Associated With Sarcomatoid or Biphasic Histology Subtype: A Series of 214 Cases From the Bio-MAPS Cohort. Clin Lung Cancer.2019 Sep;20(5):e564-75.

[109] Nguyen BH, Montgomery R, Fadia M, Wang J, Ali S. PD-L1 expression associated with worse survival outcome in malignant pleural mesothelioma. Asia Pac J Clin Oncol.

John Wiley & Sons, Ltd (10.1111); 2018 Feb;14(1):69-73.

[110] Gennen K, Käsmann L, Taugner J, Eze C, Karin M, Roengvoraphoj O, et al. Prognostic value of PD-L1 expression on tumor cells combined with CD8+ TIL density in patients with locally advanced non-small cell lung cancer treated with concurrent chemoradiotherapy. Radiat Oncol. BioMed Central; 2020 Jan 2;15(1):5-12.

[111] Shen X, Zhao B. Efficacy of PD-1 or PD-L1 inhibitors and PD-L1 expression status in cancer: meta-analysis. BMJ. 2018 Sep 10;362:k3529.

[112] Conroy JM, Pabla S, Nesline MK, Glenn ST, Papanicolau-Sengos A, Burgher B, et al. Next generation sequencing of PD-L1 for predicting response to immune checkpoint inhibitors. J Immunother Cancer. BMJ Specialist Journals; 2019 Jan 24;7(1):18.

[113] Scherpereel A, Mazieres J, Greillier L, Lantuejoul S, Dô P, Bylicki O, et al. Nivolumab or niv-olumab plus ipilimumab in patients with relapsed malignant pleural meso-thelioma (IFCT-1501 MAPS2): a multicentre, open-label, randomised, noncomparative, phase 2 trial. Lancet Oncol. 2019 Feb;20(2):239-53.

[114] Calabrò L, Morra A, Fonsatti E, Cutaia O, Amato G, Giannarelli D, et al. Tremelimumab for patients with chemotherapy-resistant advanced malignant mesothelioma: an open-label, single-arm, phase 2 trial. Lancet Oncol. 2013 Oct;14(11):1104-11.

[115] Maio M, Scherpereel A, Calabrò L, Aerts J, Cedres Perez S, Bearz A, et al. Tremelimumab as second-line or third-line treatment in relapsed malignant mesothelioma (DETERMINE): a multicentre, international, randomised, double-blind, placebo-controlled phase 2b trial. Lancet Oncol. 2017 Sep;18(9):1261-73.

[116] Alley EW, Lopez J, Santoro A, Morosky A, Saraf S, Piperdi B, et al. Clinical safety and activity of pembrolizumab in patients with malignant pleural mesothelioma (KEYNOTE-028): preliminary results from a non-randomised, open-label, phase 1b trial. Lancet Oncol. 2017 May;18(5):623-30.

[117] Desai A, Karrison T, Rose B, Tan Y, Hill B, Pemberton E, et al. OA08.03 Phase II Trial of Pembrolizumab (NCT02399371) In Previously Treated Malignant Mesothelioma (MM): Final Analysis. Journal of Thoracic Oncology. Elsevier Inc; 2018 Oct 1;13(Supplement):S339.

[118] Popat S, Curioni-Fontecedro A, Polydoropoulou V, Shah R, O'Brien M, Pope A, et al. LBA91_PRA multicentre randomized phase III trial comparing pembrolizumab (P) vs single agent chemotherapy (CT) for advanced pre-treated malignant pleural mesothelioma (MPM): Results from the European Thoracic Oncology Platform (ETOP 9-15) PROMISE-meso trial. annonc. 2019 Oct 1;30(Supplement_5).

[119] Fennell DA, Kirkpatrick E, Cozens K, Nye M, Lester J, Hanna G, et al. CONFIRM: a double-blind, placebo-controlled phase III clinical trial investigating the effect of nivolumab in patients with relapsed mesothelioma: study protocol for a randomised controlled trial. Trials. BioMed Central; 2018 Apr 18;19(1):233-10.

[120] Quispel-Janssen J, Zago G, Schouten R, Buikhuisen W, Monkhorst K, Thunissen E, et al. OA13.01 A Phase II Study of Nivolumab in Malignant Pleural Mesothelioma (NivoMes): with Translational Research (TR) Biopies. Journal of Thoracic Oncology. Elsevier; 2017 Jan 1;12(Supplement):S292-3.

[121] Okada M, Kijima T, Aoe K, Kato T, Fujimoto N, Nakagawa K, et al. Clinical

Efficacy and Safety of Nivolumab: Results of a Multicenter, Open-label, Single-arm, Japanese Phase II study in Malignant Pleural Mesohelioma (MERIT). Clin Cancer Res. 2019 Sep 15;25(18):5485.

[122] Nowak AK, Lesterhuis WJ, Hughes BGM, Brown C, Kok PS, O'Byrne KJ, et al. DREAM: A phase II study of durvalumab with first line chemotherapy in mesothelioma— First results. JCO. American Society of Clinical On cology; 2018 May 20;36 (15_suppl):8503-3.

[123] Calabrò L, Morra A, Giannarelli D, Amato G, D'Incecco A, Covre A, et al. Tremelimumab combined with durvalumab in patients with meso-thelioma (NIBIT-MESO-1): an open-label, non-randomised, phase 2 study. Lancet Respir Med. 2018 Jun; 6(6): 451-60.

[124] Disselhorst MJ, Quispel-Janssen J, Lalezari F, Monkhorst K, de Vries JF, van der Noort V, et al. Ipilimumab and nivolumab in the treatment of recurrent malignant pleural mesot-helioma (INITIATE): results of a prospective, single-arm, phase 2 trial. Lancet Respir Med. 2019 Mar;7(3): 260-70.

[125] Zeltsman M, Dozier J, McGee E, Ngai D, Adusumilli PS. CAR T-cell therapy for lung cancer and malignant pleural mesothelioma. Transl Res. 2017 Sep;187:1-10.

[126] Martinez M, Moon EK. CAR T Cells for Solid Tumors: New Strategies for Finding, Infiltrating, and Surv-iving in the Tumor Microenvironm-ent. Front Immunol. Frontiers; 2019; 10:128.

[127] Lv J, Li P. Mesothelin as a biomarker for targeted therapy. Biomark Res. BioMed Central; 2019;7(1):18-8.

[128] Zhao Y, Moon E, Carpenito C, Paulos CM, Liu X, Brennan AL, et al. Multiple injections of electroporated autologous T cells expressing a chim-eric antigen receptor mediate regress-ion of human disseminated tumor. Ca-ncer Res. 2010 Nov 15;70(22):9053-61.

[129] Zhang Z, Jiang D, Yang H, He Z, Liu X, Qin W, et al. Modified CAR T cells targeting membrane-proximal epitope of mesothelin enhances the antitumor function against large solid tumor. Cell Death Dis. Nature Publishing Group; 2019 Jun 17;10(7): 476-12.

[130] Adusumilli PS, Zauderer MG, Rusch VW, O 039 Cearbhaill RE, Zhu A, Ngai DA, et al. Abstract CT036: A phase I clinical trial of malignant pleural disease treated with regionally delivered autologous mesothelin-targeted CAR T cells: Safety and efficacy. Cancer Res. 2019 Jul 1;79(13 Supplement):CT036.

[131] Adusumilli PS, Cherkassky L, Villena-Vargas J, Colovos C, Servais E, Plotkin J, et al. Regional delivery of mesothelin-targeted CAR T cell therapy generates potent and long-lasting CD4-dependent tumor immunity. Sci Transl Med. 2014 Nov 5;6(261):261ra151-1.

[132] de Gooijer CJ, Borm FJ, Scher-pereel A, Baas P. Immunotherapy in Malignant Pleural Mesothelioma. Front Oncol. 2020;10:187.

[133] Barsky AR, Cengel KA, Katz SI, Sterman DH, Simone CB. First-ever Abscopal Effect after Palliative Radio-therapy and Immuno-gene Therapy for Malignant Pleural Mesothelioma. Cure-us. 2019 Feb 20;11(2):e4102.

[134] Kepp O, Galluzzi L, Martins I, Schlemmer F, Adjemian S, Michaud M, et al. Molecular determinants of immunogenic cell death elicited by anticancer chemotherapy. Cancer Met-astasis Rev. Springer US; 2011 Mar; 30(1):61-9.

[135] Galluzzi L, Kepp O, Kroemer G. Immunogenic cell death in radiation therapy. Oncoimmunology. 2014 Oct 27;2(10):e26536-3.

[136] Zelenay S, Reis e Sousa C. Adaptive immunity after cell death. Trends in Immunology. 2013 Jul;34(7):329-35.
[137] Dunn GP, Bruce AT, Ikeda H, Old LJ, Schreiber RD. Cancer immunoediting: from immunosurveillance to tumor escape. Nat Immunol. 2002;3(11):991-8.

[138] Schreiber RD, Old LJ, Smyth MJ. Cancer Immunoediting: Integrating Immunity's Roles in Cancer Suppression and Promotion. Science. American Association for the Advancement of Science; 2011 Mar 24;331(60 24):1565-70.

[139] Abuodeh Y, Venkat P, Kim S. Systematic review of case reports on the abscopal effect. Current Problems in Cancer. Elsevier; 2016 Jan 1;40(1):25-37.
[140] Wu L, Wu MO, la Maza De L, Yun Z, Yu J, Zhao Y, et al. Targeting the inhibitory receptor CTLA-4 on T cells increased abscopal effects in murine mesothelioma model. Oncotarget. 2015 May 20;6(14):12468-80.

[141] Bolotin DA, Poslavsky S, Mitrophanov I, Shugay M, Mamedov IZ, Putintseva EV, et al. MiXCR: software for comprehensive adaptive immunity profiling. Nat Methods. Nature Publishing Group; 2015 May; 12(5): 380-1.

[142] Mose LE, Selitsky SR, Bixby LM, Marron DL, Iglesia MD, Serody JS, et al. Assembly-based inference of B-cell receptor repertoires from short read RNA sequencing data with V'DJer. Bioinformatics. 2016 Dec15;32(24):3729-34.

[143] Selitsky SR, Mose LE, Smith CC, Chai S, Hoadley KA, Dittmer DP, et al. Prognostic value of B cells in cutaneous melanoma. Genome Med. Genome Medicine; 2019 May 25;11(1):1-11.

[144] Victora GD, Nussenzweig MC. Germinal centers. Annu Rev Immunol. Annual Reviews; 2012;30(1):429-57.

[145] Traggiai E, Becker S, Subbarao K, Kolesnikova L, Uematsu Y, Gismondo MR, et al. An efficient method to make human monoclonal antibodies from memory B cells: potent neutralization of SARS coronavirus. Nat Med. 2004 Jul 11;10(8):871-5.

[146] Kwakkenbos MJ, van Helden PM, Beaumont T, Spits H. Stable long-term cultures of self-renewing B cells and their applications. Immunol Rev. 2016 Mar;270(1):65-77.

[147] Gilbert AE, Karagiannis P, Dodev T, Koers A, Lacy K, Josephs DH, et al. Monitoring the Systemic Human Memory B Cell Compartment of Melanoma Pat-ients for Anti-Tumor IgG Antibodies. Lu S, editor. Public Library of Science; 2011 Apr 29;6(4):e19330-15.

[148] Clargo AM, Hudson AR, Ndlovu W, Wootton RJ, Cremin LA, O'Dowd VL, et al. The rapid generation of recombinant functional monoclonal antibodies from individual, antigen-specific bone marrow-derived plasma cells isolated using a novel fluorescence-based method. MAbs. Taylor & Francis; 2014 Jan;6(1):143-59.

[149] Tickle S, Howells L, O'Dowd V, Starkie D, Whale K, Saunders M, et al. A fully automated primary screening system for the discovery of therapeutic antibodies directly from B cells. J Biomol Screen. SAGE PublicationsSage CA: Los Angeles, CA; 2015 Apr; 20(4):492-7.

[150] Jin A, Ozawa T, Tajiri K, Obata T, Kondo S, Kinoshita K, et al. A rapid and

efficient single-cell manipulation method for screening antigen-specific antibody-secreting cells from human peripheral blood. Nat Med. Nature Publishing Group; 2009 Sep; 15 (9): 1088-92.

[151] Corti D, Voss J, Gamblin SJ, Codoni G, Macagno A, Jarrossay D, et al. A neutralizing antibody selected from plasma cells that binds to group 1 and group 2 influenza A hemagglutinins. Science. 2011 Aug 12;333 (6044):850-6.

[152] Walker LM, Phogat SK, Chan-Hui P-Y, Wagner D, Phung P, Goss JL, et al. Broad and potent neut-ralizing antibodies from an African donor reveal a new HIV-1 vaccine target.Science.2009 Oct 9;326(5950):285-9.

[153] Dantas-Barbosa C, de Macedo Brigido M, Maranhao AQ. Antibody phage display libraries: contributions to oncology. Int J Mol Sci. Molecular Diversity Preservation International; 2012;13(5):5420-40.

[154] Alfaleh MA, Alsaab HO, Mahmoud AB, Alkayyal AA, Jones ML, Mahler SM, et al. Phage Display Derived Monoclonal Antibodies: From Bench to Bedside. Front Immunol. Frontiers; 2020;11:1986.

[155] Rothe A, Klimka A, Tur MK, Pfitzner T, Huhn M, Sasse S, et al. Construction of phage display libraries from reactive lymph nodes of breast carcinoma patients and selection for specifically binding human single chain Fv on cell lines. Int J Mol Med. Spandidos Publications; 2004 Oct;14(4):729-35.

[156] Rouet R, Jackson KJL, Langley DB, Christ D. Next-Generation Sequencing of Antibody Display Repertoires.

[157] An F, Drummond DC, Wilson S, Kirpotin DB, Nishimura SL,

Broaddus VC, et al. Targeted drug delivery to mesothelioma cells using functionally selected internalizing human single-chain antibodies. Molecular Cancer Therapeutics. 2008 Mar 1;7(3): 569-78.

[158] Lei X, Guan C-W, Song Y, Wang H. The multifaceted role of CD146/ MCAM in the promotion of melanoma progression. Cancer Cell International. BioMed Central; 2015;15(1):3-11.

[159] de Kruijff I, Timmermans A, Bakker den M, Trapman-Jansen A, Foekens R, Meijer-Van Gelder M, et al. The Prevalence of CD146 Expression in Breast Cancer Subtypes and Its Relation to Outcome. Cancers. Multidisciplinary Digital Publishing Institute; 2018 May; 10(5):134.

[160] Olajuyin AM, Olajuyin AK, Wang Z, Zhao X, Zhang X. CD146 T cells in lung cancer: its function, detection, and clinical implications as a biomarker and therapeutic target. Cancer Cell International. BioMed Central; 2019 Sep 25;: 1-13.

[161] Bidlingmaier S, He J, Wang Y, An F, Feng J, Barbone D, et al. Identification of MCAM/CD146 as the target antigen of a human monoclonal antibody that recognizes both epithelioid and sarcomatoid types of mesothelioma. Cancer Res. American Association for Cancer Research; 2009 Feb 15;69(4): 1570-7.

[162] Beije N, Kraan J, Bakker den MA, Maat APWM, van der Leest C, Cornelissen R, et al. Improved diagnosis and prognostication of patients with pleural malignant mesothelioma using biomarkers in pleural effusions and peripheral blood samples - a short report. Cell Oncol (Dordr). Springer Netherlands; 2017 Oct;40(5):511-9.

[163] Barbas CF, Kang AS, Lerner RA, Benkovic SJ. Assembly of combinatorial antibody libraries on phage surfaces: the

gene III site. Proc Natl Acad Sci USA. National Academy of Sciences; 1991 Sep 15;88(18):7978-82.

[164] Cai X, Garen A. Anti-melanoma antibodies from melanoma patients immunized with genetically modified autologous tumor cells: selection of specific antibodies from single-chain Fv fusion phage libraries. Proc Natl Acad Sci USA. 1995 Jul 3;92(14): 6537-41.
[165] Wortzel RD, Urban JL, Philipps C, Fitch FW, Schreiber H. Independent immunodominant and immunorecessive tumor-specific antigens on a malignant tumor: antigenic dissection with cytolytic T cell clones. JI. 1983 May;130(5):2461-6.

# 14

# Extracellular Vesicles Released by *Leishmania*: Impact on Disease Development and Immune System Cells

*Rogéria Cristina Zauli, Andrey Sladkevicius Vidal,*
*Talita Vieira Dupin, Aline Correia Costa de Morais,*
*Wagner Luiz Batista and Patricia Xander*

## Abstract

*Leishmania* spp. release extracellular vesicles (EVs) containing parasite molecules, including several antigens and virulence factors. These EVs can interact with the host cells, such as immune cells, contributing to the parasite–host relationship. Studies have demonstrated that *Leishmania*-EVs can promote infection in experi-mental models and modulate the immune response. Although the immunomodula-tory effect has been demonstrated, *Leishmania*-EVs can deliver parasite antigens and therefore have the potential for use as a new diagnostic tool and development of new therapeutic and vaccine approaches. This review aims to bring significant advances in the field of extracellular vesicles and *Leishmania*, focusing on their role in the cells of the immune system.

**Keywords:** extracellular vesicles, exosomes, microvesicles, *Leishmania*, immune response, leishmaniasis

## 1. Introduction

The host–parasite communication and the parasite's intercellular interactions are crucial in the life cycle of the *Leishmania* parasites [1, 2]. In addition, several bioactive molecules released by the parasites have shown an important role in the parasite's adaptation in the host [3]. In mammalian hosts, molecules released by *Leishmania* contribute to the parasite's infectivity and the physiopathology of the leishmaniasis, acting by several mechanisms, such as subverting the immune response and favoring the intracellular multiplication of the parasite [3].

Several works have demonstrated that *Leishmania* species can release proteins and other molecules in extracellular vesicles (EVs) [4–6]. EVs is a generic term used to describe particles spontaneously released by prokaryotic and eukaryotic cells [7]. Deoxyribonucleic acid (DNA), ribonucleic acid (RNA), proteins, lipids, and cellular metabolites are present in EVs that can deliver information from one cell to another [8]. Thus, EVs are now considered a new mechanism of intercellular communication [7].

*Leishmania*-EVs carry parasites molecules, such as small RNA, heat shock proteins (HSPs), and virulence factors (glycoprotein 63 - GP63 and lipofosfoglican - LPG) [4, 5, 9]. Functional studies showed immunomodulatory and signaling-inducing activities properties of the *Leishmania*-EVs [10]. They are present in the intestinal lumen of sandflies and are regurgitated along with promastigote forms during the blood meal [6]. In addition, these particles modulate the macrophage's activation and alter the course of the parasite infection [4–6, 11]. Although immunomodula-tory properties have been demonstrated in experimental models, additional studies are necessary to better understand the role of EVs in the parasite–host relationship. Next, we describe an overview of the extracellular vesicles relevant to *Leishmania* infection and the main findings related to EVs released by *Leishmania* parasites.

## 2. Extracellular vesicles (EVs): an overview

EVs can be detected in body fluids, including urine, saliva, blood, plasma, amniotic fluid, breast milk, ascites, synovial fluid, and cerebrospinal fluid [7, 12]. Structurally, they present a spherical shape with a double layer composed of lipids and proteins and can be filled with biomolecules from the cell of origin [13]. EVs are classified based on their biogenesis, composition, and size, namely— exosomes, microvesicles (MVs), and apoptotic bodies (ABs) [8, 13]. Although MVs and exosomes show structural similarities, they are different in size, content, lipid com-position, and biogenesis [7]. ABs are released by apoptotic cells and have specific characteristics [12] that will not be covered in this review.

Exosomes present sizes between 20 and 100 nm [14]. They are formed by the internal invagination of the endosomal membrane, originating the multivesicular bodies (MVBs) [8]. After maturation, exosomes are secreted by exocytosis via fusion of MBVs with the cell surface, or they may be digested by lysosomes [14, 15]. Exosomes are rich in lipids (mainly phosphatidylserine, cholesterol, and cerami-des), nucleic acids, and proteins [8]. In addition, proteins such as endosomal sort-ing complexes required for transport (ESCRT), Alix, tumor susceptibility gene 101 (TSG101), heat shock cognate 70 (HSC70), HSP90β, HSP60 and HSP70, proteins from the annexin family, and tetraspanins (cluster of differentiation 63 - CD63, CD9, CD81, and CD82) participate in the process of formation of exosomes [8, 16]. These molecules are increased in exosomes, but they are not exclusive markers of t hese EVs types [7].

MVs are a group of EVs with a diameter between 100 and 1,000 nm [7]. They are originated from the protrusion of the cytoplasmic membrane, and they can carry molecules of cell surface such as membrane receptors, integrins, adhesins, and others [8]. Some studies have shown that structures such as actin and micro-tubules (cytoskeleton), kinesins and myosins, and soluble NSF attachment recep-tors (SNAREs) play a role in the formation of MVs [17]. However, the molecular pathway is not well understood [8, 13, 18], and specific markers of MVs have not yet been described. The releasing of MVs and exosomes occurs under physiological cell conditions, but the quantity and content can be altered after stimuli, such as low oxygen and nitrogen content, oxidative stress, among others [4, 5, 19].

Different vesicle isolation techniques have been performed; however, centrifu-gation/ultracentrifugation and size exclusion chromatography are the most commonly used [7]. Flow cytometry, Western blotting, nanoparticle tracking technique (NTA), mass spectrometry, and electron microscopy have been used to quantify and better characterize the isolated EVs (exosomes and/or MVs) [7]. The inclusion of new methodologies and the discovering of specific EVs markers will bring a new perspective to understand the role of these nanoparticles in the biology and the pathophysiology of several diseases. In addition, there is a great expectation of the applications of EVs in diagnostics, treatments, and vaccine development.

Currently, there is a consensus that EVs play an important role in cell–cell communication being a vehicle for transporting molecules between cells, even cross-kingdom [8, 18, 20]. The effects on the recipient cells depend on the cell type, the origin of EVs, their content, and EVs can act locally and/or systemically. The changes in the recipient cells include modulation of the intracellular signaling pathways, gene regulation, post-transcriptional regulation, activation, or inhibition of different cell types [21–23]. After target cell recognition, EVs can interact with surface receptors, followed by fusion with the plasma membrane for releasing their content, and signaling different intracellular events. However, EVs can also be endocytosed by target cells or collapse after their secretion, delivering their contents into the intracellular space [8, 15].

In parasitic diseases, EVs have brought an exciting field to investigate since they can act as mediators in parasite–host interaction, allowing the transfer of virulence factors and effector molecules from the parasites to the host [24–26]. Parasites EVs are related to the pathogen adhesion, the spread of the parasites, and play a role in regulating the host's immune system. In addition, immune cells infected and/or stimulated with parasite components can release EVs [23] containing messenger RNA (mRNA), small noncoding RNAs (microRNA), chromosomal and mitochondrial DNA, retrotransposons, parasites antigens, and major histocompatibility complex (MHC) I and II [23, 27]. The effects in immunity are diverse, including modulation of innate immune response and antigen presentation.

The production and releasing of EVs by parasites or parasitized cells have been described and characterized in several parasitic infections [25]. For example, in *Leishmania*, several biological markers and virulence factors have been described in EVs released by the parasites [10, 28]. Thus, EVs released by these pathogens can have a role in the disease progression and the host's immune response to the parasite, contributing to the strategy to bypass the immune system.

## 3. EVs released by *Leishmania spp*

*Leishmania* species can release proteins and other molecules in EVs. Although the mechanisms for exosome/MVs secretion in *Leishmania* are still unclear, proteomics analysis of EVs has shed light on the functions and properties of these particles. Initial work showed that *Leishmania donovani* could use EVs as a protein transport vehicle [29]. Additional studies confirmed that *L. donovani* releases EVs. *Leishmania major*, *Leishmania mexicana*, and *Leishmania amazonensis* also used EVs as an important mechanism for protein secretion [4, 5, 30]. The presence of EVs in the intestinal lumen of sandflies and their release together with the parasites during the blood meal reinforce the hypothesis that these EVs contribute to the process of infection and development of leishmaniasis [6].

The release of EVs by *Leishmania* is related to the temperature. Promastigotes of *L. mexicana* and *L. donovani* increased the release of EVs after parasite cultivation at 37°C (mammalian host temperature), compared to the EVs obtained from parasites incubated at 26°C (vector temperature) [30]. Furthermore, to *L. donovani*, differ-ences in the content of the EVs obtained at 37°C and 26°C [4] were also observed, suggesting a possible parasite strategy for establishment in the host. However, *L. amazonensis* showed a different pattern in EVs releasing since a higher number of particles were detected after cultivation at 26°C, compared to the parasite incubated at 34°C or 37°C [5]. Altogether these observations suggest that *Leishmania* species can adapt differently to the release of EVs.

Proteomic studies showed the presence of the metalloprotease GP63 in EVs released by *Leishmania* cultivated *in vitro* and by the parasite infecting sandflies. GP63 is the main surface glycoprotein of *Leishmania* and is considered a virulence factor since it contributes to the parasite escape of immune response [31–34]. Evaluating the proteomic profile of EVs released by *Leishmania infantum* in three different phases (logarithmic, stationary, and metacyclic stages) showed that the metacyclic phase had a higher abundance of GP63. In contrast, EVs of parasites in the logarithmic phase had the lowest abundance [35]. In a similar approach, higher concentrations of GP63 were detected in EVs released by *L. infantum* in the stationary phase while parasites in the logarithmic phase showed enrichment of ribosomal proteins [36]. However, proteomic analysis of EVs from *Leishmania infantum chagasi* showed no significant biological differences in EVs released by parasites in logarith-mic or stationary phases [37].

Besides GP63, other proteins have already been identified in *L. donovani*-EVs, such as elongation factor-1α (EF-1α), fructose-1,6-bisphosphate aldolase FBA, HSP70, and HSP90 [4]. A comparative study of *L. infantum*-EVs from drug-resistance parasites identified differences in their morphology, size, distribution, and protein content. Identifying proteins related to drug resistance in EVs from resistant parasites can bring new possibilities to predict prognostics and treatments in leishmaniasis [38].

The presence of small noncoding RNAs was identified in EVs released by *L. donovani* and *Leishmania braziliensis*, suggesting the regulatory role of these EVs in the host cells [39]. Additional studies to address the EVs content from different *Leishmania* species may clarify the role of these particles in visceral and cutaneous leishmaniasis. Furthermore, these studies may provide the use of *Leishmania*-EVs in diagnostics, the development of a vaccine, and promising therapeutic alternatives.

## 4. *Leishmania*-EVs and immune response

Some evidence have pointed that *Leishmania*-EVs present immunomodulatory effects, altering the immune response and contributing to the disease progression. The treatment of human monocytes with *L. donovani*-EVs induced the production of interleukin 10 (IL-10) and inhibited the tumor necrosis factor-alpha (TNF-α) production, even after challenging with interferon-gamma (IFN-γ) [11]. Similar effects were observed in dendritic cells (DC) treated with these EVs since the production of cytokines IL-12p70, TNF-α and IL-10 were inhibited and there was impaired in the ability of these cells to stimulate the differentiation naive CD4 T lymphocytes into T helper 1 (Th1) profile [11]. On the other hand, EVs released by *L. amazonensis* increased the expression of IL-10 and IL-6 in bone marrow-derived macrophages (BMDM) [5]. In fact, EVs released by different *Leishmania* species seem to induce different responses in human macrophages [40]. EVs from *L. infantum* and *L. braziliensis* failed to induce an inflammatory response in human macrophages. However, *L. amazonensis*-EVs stimulated human macrophages to produce nitric oxide (NO), TNF-α, IL-6, and IL-10 via Toll-like receptor 4 (TLR4) and TLR2 (**Figure 1A**) [40].

Few studies have proposed mechanisms of intracellular signaling pathways activated by *Leishmania*-EVs into phagocytes cells. EVs released by *L. amazonensis* amastigotes containing DNA fragments were capable of inducing the CD200 expression in macrophages [41]. The high expression of this molecule leads to the inhibition of NO production, contributing to the parasite survival [41]. In addition, evidence suggests that the composition of EVs can influence the outcome of cell

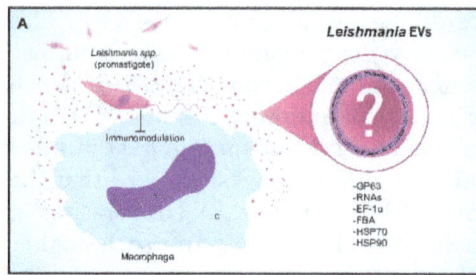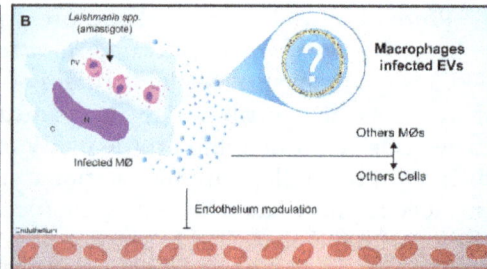

**Figure 1.**

*Leishmania EVs and their influence on the modulation of immune and endothelial cells. (A) Macrophage modulation by EVs released by Leishmania spp. promastigotes. (B) Macrophages infected with Leishmania spp. release EVs with modulating activities. C - cytoplasm; N - nucleus; PV - parasitophorous vacuole; Mɸ(s) – Macrophages.*

signaling. *Leishmania* EVs-containing *Leishmania* RNA virus (LRV1) released by *Leishmania guyanensis* trigger TLR3/TRIF (TIR domain-containing adaptor inducing interferon-β signaling), inducing inflammatory cytokines (pro-IL-1b, TNF-a, and IL-12), and the autophagy by impairing NLRP3 (NOD-, LRR- and pyrin domain-containing protein 3) inflammasome network [42, 43] (**Figure 1B**). Thus, these initial studies demonstrated a refined and complex intracellular signaling pathway induced by EVs, which depends on the species and evolutionary form that is releasing the EVs and the presence or absence of *Leishmania* virus.

Besides macrophages and DCs, *Leishmania*-EVs can modulate other immune cells. EVs released by *L. infantum* inhibited the expansion of peripheral iNKT (Invariant Natural Killer T) cells and the production of IL-4 and IFN-γ by this cell type[44].

Experiments using CD1d specific ligands (glycolipid α-GalactosylCeramide (α-GalCer) suggest that lipids present in *L. infantum*-EVs and other exocomponents released by the parasites may compete for the CD1 binding site, inhibiting iNKT activation [44]. In addition, our group showed that murine B-1 cells (a subtype of B lymphocytes) stimulated with EVs released by *L. amazonensis* produced higher levels of NO, compared to non-stimulated B-1 cells [45]. The increase in the expression of TLR-9,

TNF -α, and transcriptional factors related to the differentiation of B-1 cells to phagocytes are important changes observed in B-1 cells treated with *L. amazonensis*-EVs [45]. These data suggest that *Leishmania*-EVs participate in the modulation of different cells and different levels of the immune response. Interestingly, some mechanisms seem conserved between species, but some specifies are related to *Leishmania* species making comparative studies necessary.

In a mammalian host, *Leishmania* is an intracellular parasite. Thus, studying changes in infected cells can provide important information about the parasite's biology. Silverman et al. [4] showed *Leishmania* exosomes and exosomal proteins in the cytosolic compartment of infected macrophages. In addition, EVs released by macrophages infected with *L. mexicana* containing GP63, and this finding instigated the investigation to uncover the role of these EVs in immunity [46]. Naïve macrophages exposed to EVs from *L. mexicana*-macrophages infected cells induced the activation of mitogen-activated protein (MAP) kinases (except c-Jun N-terminal kinase - JNK) and the nuclear translocation of nuclear factor-κB (NF-κB) and activator protein 1 (AP-1) [46]. BMDM infected with *L. amazonensis* released EVs which were able to activate naive macrophages to produce proinflammatory cytokines IL-12, IL-1β, and TNF-α, contributing both to modulate the immune system in favor of a Th1 immune response and to the elimination of the *Leishmania*, leading, therefore, to the control the infection [47] (**Figure 1B**).

Thus, infected macrophages are able to release EVs that deliver information to activate naïve macrophages, contributing to activate an innate immune response.

Evidence suggests that EVs released by *Leishmania*-infected cells can stimu-late different cells, promoting a response against the parasite. EVs released by macrophages infected with *L. donovani* stimulated endothelial cells to produce granulocyte colony-stimulating factor (G-CSF)/CSF-3, and vascular endothe-lial growth factor A (VEGF-A), promoted an increase in epithelial cell migra-tion and induced endothelial cell tube formation [48] (**Figure 1B**). A study with EVs released by B-1 cells infected with *L. amazonensis* showed the impact of these EVs on naive macrophages activation and the protective effect on the experimental infection with the parasite [49]. Macrophages treated with EVs from infected peritoneal B-1 cells alter the expression of inducible nitric oxide

synthase (iNOS), IL-6, IL-10, and TNF-α [49]. Overall, these studies demon-strated that *Leishmania* infection changes the content of EVs from infected cells and suggest that these EVs participate in the activation of immune and nonim-mune cells, actively participating in the pathophysiology of the *Leishmania* infection.

## 5. EVs and leishmaniasis progression

Experimental models have contributed to better understanding the role of EVs in the leishmaniasis progression. The treatment of mice with *L. donovani*-EVs before the parasite infection exacerbated the infection and induced IL-10 production in the spleen [11]. Furthermore, mice treated with *L. major*-EVs before challenge with the parasite showed an increased frequency of IL-4-producing CD4 + T cells in both the spleen and lymph nodes, leading to disease exacerbation [11]. These find-ings suggest that *Leishmania* EVs are predominantly immunosuppr-essive and favor the parasite. In fact, our group demonstrated that *L. amazonensis* EVs co-injected with the parasite led to disease exacerbation with a predominance of Th2 response in BALB/c mice [5]. Similar results were observed for *L. major*, but the co-injection of the parasite and related EVs induced an increase in the expression of IL-17 and IL-4 [6].

Changes in the content of EVs may impact the immune response and disease progression [9, 11]. Studies performed with genetically modified parasites showed that in a mouse model of air pouch formation (murine air pouch injection) EVs derived from *L. major* GP63 knockout (KO) (*L. major* GP63$^{-/-}$) induced greater recruitment of inflammatory cells, compared to EVs derived from wild parasites [9]. Furthermore, EVs derived from *L. donovani* exhibited an immunosuppressive effect and exacerbated the disease in animals challenged with the parasite, but EVs derived from *L. donovani* HSP100 KO (*L. donovani* HSP100$^{-/-}$) were able to induce a pro-inflammatory response and did not exacerbate the disease [11]. Thus, the hypothesis that EVs derived from parasites with different virulence profiles (viru-lent and attenuated) present relevant alterations in their protein content and can induce distinct immune responses in an experimental immunization model cannot be discarded.

The relevance of EVs in *Leishmania* infection's biology was shown by the demonstration that *Leishmania* promastigotes release EVs in the sandflies [6]. The experimental infection with *L. major* in the presence of EVs released by the parasite in the vector led to higher lesion size and parasite load, associated with impaired effector immune response [6]. Taken together, the *in vivo* studies suggest that EVs released by *Leishmania* participate in the infection, favoring the establishment of the parasite and the progression of the disease.

## 6. Conclusions

The knowledge acquired studying EVs has allowed understanding that these particles are related to intercellular communication and cross-kingdom relationship. The release of these EVs by *Leishmania* is related to initial infection, modulation of the immune system, and disease progression in the host (**Table 1**). However, several aspects of the biology and physiology of these molecules still need to be better investi-gated. Would releasing these EVs into the vector be related to the parasite's adaptation to that environment? Can EVs contribute to parasite multiplication in the vector? Is there population regulation and/or transfer of resistance factors and immune response escape by EVs between different *Leishmania* species? Do these transfers occur in the vector and/or in the mammalian host? Can vesicles released by *Leishmania* be used for the development of vaccines and new diagnostic approaches? Thus, the field of EVs released by *Leishmania* and other pathogens is fascinating and, there will be signifi-cant advances and contributions to the area in the future with the discovery of new therapeutic targets and new players in the host–parasite relationship.

| *Leishmania* species | Biological function | Reference |
|---|---|---|
| *L. donovani* | • Increased IL-10 and inhibited TNF-α production by human monocytes;<br>• Inhibited IL-12p70, TNF-α, and IL-10 production by DC;<br>• Impaired the ability of DC to drive T cells differentiation into Th1;<br>• In experimental infection: exacerbated the infection; promoted IL-10 production in the spleen. | [11] |
| *L. amazonensis* | • Increased the expression of IL-10 and IL-6 in BMDM;<br>• In experimental infection: led to disease exacerbation with a predominance of Th2 response in BALB/c mice; | [5] |
| | • Increased the production of NO, TNF-α, IL-6, and IL-10 via TLR4 and TLR2 by human monocytes; | [40] |
| | • In B-1 cells: increased NO production; increased expres-sion of TLR-9 and TNF-α; induced the expression of factors related to myeloid commitment; | [45] |
| | • Increased the CD200 expression and inhibited the NO production (EVs released by amastigotes) | [41] |
| *L. guyanensis* infected with *Leishmania* RNA Virus (LRV1) | • Triggered TLR3/TRIF signaling;<br>• Impaired NLRP3 inflammasome network | [42] |
| *L. infantum* | • Inhibited iNKT activation and production of IL-4 and IFN-γ by these cells; | [44] |
| *L. major* | • In experimental infection:<br>• Increased the disease progression;<br>• Increased the expression of IL-17 and IL-4 | [10] |

**Table 1.**
*Biological effects of the EVs released by different Leishmania species.*

## Acknowledgements

This work was supported by Fundação de Amparo à Pesquisa do Estado de São Paulo (grant number 2019/21614-3). Scholarships were provided by the Fundação de Amparo à Pesquisa do Estado de São Paulo (2021/01556-9), Conselho Nacional de Desenvolvimento Científico e Tecnológico (CNPq), and Coordenação de Aperfeiçoamento de Pessoal de Nível Superior (CAPES).

## Author details

Rogéria Cristina Zauli[1,2] , Andrey Sladkevicius Vidal[2] , Talita Vieira Dupin[2],

Aline Correia Costa de Morais[2], Wagner Luiz Batista[2] and Patricia Xander[2*]

1 Technical Support Center for Teaching, Research and Extension (NATEPE), Federal University of São Paulo, Campus Diadema, Diadema, Brazil

2 Laboratory of Cellular Immunology and Biochemistry of Fungi and Protozoa, Department of Pharmaceutical Sciences, Federal University of São Paulo, Campus Diadema, Diadema, Brazil

*Address all correspondence to: patricia.xander@unifesp.br

# References

[1] Burza S, Croft SL, Boelaert M, Leishmaniasis. Lancet. 2018;**392**: 951-970. S0140- 6736(18) 31204-2

[2] Scott P, Novais FO, Cutaneous leishmaniasis: Immune responses in protection and pathogenesis. Nature Reviews Immunology. 2016;**16(9)**: 581-592.

[3] de Morais CG, Castro Lima AK, Terra R, dos Santos RF, Da-Silva SA, Dutra PM. The Dialogue of the Host-Parasite Relationship: *Leishmania* spp. and *Trypanosoma cruzi* Infection.

[4] Silverman JM, Clos J, de'Oliveira CC, Shirvani O, Fang Y, Wang C, et al. An exosome-based secretion pathway is responsible for protein export from *Leishmania* and communication with macrophages. Journal of Cell Science. 2010; **123**: 842-852.

[5] Barbosa FMC, Dupin TV, Toledo MDS, Reis NFDC, Ribeiro K, Cronemberger-Andrade A, et al. Extracellular vesicles released by *Leishmania (Leishmania) amazonensis* promote disease progression and induce the production of different cytokines in macrophages and B-1 cells. Frontiers in Microbiology. 2018; **9**:3056.

[6] Atayde VD, Aslan H, Townsend S, Hassani K, Kamhawi S, Olivier M. Exosome secretion by the parasitic protozoan *Leishmania* within the sand fly midgut. Cell Reports. 2015;**13** (5): 957- 967.

[7] Théry C, Witwer KW, Aikawa E, Alcaraz MJ, Anderson JD, Andriantsitohaina R, et al. Minimal information for studies of extracellular vesicles 2018 (MISEV2018): A position statement of the International Society for Extracellular Vesicles and update of the MISEV2014 guidelines. Journal of Extra cellular Vesicles. 2018; 7(1): 1535750.

[8] van Niel G, D'Angelo G, Raposo G. Shedding light on the cell biology of extracellular vesicles. Nature Reviews Molecular Cell Biology. 2018;**19**(4): 213-228. DOI: 10.1038/nrm.2017.125

[9] Hassani K, Shio MT, Martel C, Faubert D, Olivier M. Absence of metalloprotease GP63 alters the protein content of *Leishmania* exosomes. PLoS ONE. 2014;**9**(4):e95007. DOI: 10.1371/journal.pone.0095007

[10] Atayde VD, Hassani K, da Silva Lira Filho A, Borges AR, Adhikari A, Martel C, et al. *Leishmania* exosomes and other virulence factors: Impact on innate immune response and macrophage functions. Cellular Immunology. 2016;**309**:7-18.

[11] Silverman JM, Clos J, Horakova E, Wang AY, Wiesgigl M, Kelly I, et al. *Leishmania* exosomes modulate innate and adaptive immune responses through effects on monocytes and dendritic cells. Journal of Immunology. 2010; **185**(9):5011-5022. DOI: 10.4049/jimmunol.1000541

[12] Battistelli M, Falcieri E. Apoptotic bodies: Particular extracellular vesicles involved in intercellular communication. Biology (Basel). 2020;**9**(1):21.

[13] Raposo G, Stoorvogel W. Extracellular vesicles: Exosomes, microvesicles, and friends. The Journal of Cell Biology. 2013;**200**:373-383.

[14] Tkach M, Théry C. Communication by extracellular vesicles: Where we are

and where we need to go. Cell 2016; **164**(6):1226-1232. DOI: 10.1016/j. cell.2016.01.043

[15] Meldolesi J. Exosomes and ectosomes in intercellular communication. Current Biology. 2018;**28**(8): R435-RR44. DOI: 10.1016/j. cub.2018. 01.059

[16] Kowal J, Arras G, Colombo M, Jouve M, Morath JP, Primdal-Bengtson B, et al. Proteomic comparison defines novel markers to characterize heterogeneous populations of extracellular vesicle subtypes. Proceedings of the National Academy of Sciences of the United States ·of America.2016;**113**(8):E968-E977.

[17] Cai H, Reinisch K, Ferro-Novick S. Coats, tethers, Rabs, and SNAREs work together to mediate the intracellular destination of a transport vesicle. Developmental Cell. 2007;**12**(5):671-682.

[18] Yáñez-Mó M, Siljander PR, Andreu Z, Zavec AB, Borràs FE, Buzas EI, et al. Biological properties of extracellular vesicles and their physiological functions. Journal of Extracellular Vesicles.

[19] Gavinho B, Sabatke B, Feijoli V, Rossi IV, da Silva JM, Evans-Osses I, et al. Peptidylarginine deiminase inhibition abolishes the production of large extracellular vesicles from *Giardia intestinalis*, Affecting host-pathogen interactions by hindering adhesion to host cells, Frontiers in Cellular Infection Microbiology. 20 20;**10**:417.

[20] Schorey JS, Cheng Y, Singh PP, Smith VL. Exosomes and other extracellular vesicles in host-pathogen interactions. EMBO Reports. 2015; **16**(1): 24-43.

[21] Campos JH, Soares RP, Ribeiro K, Andrade AC, Batista WL, Torrecilhas AC. Extracellular vesicles: Role in inflammatory responses and potential uses in vaccination in cancer and infectious diseases. Journal of Immunology Research.

[22] Dong G, Filho AL, Olivier M. Modulation of host-pathogen communication by extracellular vesicles (EVs) of the protozoan parasite. Frontiers in Cellular and Infection Microbiology. 2019;**9**:100.

[23] Khosravi M, Mirsamadi ES, Mirjalali H, Zali MR. Isolation and functions of extracellular vesicles derived from parasites: The promise of a new era in immunotherapy, vaccination, and diagnosis. International Journal of Nanomedicine. 2020; **15**: 2957-2969.

[24] Montaner S, Galiano A, Trelis M, Martin-Jaular L, Del Portillo HA, Bernal D, et al. The role of extracellular vesicles in modulating the host immune response during parasitic infections. Frontiers in Immunology. 2014;**5**:433. DOI: 10.3389/fimmu.2014.00433

[25] Marcilla A, Martin-Jaular L, Trelis M, de Menezes-Neto A, Osuna A, Bernal D, et al. Extracellular vesicles in parasitic diseases. Journal of Extraclluar Vesicles. 2014;**3**:25040. DOI: 10.34 02/jev.v3.25040

[26] Soares R, Xander P, Costa A, Marcilla A, Menezes-Neto A, Del Portillo H, et al. Highlights of the São Paulo ISEV workshop on extracellular vesicles in cross-kingdom communication. Journal of Extracellular Vesicles. 2017;**6**(1):1407213.

[27] Jeppesen DK, Fenix AM, Franklin JL, Higginbotham JN, Zhang Q, Zimmerman LJ, et al.

Reassessment of exosome composition. Cell. 2019;**177**(2):428-445.

[28] Lambertz U, Silverman JM, Nandan D, McMaster WR, Clos J, Foster LJ, et al. Secreted virulence factors and immune evasion in visceral leishmaniasis. Journal of Leukocyte Biology.

[29] Silverman JM, Chan SK, Robinson DP, Dwyer DM, Nandan D, Foster LJ, et al. Proteomic analysis of the secretome of *Leishmania donovani*. Genome Biology. 2008;**9**(2):R35. DOI: 10.1186/gb-2008-9-2-r35

[30] Hassani K, Antoniak E, Jardim A, Olivier M. Temperature-induced protein secretion by *Leishmania mexicana* modulates macrophage signalling and function.

[31] Gomez MA, Contreras I, Hallé M, Tremblay ML, McMaster RW, Olivier M. *Leishmania* GP63 alters host signaling through cleavage-activated protein tyrosine phosphatases. Sci Signal. 2009;**2**(90):ra58.

[32] Hallé M, Gomez MA, Stuible M, Shimizu H, McMaster WR, Olivier M, et al. The *Leishmania* surface protease GP63 cleaves multiple intracellular proteins and actively participates in p38 mitogen-activated protein kinase inactivation. The Journal of Biological Chemistry. 2009;**284**(11):6893-6908. DOI: 10.1074/jbc.M805861200

[33] Isnard A, Shio MT, Olivier M. Impact of *Leishmania* metalloprotease GP63 on macrophage signaling. Frontiers in Cellular and Infection Microbiology. 2012;**2**:72.

[34] Olivier M, Atayde VD, Isnard A, Hassani K, Shio MT. *Leishmania*

virulence factors: Focus on the metalloprotease GP63. Microbes and Infection. 2012;**14**(15):1377-1389.

[35] Marshall S, Kelly PH, Singh BK, Pope RM, Kim P, Zhanbolat B, et al. Extracellular release of virulence factor major surface protease via exosomes in *Leishmania infantum* promastigotes. Parasites & Vectors. 2018;**11**(1):355.

[36] Santarém N, Racine G, Silvestre R, Cordeiro-da-Silva A, Ouellette M. Exoproteome dynamics in *Leishmania infantum*. Journal of Proteomics. 2013;**84**:106-118. DOI: 10.1016/j. jprot. 2013.03.012

[37] Forrest DM, Batista M, Marchini FK, Tempone AJ, Traub-Csekö YM. Proteomic analysis of exosomes derived from procyclic and metacyclic-like cultured *Leishmania infantum chagasi*. Journal of Proteomics. 2020; **227**:103902. DOI: 10.1016/j. jprot. 2020.103902

[38] Douanne N, Dong G, Douanne M, Olivier M, Fernandez-Prada C. Unravelling the proteomic signature of extracellular vesicles released by drug-resistant *Leishmania infantum* parasites. PLoS Neglected Tropical Diseases. 2020;**14**(7):e0008439.

[39] Lambertz U, Oviedo Ovando ME, Vasconcelos EJ, Unrau PJ, Myler PJ, Reiner NE. Small RNAs derived from tRNAs and rRNAs are highly enriched in exosomes from both old and new world *Leishmania* providing evidence for conserved exosomal RNA Packaging. BMC Genomics. 2015;**16**:151. DOI: 10.1186/s12864-015-1260-7

[40] Nogueira PM, de Menezes-Neto A, Borges VM, Descoteaux A, Torrecilhas AC, Xander P, et al. Immunomodulatory Properties of *leishmania* extracellular vesicles during

host-parasite interaction: Differential activation of TLRs and NF-κB translocation by dermotropic and viscerotropic species. Frontiers in Cellular and Infection Microbiology. 2020;**10**:380.

[41] Sauter IP, Madrid KG, de Assis JB, Sá-Nunes A, Torrecilhas AC, Staquicini DI, et al. TLR9/MyD88/TRIF signaling activates host immune inhibitory CD200 in *Leishmania* infection. JCI Insight. 2019;**4**(10). DOI: 10.1172/jci.insight.126207

[42] de Carvalho RVH, Lima-Junior DS, da Silva MVG, Dilucca M, Rodrigues TS, Horta CV, et al. *Leishmania* RNA virus exacerbates Leishmaniasis by subverting innate immunity via TLR3-mediated NLRP3 inflammasome inhibition. Nature Communications.

[43] Olivier M, Zamboni DS. *Leishmania Viannia guyanensis*, LRV1 virus and extracellular vesicles: A dangerous trio influencing the faith of immune response during mucocutaneous leishmaniasis. Current Opinion in Immunology.

[44] Belo R, Santarém N, Pereira C, Pérez-Cabezas B, Macedo F, Leite-de-Moraes M, et al. Exoproducts Inhibit Human Invariant NKT Cell Expansion and Activation. Frontiers in Immunology. 2017;**8**:710. DOI: 10.3389/fimmu.2017.00710

[45] Reis NFC, Dupin TV, Costa CR, Toledo MDS, de Oliveira VC, Popi AF, et al. Promastigotes or extracellular vesicles modulate B-1 cell activation and differentiation. Frontiers in Cellular and Infection Microbiology. 2020;**10**:573813.

[46] Hassani K, Olivier M. Immunomodulatory impact of

*leishmania*-induced macrophage exosomes: A comparative proteomic and functional analysis. PLoS Neglected Tropical Diseases. 2013;**7**(5):e2185.

[47] Cronemberger-Andrade A, Aragão-França L, de Araujo CF, Rocha VJ, Borges-Silva MaC, Figueira CP, et al. Extracellular vesicles from *Leishmania*-infected macrophages confer an anti-infection cytokine-production profile to naïve macrophages. PLoS Neglected Tropical Diseases. 2014;**8**(9):e3161. DOI: 10.1371/journal. pntd.0003161

[48] Gioseffi A, Hamerly T, Van K, Zhang N, Dinglasan RR, Yates PA, et al. Leishmania-infected macrophages release extracellular vesicles that can promote lesion development. Life Science Alliance. 2020;**3**(12): e202000742.

[49] Toledo MDS, Cronemberger-Andrade A, Barbosa FMC, Reis NFC, Dupin TV, Soares RP, et al. Effects of extracellular vesicles released by peritoneal B-1 cells on experimental *Leishmania (Leishmania) amazonensis* infection. Journal of Leukocyte Biology. 2020;**108**(6):1803-1814. DOI: 10.1002/ JLB.3MA0220-464RR

# Permissions

All chapters in this book were first published by InTech Open; hereby published with permission under the Creative Commons Attribution License or equivalent. Every chapter published in this book has been scrutinized by our experts. Their significance has been extensively debated. The topics covered herein carry significant findings which will fuel the growth of the discipline. They may even be implemented as practical applications or may be referred to as a beginning point for another development.

The contributors of this book come from diverse backgrounds, making this book a truly international effort. This book will bring forth new frontiers with its revolutionizing research information and detailed analysis of the nascent developments around the world.

We would like to thank all the contributing authors for lending their expertise to make the book truly unique. They have played a crucial role in the development of this book. Without their invaluable contributions this book wouldn't have been possible. They have made vital efforts to compile up to date information on the varied aspects of this subject to make this book a valuable addition to the collection of many professionals and students.

This book was conceptualized with the vision of imparting up-to-date information and advanced data in this field. To ensure the same, a matchless editorial board was set up. Every individual on the board went through rigorous rounds of assessment to prove their worth. After which they invested a large part of their time researching and compiling the most relevant data for our readers.

The editorial board has been involved in producing this book since its inception. They have spent rigorous hours researching and exploring the diverse topics which have resulted in the successful publishing of this book. They have passed on their knowledge of decades through this book. To expedite this challenging task, the publisher supported the team at every step. A small team of assistant editors was also appointed to further simplify the editing procedure and attain best results for the readers.

Apart from the editorial board, the designing team has also invested a significant amount of their time in understanding the subject and creating the most relevant covers. They scrutinized every image to scout for the most suitable representation of the subject and create an appropriate cover for the book.

The publishing team has been an ardent support to the editorial, designing and production team. Their endless efforts to recruit the best for this project, has resulted in the accomplishment of this book. They are a veteran in the field of academics and their pool of knowledge is as vast as their experience in printing. Their expertise and guidance has proved useful at every step. Their uncompromising quality standards have made this book an exceptional effort. Their encouragement from time to time has been an inspiration for everyone.

The publisher and the editorial board hope that this book will prove to be a valuable piece of knowledge for researchers, students, practitioners and scholars across the globe.

# List of Contributors

**Wendy M. Toyofuku**
Centre for Innovation, Canadian Blood Services, University of British Columbia, Vancouver, BC, Canada
Centre for Blood Research, University of British Columbia, Vancouver, BC, Canada

**Mark D. Scott and Xining Yang**
Centre for Innovation, Canadian Blood Services, University of British Columbia, Vancouver, BC, Canada
Centre for Blood Research, University of British Columbia, Vancouver, BC, Canada
Department of Pathology and Laboratory Medicine, University of British Columbia, Vancouver, BC, Canada

**Duncheng Wang**
MD Anderson Cancer Center, Houston, Texas, USA

**Tsung-Meng Wu and Yu-Sheng Wu**
Department of Aquaculture, National Pingtung University of Science and Technology, Pingtung, Taiwan

**Shiu-Nan Chen**
Department of Life Science, National Taiwan University, Taipei, Taiwan

**Matilde Otero-Losada and Lucas Udovin**
Institute of Cardiological Research, University of Buenos Aires, National Research Council, ININCA, UBA-CONICET, Buenos Aires, Argentina

**Meenakshi Singh and Selma Z. D'Silva**
HLA and Immunogenetics Laboratory, Tata Memorial Hospital, Mumbai, India

**Maria-Isabel Leyva-Carmona**
Institute of Social Security and Services of State Workers (ISSSTE), Mexico City, Mexico

**María Inés Herrera and Francisco Capani**
Institute of Cardiological Research, University of Buenos Aires, National Research Council, ININCA, UBA-CONICET, Buenos Aires, Argentina
Pontifical Catholic University of Argentina, Buenos Aires, Argentina

**Daping Fan**
Department of Cell Biology and Anatomy, University of South Carolina School of Medicine, Columbia, SC, USA

**Samir Raychoudhury and Walden Ai**
Department of Biology, Chemistry and Environmental Health Science, Benedict College, Columbia, SC, USA

**Daniella Insuela, Diego Coutinho, Marco Martins and Maximiliano Ferrero**
Laboratory of Inflammation, Oswaldo Cruz Institute, Oswaldo Cruz Foundation (FIOCRUZ), Rio de Janeiro, Brazil

**Vinicius Carvalho**
Laboratory of Inflammation, Oswaldo Cruz Institute, Oswaldo Cruz Foundation (FIOCRUZ), Rio de Janeiro, Brazil
National Institute of Science and Technology on Neuroimmunomodulation (INCT-NIM), Brazil

**Carlos Melero Moreno**
Institute for Health Research (i+12), Hospital Universitario 12 de Octubre, Madrid, Spain

**Marta Corral Blanco and Rocío Magdalena Díaz Campos**
Institute for Health Research (i+12), Hospital Universitario 12 de Octubre, Madrid, Spain
Pneumology Service, Hospital Universitario 12 de Octubre, Madrid, Spain

**Rodolfo Alberto Kölliker Frers**
Institute of Cardiological Research, University of Buenos Aires, National Research Council, ININCA, UBA-CONICET, Buenos Aires, Argentina
Hospital Ramos Mejía, Buenos Aires, Argentina

**Abhishweta Saxena**
Department of Transfusion Medicine, Homi Bhabha Cancer Hospital, Varanasi, India

**Maria-de-Lourdes Irigoyen-Coria**
Lindavista Integral Specialized Clinics Laboratory (LCEIL), Mexican Social Security Institute (IMSS), Mexico City, Mexico

**Hasan Akbaba**
Faculty of Pharmacy, Ege University, Izmir, Turkey

**Sabrina Porta, Vanesa Cosentino and Eduardo Kerzberg**
Hospital Ramos Mejía, Buenos Aires, Argentina

**Samuel Moreno-Olivares**
Mexican Social Security Institute (IMSS), Mexico City, Mexico

**David Solis-Hernandez**
National Autonomous University of Mexico (UNAM) and Lindavista Integral Specialized Clinics Laboratory (LCEIL), Mexico City, Mexico

**Oksana O. Shevchuk**
I. Horbachevsky Ternopil State Medical University, Ternopil, Ukraine

**Elisaveta A. Snezhkova, Veronika V. Sarnatskaya, Kvitoslava I. Badakhivska, Larysa A. Sakhno, Vasyl F. Chekhun and Volodymyr G. Nikolaev**
R.E. Kavetsky Institute of Experimental Pathology, Oncology and Radiobiology of National Academy of Science of Ukraine, Kyiv, Ukraine

**Guida Giuseppe and Antonelli Andrea**
Allergy and Pneumology Unit, A.S.O Santa Croce and Carle, Cuneo, Italy

**Judie Noemie Hoilat**
Alfaisal University College of Medicine, Riyadh, Saudi Arabia

**Mohamad Fekredeen Ayas**
Ascension St. John Hospital, Detroit, United States of America

**Anatoliy G. Bilous**
Institute of General and Inorganic Chemistry of National Academy of Science of Ukraine, Kyiv, Ukraine

**Vilma-Carolina Bekker-Mendez and Cecilia Rosel-Pech**
Biomedical Research Unit Hospital of CMN Infectology "La Raza" IMSS, Mexico City, Mexico

**Gilles Jadd Hoilat, Sana Riaz and Divey Manocha**
State University of New York Upstate Medical University, Syracuse, United States of America

**Fabio Nicolini and Massimiliano Mazza**
Immunotherapy, Cell Therapy and Biobank (ITCB), IRCCS Istituto Romagnolo per lo Studio dei Tumori (IRST) "Dino Amadori", Meldola, Italy

**Rogéria Cristina Zauli**
Technical Support Center for Teaching, Research and Extension (NATEPE), Federal University of São Paulo, Campus Diadema, Diadema, Brazil
Laboratory of Cellular Immunology and Biochemistry of Fungi and Protozoa, Department of Pharmaceutical Sciences, Federal University of São Paulo, Campus Diadema, Diadema, Brazil

**Andrey Sladkevicius Vidal, Talita Vieira Dupin, Aline Correia Costa de Morais, Wagner Luiz Batista and Patricia Xander**
Laboratory of Cellular Immunology and Biochemistry of Fungi and Protozoa, Department of Pharmaceutical Sciences, Federal University of São Paulo, Campus Diadema, Diadema, Brazil

www.ingramcontent.com/pod-product-compliance
Lightning Source LLC
Chambersburg PA
CBHW080409190526
45161CB00003B/181